THE MENTAL HEALTH CLINICIAN'S WORKBOOK

Also from James Morrison

Diagnosis Made Easier, Second Edition:
Principles and Techniques for Mental Health Clinicians

DSM-5 Made Easy: The Clinician's Guide to Diagnosis

The First Interview, Fourth Edition

Interviewing Children and Adolescents, Second Edition:
Skills and Strategies for Effective DSM-5 Diagnosis
James Morrison and Kathryn Flegel

When Psychological Problems Mask Medical Disorders, Second Edition:
A Guide for Psychotherapists

The Mental Health Clinician's Workbook

Locking In Your Professional Skills

JAMES MORRISON

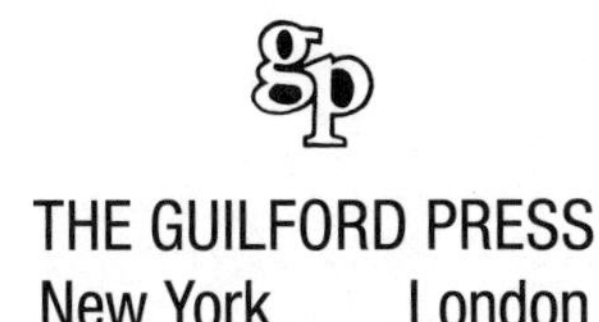

THE GUILFORD PRESS
New York London

A Division of Guilford Publications, Inc.
370 Seventh Avenue, Suite 1200, New York, NY 10001
www.guilford.com

Printed in the United States of America

This book is printed on acid-free paper.

Last digit is print number: 9 8 7 6 5 4 3 2

Library of Congress Cataloging-in-Publication Data

Names: Morrison, James R., author.
Title: The mental health clinician's workbook : locking in your professional skills / James Morrison.
Description: New York, NY : The Guilford Press, [2018] | Includes bibliographical references and index.
Identifiers: LCCN 2017055918| ISBN 9781462534852 (hardcover : alk. paper) | ISBN 9781462534845 (paperback : alk. paper)
Subjects: | MESH: Mental Disorders—diagnosis | Interview, Psychological—methods | Diagnosis, Differential | Problems and Exercises
Classification: LCC RC469 | NLM WM 18.2 | DDC 616.89/075—dc23
LC record available at https://lccn.loc.gov/2017055918

To the memory of Alan Carl Morrison, 1987–2014

About the Author

James Morrison, MD, is Affiliate Professor of Psychiatry at Oregon Health and Science University in Portland. He has extensive experience in both the private and public sectors. With his acclaimed practical books—including *Diagnosis Made Easier, Second Edition*; *DSM-5 Made Easy*; *The First Interview, Fourth Edition*; *Interviewing Children and Adolescents, Second Edition;* and *When Psychological Problems Mask Medical Disorders, Second Edition*—Dr. Morrison has guided hundreds of thousands of mental health professionals and students through the complexities of clinical evaluation and diagnosis.

Contents

Introduction

I have chosen the title of this book with some care, rejecting the alternative *Casebook* as not quite conveying what I've tried to do. Of course, I hope the many case histories you'll encounter here will help you along the road to a better understanding of how a mental health clinician evaluates a patient. But mostly, because we all learn better by doing, I ask you at many, many points in the course of these discussions to lean in and work through the material. There are lots of boxes to check off, and lots of stuff to write down.

Each of these fictionalized histories is constructed to encourage you to think about the processes of obtaining information from and concerning patients, and about the process of making a diagnosis. To a degree, each discussion builds on what has come before; that is, I intend these cases to be read serially. Each of the 26 cases in my "alphabet" of patients (note that, in naming them, I've started with A and marched right through to Z) features a different individual with different problems, and each comprises a series of Steps and Notes, as well as some additional features.

- Steps (which are numbered) contain the life stories of the patients, and ask for your input about their evaluation. At the end of each Step, I pose a question about the material. Usually I try to provide a number of choices for your response. That's because I don't want to put you in the position of having to guess from the universe of possible responses what I'm thinking. OK, once in a while, multiple choices may not be possible, or may even prove counterproductive. But I'll try to keep those instances to a minimum.

- Notes (which are given capital letters) discuss the answers to the questions I've asked throughout the Steps in each case.

- The Takeaway briefly summarizes what I've hoped to accomplish in each case, especially which principles, rules, and diagnoses have been covered.

- In a number of Rants, you'll find special issues—overdiagnosis of some disorders, for example—that ruffle (or sometimes smooth) my feathers. I have attempted to resurrect and address every one of these enemies of good diagnostic practice, so that perhaps they will begin to bother you, too—enough that you will avoid them.

• And in a series of Break Time discussions, I've indulged some of my other interests. Mostly, though these brief discussions are all related to mental health issues, I've tried not to involve actual interview techniques and diagnostic criteria. OK, sometimes I've failed utterly. You can indulge me or ignore me as you wish; obviously, what you do on your break is your business!

• Supporting literature for each chapter is included in the "References and Suggested Reading" section at the end of the book. I've included each reference specifically mentioned in the text, plus others that I think are just plain interesting. As often as possible, I've featured those that offer free full text—either through a specific website that I've listed, or through the U.S. National Library of Medicine's PubMed database. For the latter, just enter the full title of the article into the PubMed search box and press the button.

• Finally, anyone who wants to look up to see where I've deployed a particular interviewing issue, diagnostic principle, or main diagnosis can refer to the three (rather boring) tables in the Appendix. There I've listed them by case, with page references to three of my other books.

However, you'll find little in these pages about treatment options. That's because I've intended this book as an introduction to the science and art of interacting with patients, in the service of two goals: forming a relationship, and obtaining the information needed to make a diagnosis. For treatment issues, many texts and monographs are available. I've mentioned a couple of my favorites in the References.

How might you use this book? Let me count the ways.

- You could use it as an exercise book when learning to do mental health interviews or reviewing the basics of diagnosis. This might take place either in a classroom or as a self-study effort.
- You could instead put it to use as a self-study guide to the mental health issues and principles I've talked about in my other books.
- You might employ it as a review guide in preparing for various qualifying exams.
- Or you might use it as a stand-alone book, without reference to some of the other materials cited. But I think that would be passing up a good opportunity.
- Finally, you could treat it as a storybook and just read right through without trying to complete the exercises. I suspect some readers will be tempted to do just that. But I predict that they will take less away from their experience than will those who put in the effort to do the exercises as they engage with the material.

Whatever your needs, I do hope that before reading each Note, you will take time to think about the possible answer(s) you could give to the question posed in the preceding Step, and to write down your choice(s). Only then should you compare your choice(s) with what I've written. I believe that through this active learning mode, you'll get the very most out of the time you spend with this workbook. Of course, you could just read the stories and questions in the Steps, and then read my answers in the Notes, without ever really engaging with the active learning process. You could get through the text a lot faster that way, but I think you'd take much less away from your experience.

One more caution: When I get a new book, I'm sometimes tempted to tear right through it in just a few marathon sessions. But in this case, please don't follow my lead. Rather, do as I *say* and practice moderation; I think you'll get more out of this book if you take it in small bits. For one thing, you'll fall into the habit of thinking in terms of a differential diagnosis; for another, you'll remember the steps to a diagnosis better if you repeat them on many different days, rather than doing it all at once.

Finally, let me confess that many of the ideas expressed herein are issues I would have liked to set forth right at the beginning. But if I had, the case of Abby would have taken up more than half the book, and the rest would be review. This is another way of saying that some of what you read in later chapters might have been good to know earlier. That's just the way with workbooks: They're a lot of work, for both the reader and the writer.

I am indebted to Hans J. Markowitsch at Bielefeld University in Germany, and to David Barnard at Oregon Health and Science University, for their assistance in the preparation of the material in this book. I am also indebted to the many people at The Guilford Press who have labored, sometimes under duress (caused by me!) to bring this and my other books to fruition. I especially have in mind Kitty Moore, Marie Sprayberry, Anna Brackett, Judith Grauman, Carolyn Graham, Katherine Lieber, Martin Coleman, David Mitchell, and Seymour Weingarten.

I want to express gratitude to my first readers, Mary Morrison and Kitty Moore, for their careful reading and many excellent suggestions. And I especially thank my friend and colleague JoAnne Renz for reading and commenting on every chapter of the penultimate draft. Her many valuable suggestions have improved the text remarkably. In the end, of course, any errors of fact or infelicities of expression are entirely my own responsibility.

1

Good Beginnings—Abby

Step 1

"This school's right for me. I know it in my heart." That's how Abby begins her story.

Indeed, Abby's first few weeks at college seemed to go swimmingly. She enjoyed her classes—she even excelled in the challenging humanities course all freshmen had to take—and she'd begun a relationship with a fellow biology major, now in his second year at the school. She'd telephoned her mother a couple of times, but so far hadn't shared any of her anxieties.

Abby's high school grades and extracurricular work had earned her a full scholarship. Indeed, as she elaborates now on her successes (even "blessings," she calls them, though she later acknowledges that she doesn't think she is a believer), you might be tempted to ask, "What are you even doing here in my office?"

Or would that be a mistake? Just what *should* you say at this point?

- ☐ As suggested above, ask frankly, "Why are you here?"
- ☐ Suggest that you'd like Abby to focus on her recent experiences (in other words, what's happened to her since she came to college).
- ☐ Or just keep quiet and let her talk.

Note A

Wouldn't you just know—the first question in the book, and it's a trick! I'd feel ashamed, if it weren't that I want to drive home the importance of listening to what patients have to say. It's a point I'll make time and again, so be prepared for a little parentalistic* redundancy.

In my view, asking *anything* would be a mistake when you have a patient who is intelligent, motivated (Abby has appeared at the office more or less under her own steam), and is pouring forth a stream of information without prompts from you. OK, maybe she's telling more than you want to know right now, but it's all stuff you'll need eventually. Consequently, I'd let her come around to the point in her own time.

From every patient you encounter, you want a fair sample of what I call *free speech.* That's the uninterrupted production of thoughts, ideas, feelings, and fears—whatever mental or emotional content that has impelled the patient to your door. Free speech gives you the opportunity to hear what's important to your patient, and it provides *you* the opportunity to listen for two sorts of speech characteristics.

1. The first is the person's speech cadences and tonal variations (termed *prosody*). For instance, do you detect the slow, hesitant beat of the depressive voice? Or a flattened, devoid-of-emotion tone that may also signal depression, but can even indicate psychosis?
2. The second is *flow of thought.* Does one idea emerge naturally from the one before? Do you note any irrelevancies in the speech—perhaps a skipping from one concept to the next, so that the two ideas appear unconnected? Whatever you hear, even a few moments of free speech can provide a good start for most mental health interviews.

So for now, to encourage a longer run of free speech, if you need to say anything at all, it should be something wonderfully open-ended and encouraging, such as the clinician's classic comment "Tell me more."

Stay tuned: We'll talk more about these issues later on in the book. And for the rest of this case presentation, I'll stay out of the way. I'm not setting a precedent for future discussions (far from it; mostly, I'll interrupt until you may wish otherwise), but I'd like to start out with something a little simple, something clean and clear—in short, a good beginning.

Step 2

In the following narrative (as in similar case material in several later chapters of this book), some of the material is underlined and given superscript numbers ([1]). We'll use those bits to answer the questions in Note D.

> As Abby's story unfolds, you can see how things began to go awry. Some issues were minor—just before the Thanksgiving break, she'd gotten back a test paper that bore

*Yes, I *know* the word is "paternalistic." Each of my half-dozen or so dictionaries lists it that way; even Gail Collins used it in one of her *New York Times* columns, for Pete's sake. But I prefer my own almost-neologism (and perfect anagram), partly for its stick-in-the-eye challenge to maintain vigilance for fairness in communication.

a grudging C+ grade ("I thought I knew that material like the home screen on my phone!"). She'd also developed a swimsuit rash that wouldn't go away.

And she found that she'd stepped up her use of Xanax. During her senior year of high school, her doctor back home had prescribed it for anxiety attacks she'd had before taking several exams. Things had eventually settled down; she'd aced the SATs and had been accepted at several high-ranking colleges and universities. Her first-choice school had offered her a full ride, and 6 months later, here she was with an honors schedule, two roommates, and a boyfriend.

Her relationship with Denis had started off just fine. The two biology majors became acquainted at a mixer during the first week of school. They'd rapidly bonded over a discussion of evolution and biodiversity—and a bottle of homemade dandelion wine. "He said it was vintage July," Abby reports with amusement. They'd since become nearly inseparable, studying and eating together and indulging in a little enthusiastic, but careful, snogging—Abby admitted she'd had no experience with "real sex" and wasn't yet quite ready to commit. With his sophomore-year experience, Denis guided Abby through the maze of college life. With the sensibilities derived from a working-class upbringing, she drew him into her after-hours world of protests and community service. Together, on the campus radio station, they started a call-in program about science.

All of this took place back in the fall, when Abby was still functioning well. But as the holidays loomed, she noticed that her mood was "trending downward[1] with the temperature." At first, she only experienced a mild overall fogginess, as though the world were gradually losing its color; later, reality asserted itself, and she finally admitted that the gloom was internal.[1]

Her attention in class faded.[2] "Even my microscope lost focus," she offers, with only the trace of a smile. Her ability to concentrate[2] on her studies took "an enormous hit," and her grades began a downward spiral. She tried to shrug it off, telling herself that she didn't give a damn that she felt she'd never achieve her goals, "whatever they might have been."

Her interest in other things[3]—her political involvement, her physicality with Denis—had "sputtered into the void."[3] Denis had invited her to a conference on evolutionary biology just across town, but she begged off, saying she was "way too tired."[4] Instead, she spent that weekend sleeping,[5] venturing out only once on a Sunday to get some breakfast—"It was only coffee, I'm living on coffee."

In barely a month, she had shed 10 pounds[6] ("I was hardly fat and didn't need to lose weight, but I just didn't feel hungry"), so she'd visited the student health service. After the nurse practitioner pronounced her "thin but sound," she'd returned to her room and to bed, and she'd cried. "I've done a lot of that recently—crying,"[7] she says as she helps herself to another tissue.

And so, last weekend, among her roommate's cosmetics she found a bottle of aspirin. "I swallowed one, then another. Then I just kept on swallowing," she explains, until she'd finished the bottle,[8] which had originally contained 100 tablets. She didn't call Denis or anyone else. "I thought I'd done the job,[8] and I just lay down to wait." Denis repeatedly texted her from the conference. When he finally returned, aware that her roommates were both away for the weekend, he persuaded a security guard to open her door.

The 911 call resulted in a trip to the emergency room, where she was intubated and relieved of her stomach contents, including most of the aspirin. When a nurse suggested that she'd been in no serious danger, she wept. "You mean, I went through all that without even the hope of success? I feel so worthless—about as useless[9] as those frogs we're always sacrificing."

After 3 days in the hospital, she'd been judged no longer a danger to herself and released. Denis had taken her home, and later driven her to this appointment.

Now you're ready to make a diagnosis. But wait! Have we forgotten anything? You could look back through this history and write down whatever you think you might still find useful in making a diagnosis . . .

. . . but, actually, I've already done some of the hard work for you. Just below is a brief outline of the classes of information that are needed. All I'm asking you to do is to put a checkmark beside those items for which we've already obtained information.

- ☐ Chief complaint
- ☐ History of the present illness
- ☐ Personal and social history
  - ☐ Early childhood relationships
  - ☐ Family history
  - ☐ Schooling
  - ☐ Sexual and marital history
  - ☐ Employment history
  - ☐ Military experience
  - ☐ Legal issues
  - ☐ Religion
  - ☐ Leisure activities and interests
- ☐ Substance use
- ☐ Medical history and review of systems
- ☐ Mental status evaluation (MSE)

Rant

Later in the book, we'll deal in greater detail with the issue of identifying suicide risk. For right now, let's just quickly note two ways to assess the seriousness of a suicide attempt: its physical effects and its psychological implications.

A physically serious attempt is one that results in significant bodily harm—or might have, if an intervention had not occurred. Examples would be profound loss of blood from a slashed major blood vessel, deep coma due to an overdose, and a gunshot wound to the chest. Swallowing a potentially lethal overdose that was treated effectively is something else we would consider physically serious. On the other hand, because minor scratches on the wrist or four to five ingested aspirin tablets pose no actual risk to the patient, we wouldn't consider them physically serious.

Psychological seriousness speaks to the patient's state of mind around the time of the attempt. In the "serious" column, I'd include someone who took pains to avoid discovery, a patient who laments the failure of an attempt, and one who expresses an intent to "do a better job next time." Based on her Step 2 statement, we'd place Abby's attempt in the psychologically serious category.

Obviously, we should take the utmost care in planning future services for any patient who has made an attempt we'd rate as serious on *either* of these dimensions—physical or psychological.

Note B

I've actually either glossed over or completely left out a lot of material. It's not that I consider the left-out bits unimportant (far from it), but at this early point in the book, I want to focus on a few broad principles. Later on, we'll get down on all fours and wrestle with the details of other patients' histories. For now, let's just outline the information we must consider in every mental health evaluation we do. Here is the list again; what's missing from Abby's story I've left without checkmarks:

- ☑ Chief complaint
- ☑ History of the present illness
    - ☐ Personal and social history
    - ☐ Early childhood relationships
    - ☐ Family history
    - ☑ Schooling
    - ☑ Sexual and marital history
    - ☐ Employment history
    - ☐ Military experience
    - ☐ Legal issues
    - ☑ Religion
    - ☑ Leisure activities and interests
- ☐ Substance use
- ☐ Medical history and review of systems
- ☐ MSE

You'll notice that over half the list is checkmark-free, so there's obviously a lot of work to do before we can completely sort out Abby's history. For right now, here's a bit more to work with.

Step 3

Abby's early childhood was "pretty close to idyllic." She was the second of three children born to a husband and wife who worked together at home; among the couple's other occupations, they edited and produced a newsletter about making jewelry. As a result, Abby and her two brothers enjoyed a lot of attention from both their mother and father—not to mention "a substantial collection of uncles, aunts, and cousins." As a child, she always felt wanted and loved, cared for and secure.

The family never moved. When Abby headed off to college, she left behind the house she'd lived in since she was 2 days old. To her knowledge, the only relative who had experienced mental illness was a great-uncle who became depressed at some point during middle age and hanged himself with his bathrobe sash.[10] "He was a drinker, I'm told," Abby says. She claims that she's never abused substances,[11] including alcohol and street drugs. And throughout her life so far, her physical health has been superb.[12]

Now you have the basic facts in Abby's case—not all of them, but as many as I plan to give you. So the question is "What's wrong?" And by that, I mean "What general area of mental disorder should we investigate for Abby?"

Let's operationalize the question: What chapter of a guide to mental disorders, such as the *Diagnostic and Statistical Manual of Mental Disorders,* fifth edition (DSM-5), bears investigation? Although this is one of those places where a list of choices might not be absolutely necessary (I've given quite a few hints), let's make a list of them anyway. It might come in handy later on.

The possible chapters are those that concern these groups of disorders, the names of which I have slightly condensed:

- Neurodevelopmental disorders (those seen first in children)
- Schizophrenia and other psychotic disorders
- Mood (depressive and bipolar) disorders
- Anxiety disorders
- Obsessive–compulsive disorders
- Trauma- and stressor-related disorders
- Dissociative disorders
- Somatic symptom disorders
- Feeding and eating disorders
- Elimination disorders
- Sleep–wake disorders
- Sexual dysfunctions
- Gender dysphoria
- Disruptive, impulse-control, and conduct disorders
- Substance-related and addictive disorders
- Neurocognitive disorders
- Personality disorders
- Paraphilic disorders

And the chapter you'd turn to first is this one: ____________________

Note C

That exercise was fairly easy: Almost everything Abby has experienced and talked about, from the beginning of her story, suggests the area of mood disorders. Much of what she has told us so far involves her feelings of being sad and losing interest in things she cares about deeply. I think we can safely say that she has the principal prerequisites for entry into the depressive disorder ballpark: depressed mood and affect. Depressive symptoms are chock-a-block throughout Abby's history.

However, it is worthwhile to consider other possibilities, and that's why I've asked you to look at the other DSM-5 chapters. An important part of being a clinician who makes diagnoses is to think beyond that which is obvious—to consider issues that, at first blush, may seem obscure. I can assure you that by the time you've read this book clear through, you will have heard this message again.

So far, this is pretty routine stuff. But now let's step off into the weeds of the diagnostic process.

Step 4

In Abby's history, what *inclusion* features do we find that support a diagnosis of some sort of depression?

With all those underlinings and superscript numbers in Steps 2 and 3, I've tried to make this easy. Just check the boxes of the underlined passages that you believe serve to include Abby in this category of disorder.

☐ 1	☐ 2	☐ 3	☐ 4	☐ 5	☐ 6
☐ 7	☐ 8	☐ 9	☐ 10	☐ 11	☐ 12

Note D

Here are the numbers I'd choose: 1, 2, 3, 4, 5, 6, 8, and 9. And here's my rationale.

Whereas I call these the *inclusion* symptoms of a depressive episode, DSM-5 refers to them as the *criterion* symptoms. Nearly every DSM-5 diagnosis has inclusion/criterion symptoms of one sort or another. Usually they will be the first ones mentioned—the *A criteria* (so called because they are usually grouped in a criteria list under the letter A)—in the sets of diagnostic requirements. By whatever name, they constitute much of the catalog of misery that haunts anyone who suffers from serious mental disorder.

Specifically, you should have noted that Abby complained of these things:

- Low mood (1)
- Trouble concentrating (2)
- Loss of interest in things she formerly enjoyed (DSM-5 requires either low mood or loss of interest for a major depressive episode; 3)
- Fatigue (4)
- Problems with sleep (usually it's some form of insomnia, though Abby seemed to sleep excessively; 5)
- Change in appetite and/or weight (Abby, like the classic depressed person, complained of anorexia and weight loss, though some patients eat a lot and gain weight in response to low mood; 6)
- Alarming thoughts of death and suicidal ideas (8)
- Feelings of worthlessness (or inappropriate guilt; 9)

I didn't include crying spells (7). Episodes of crying are hardly specific to mood disorders (tears can also indicate anger, frustration, grief, or joy). And we've noted no change in

Abby's psychomotor activity; that's also an inclusion symptom of depression. In depression, activity change will usually be a slowing of voluntary movement, but sometimes it is the opposite—agitation that can become quite profound and distressing, even just to witness.

And now I'll point out two other aspects of these inclusion symptoms. First, each must represent a change of functioning from the person's usual state; second, two of them must be present most of the day, and all but two must occur nearly every day. Those are qualities that we'd have to investigate a bit further, to assure that Abby's symptoms are indeed serious enough to punch her ticket of admission to the chapter on depression.

Just below, I've dropped in a convenient table that lists all nine of the inclusion symptoms or A criteria for an episode of major depression. It makes clear which symptoms the "all day, most of every day" strictures apply to.

If you like to count things, Abby has eight of DSM-5's A criteria for a major depressive episode; she lacks only changes in psychomotor activity. And maybe we just didn't spend quite long enough digging for information relevant to that remaining symptom. (We don't note that she has experienced guilt feelings, but she has complained of feeling worthless; that works for this criterion.) In any event, of the DSM-5 inclusion symptoms for a major depressive episode, she easily has the stated minimum of five, and then some.

Rant

In the first paragraph of Note C is an issue I don't want to gloss over. That is, what is the difference between *mood* and *affect*? Various clinicians and writers use them differently. Some will make an analogy to the difference between *climate* (which is relatively stable) and *weather* (here today, gone tomorrow), but that seems a bit casual. I prefer to explain the difference this way: Mood is how someone *claims* to feel, whereas affect is the way the person *appears* to feel. If Andrew says that he feels sad and gloomy, then his stated *mood* is one of depression. If he weeps, his shoulders slump, and the corners of his mouth turn down, then his appearance (*affect*) is also depressed.

Inclusion Symptoms for a Major Depressive Episode

Symptom	Nearly every day?	Most of day?
Depressed mood	✓	✓
Loss of interest or pleasure in most activities	✓	✓
Change of appetite or weight	✓	
Increased or decreased sleep	✓	
Psychomotor retardation or agitation	✓	
Fatigue or low energy	✓	
Feeling worthless or guilty	✓	
Trouble concentrating or thinking	✓	
Repeated thoughts of death or suicidal ideas		

Step 5

Now please write down the possibilities you see for Abby's diagnosis. What's wrong seems blindingly obvious, doesn't it? But that's one of the problems we all have as diagnosticians: the too-ready acceptance at face value of a seemingly crystal-clear, first-blush assessment that practically leaps from our pens and computers. Rather, what I'd like from you now is not a *diagnosis,* but a broad *differential diagnosis*—a list of all the conditions that *could* conceivably have caused a given set of signs and symptoms. Below, I've left enough lines to accommodate each of the diagnoses on my differential list for Abby.

By the way, if you're stuck for ideas as to disorders you should include in the differential diagnosis, you could turn to the listing I've made in the Appendix (see Table 3 there). It includes every disorder I've considered anywhere in this book. Uh-oh, it can also serve as a differential list for each of our 26 patients, so if you use the Table 3 listing for suggestions, be sure to look only at the first two columns and disregard my X's. I'd like you to do your own thinking.

____

____

____

____

____

____

____

____

Now compare what you've written to the answer I've given in Note E to my own question.

Note E

If you didn't write down a minimum of two or three different possible diagnoses, take a moment to go back and do so now, before you read my take on what ails Abby. (To make them stand out from other lists, throughout this book I'll use a different type of bullet to denote items in a differential diagnosis.)

◊ Substance/medication-induced mood disorder
◊ Depressive disorder due to another medical condition
◊ Major depressive disorder
◊ A bipolar disorder, current episode depressed
◊ Persistent depressive disorder (dysthymia)

◊ Premenstrual dysphoric disorder
◊ Adjustment disorder with depressed mood
◊ Schizoaffective disorder
◊ Personality disorder (such as borderline)

Some of the items in this list do indeed seem somewhat over the top—such as schizoaffective disorder, when we've heard nothing from Abby that would suggest psychosis. In my own defense, I'd point out that there's still a lot missing from her history.

The idea of creating a *broad* differential diagnosis for every patient may be the best diagnostic advice you'll ever receive. Indeed, I'll give it so often that either you'll become terminally sick of it and chuck this book across the room, or it'll sink in and you'll embrace my nagging as intended—something for your own good. Creating a broad differential diagnosis is one of my *diagnostic principles,* which are important ideas to keep in mind whenever you go about diagnosing a patient. I promise to pester you unmercifully about it.

The reason for a differential diagnosis is, of course, that before you can diagnose anything, you must think of it first. And a wide-ranging differential diagnosis is how clinicians force themselves to consider disorders that may not occur very often, but that occasionally turn out to be the cause for a given patient's symptoms—let's call it the "blue moon" approach to diagnosis.

At the very top of the differential lists I construct will be disorders related to the use of substances and those caused by physical illness. That's *not* because they are so terribly common; in fact, they occur far less often than major mental disorders such as, say, schizophrenia and bipolar disorders. But when an example does come around, you want to know about it as soon as possible. Otherwise, you risk dire consequences.

Suppose, for example, that Abby had recently begun using a hormonal contraceptive. We'd have to consider the possibility that it was in part responsible for her deteriorating mood. In such a case, adding yet another chemical (such as an antidepressant drug) could be not only ineffective, but irresponsible: It could make her worse. And if her depression had begun as a symptom of some physical condition—the consequence of Lyme disease, perhaps—directly attacking her mood might leave her still sick, with the physical ailment unaddressed. The act of diagnosing a mental health condition carries with it certain responsibilities; one of them is to consider all the possibilities.

The list of medications that have been associated with depressive symptoms is long; you can look it up in a textbook or a reliable online source. But you don't have to memorize the list; it's enough *always* to put the possibility of a substance at the top of your differential diagnosis, and to ask *every* patient about the use of alcohol, street drugs, and medications, including over-the-counter medications. And as far as physical illnesses are concerned, a huge number of these can cause mental symptoms—way too many to memorize. You can consult lists for details, but it is vital to ensure that medical conditions have been considered for every patient who has mental or behavioral symptoms.

Each of the remaining disorders on my differential diagnosis is there because depressive mood appears prominently among its symptoms. Note that always being alert for depressive disease is another important diagnostic principle.

Step 6

With a broad-ranging differential diagnosis in hand, it's time to select our *best diagnosis*. That's the one that stands out from all those possibilities, the one we judge most likely to account for a patient's signs and symptoms—even though it may not appear at the top of our differential diagnosis. It's the one for which we would then proceed to formulate an initial treatment plan.

How do the facts of Abby's history stack up against the various elements we've identified in her differential diagnosis? To help structure your work, I've provided some capsule evaluations you can use to think about these conditions as they might apply to Abby. But please feel free to add any thoughts of your own. (In fact, if you think your ideas are better than mine, send me an email: morrjame@ohsu.edu. I'd love to hear from you.).

a. No evidence, or even evidence to the contrary, but must keep alert for future developments.
b. Inclusion symptoms sufficient, but more information is needed to rule it in.
c. Seems a dead cert!
d. Insufficient inclusion symptoms.
e. Something wrong in the pattern of symptoms.
f. No chance—totally rule this one out.

Now, starting at the top of the list in Note D, jot down your thoughts about the suitability of each diagnosis. Then compare your thinking with mine in Note F.

Substance/medication-induced mood disorder: ______________________

Depression due to another medical condition: ______________________

Major depressive disorder: ______________________

A bipolar disorder, current episode depressed: ______________________

Persistent depressive disorder (dysthymia): ______________________

Premenstrual dysphoric disorder: ______________________

Adjustment disorder with depressed mood: ______________________

Schizoaffective disorder: ______________________

Personality disorder: ______________________

Note F

The last step in our search for truth is to move methodically through the differential list, ruling out possibilities until we're left with the one most likely to survive the test of time. In so doing, we need to keep in mind that the diagnosis of a mood disorder is about two things: symptoms, and how they are arranged into patterns. (Sure, that pretty well describes all diagnoses; here, we'll see how it plays out with a depressive disorder.)

We've already agreed (in Note C) that Abby has plenty of the symptoms typical of depression—low mood, poor appetite, sleep problems, and so forth. Indeed, from these symptoms alone, she appears to qualify for a diagnosis of major depressive disorder—the most common mood disorder diagnosis, one that is used by nearly every clinician countless times in evaluating new patients. It would be so easy just to say, "Yep, that's what's wrong with Abby!" and move on to consider what to do about it.

But that would do a disservice to her and to every other patient we might ever evaluate. That's because, sure, often the diagnosis will be major depressive disorder, but sometimes a different etiology will be responsible for the symptoms. So each time we evaluate a patient, we must carefully pore over a few lines of fine print to certify that something else doesn't explain the symptoms better.

In later chapters, we're going to examine carefully the additional requirements we need to evaluate before making any definitive diagnosis. But I think that for now, we've crammed about enough into one case history. So let me just go through my thinking about the other disorders on the list.

- We have information that Abby did not drink alcohol or use drugs to any significant extent. And we've noted that her physical health is excellent (so we'll assume that she's suffered no recent tick bites, her thyroid is in good working order, and so forth). In any event, for the purposes of this exercise, let's stipulate that her mood disorder isn't due to substance use or another medical illness, and discard the first two elements on our differential. Using the lettered choices in Step 6, I'd choose a for each of them.

- A bipolar disorder, current episode depressed? It could be, but we know of no history of mania or hypomania. We could only diagnose bipolar disease at some time in the future if Abby should develop manic or hypomanic symptoms. Choice b.

- Persistent depressive disorder (or dysthymia, as clinicians used to refer to it)? Nope. Abby's been ill for only a few weeks, not the minimum of 2 years required for chronic depression. And really, when you think about it, her symptoms have been more numerous and more serious than most cases of persistent depressive disorder. The 2-year minimum is the deal breaker. Choice e.

- Premenstrual dysphoric disorder? Uh-oh, we don't find anything about Abby's menstrual cycle in our history. That's a sin of omission that we should correct the next time we speak with Abby. But we can already note that there doesn't seem to be any rhythmicity to her depressive symptoms, and that would be required for a diagnosis of premenstrual dysphoric disorder. Choice d.

- Adjustment disorder? That would be a stretch, because there hasn't been any clear-cut stressor that might have caused her depressive symptoms. Also, the criteria for adjustment disorder clearly require us first to rule out other mood disorders. So yet another possibility goes down. Choice d.

- Schizoaffective disorder? Nice try, but no psychotic symptoms. Choice d.

- Personality disorder, then? In a later chapter, we'll have a really good conversation about when it's appropriate to diagnose a personality disorder. For right now, let me just refer you to another of my diagnostic principles: Avoid diagnosing a personality disorder when your patient is acutely ill with a major mental disorder. Yep, d.

And so we've come to the bottom of the list; now we can confidently say that Abby most likely has major depressive disorder. (Even so, I still wouldn't say it's certain, but it's good enough to choose as our best diagnosis.) This is her first episode (maybe it will be her only episode). We'll have to leave treatment to her own clinicians. Major depressive disorder will come up in this book again and again, inasmuch as it is encountered in a huge variety of guises, in countless patients every year, worldwide.

The Takeaway

We've used Abby's case to illustrate some of the basic steps in interviewing patients, thinking about diagnosis, and ruling specific disorders in or out. Specifically, we've discussed free speech (my favorite interview technique, because it allows patients to speak at length about issues of concern); the importance of the differential diagnosis; and some specific conditions that need to be excluded in pursuing a diagnosis of major depressive disorder. Specific MSE issues we've encountered include speech cadence and prosody, and abnormalities in flow of thought. We've mentioned a couple of diagnostic principles: Always consider depressive disease (because it is so common), and avoid diagnosing personality disorder in the face of a major mental disorder. And I've provided a Rant about the definitions of *mood* and *affect*, and how they differ.

Break Time

Can I start by emphasizing the importance of having hobbies and avocations that extend beyond your professional interests? No matter how much you love the work you do, I'll bet that when you are on vacation, you don't intend to write up old case histories or practice creating differential diagnoses. Neither activity is likely to relax you or to provide the perspective on life that will contrast with your actual job.

Rather, during evenings and weekends, I hope you gravitate to something that gives you a breather from the daily provision of health care services. You can choose all sorts of wonderful things to do—collecting stuff, gardening, photography, extreme sports (OK, maybe just walking or bike riding), reading, watching movies. Go ahead, indulge yourself. (If you cannot stand to divorce yourself from work completely, maybe you could collect stamps or read books with subject matter related to mental health issues.)

Relaxation is vital for people of our professions. You need it, and your patients will benefit from it. And I've prescribed it.

2

Complaint Department—Brad

Step 1

"My boss made me promise I'd give you this." Wearing a smile that seems a bit skewed, Brad holds out a sealed envelope. "In truth, I'm kinda worried about *him*. He's been acting secretive and, well, weird. I think he's even had me followed." Again, that lop-sided smile.

"I hope he's OK," Brad remarks as you tear open the envelope. Inside is a second envelope, and inside *that* is a handwritten note on letterhead stationery. It begins:

> *To Whom It May Concern: This will introduce Brad Fuller, my employee of the last 3 years. In the past 2 or 3 months, he has been behaving peculiarly. Several times, I've caught him looking at the underside of his desk (for microphones?)* . . .

In effect, you've been handed *two* chief complaints:

1. Brad's opening statement of concern *about* his boss, on the one hand . . .
2. . . . and the note *from* his boss about Brad, on the other.

Which do you ultimately write down? Which do you explore?

Note A

I suspect that your answer is the same as mine: You'd record both of them. Each has something to offer the investigating diagnostician's quest for truth. To a degree, you'll pursue them both.

The *chief complaint* is a vehicle for conveying the face of a case history—usually, whatever behavior or emotion the patient (or someone else) regards as a call to action. In the case of Brad, there's a conflict between what he thinks is going on and what someone else (his boss) perceives. Based on our current information, we cannot make a fair decision regarding the veracity of either of these opposing points of view. Indeed, even if we could state with certainty which one was correct, we'd want to pursue the information in each, to broaden our understanding of the situation. And we'd certainly want to preserve them both in our writeup.

Of course, this gets us ahead of ourselves; we're a long way from writing up Brad's case. So let's get back to the interview.

Step 2

With a shake of his head and a curled lip, Brad continues, "I'll bet it starts 'To Whom It May Concern.' Steve—my boss—likes that expression. He thinks it shows class."

The note continues:

> *. . . (for microphones?) When I've asked about it, he either ignores me or gets mad. No actual shouting, but I can tell he's pretty upset.*
>
> *Brad has shown some other peculiar behaviors. He's begun parking in the farthest corner of the company lot, away from all other vehicles. On break, instead of gathering with coworkers in the staff room as he used to, he goes outside (he doesn't smoke). Sometimes, when I've watched him as he walks back and forth, he seems to be muttering to himself. His colleagues have started talking about him, and, frankly, his behavior is interfering with the office workflow. He needs to get an evaluation, maybe treatment, before he can come back to work.*

In response to questions, Brad denies talking to himself, says that he's just fine, and then reiterates that it's Steve who has the problem. Brad doesn't feel depressed or anxious, he says. He just wants to do his job, and he wishes people would "stop making a big deal over me."

Hired right out of college, Brad has worked for this import–export company for 2 years. He's responsible for invoicing and billing, and he sits at a desk right in the main office. His boss values him in part because he's so good at dealing with people who have complaints. Usually it's about bills, but sometimes it concerns the condition of the merchandise they have received. Brad admits that he's made no real friends at work, but says that this doesn't bother him; he has "other outlets" for friendship.

Though he's never been married, he was briefly engaged last summer. "She decided—*we* decided—to see other people while we're still young," he remarks calmly. He has no girlfriend now. He does have a lot of nieces and nephews who live near the small apartment he rents, just a few blocks from his parents' home. He has supper with relatives once or twice a week. He enjoys skiing and the movies; he doesn't drink or use drugs.

This is Brad's first contact with the mental health care system; indeed, he's never been seriously ill in any way. He gets a flu shot each fall and takes a single multivitamin tablet every morning with his orange juice. He doesn't know of any relatives who have ever had emotional problems, "though, to be truthful, I've never asked."

"I wish you'd speak with my boss," Brad says. "But change the focus: *He* seems to be having some sort of problem. Quite frankly, I'm not sure I want to work for someone who's that unstable."

So here you are, still with two radically different stories: one from a normal-appearing patient, the other from a supposedly reliable informant. You've concluded that something must be wrong, but you aren't sure what it is. Your own observations don't go far toward resolving the apparent contradictions. How do you proceed?

Let's make this just a little easier with a dichotomy:

- ☐ Would you confront the patient with your uncertainty? If so, how would you phrase it?
- ☐ Or would it be better to find another informant?

Note B

Of course, one approach would be to point out the discrepancy and ask for help. Framing the question in terms of *your* inability to understand (rather than some defect in the patient's story) might help preserve what rapport you've managed to create during the brief interview so far. Still, however, you would risk erecting a barrier to trust.

In an instance such as this one, another method might have a better chance at success. That would be to get the view of another person, someone who has known the patient for a long time. In short, obtain collateral information.

It's pretty obvious that you'd want to choose someone who is likely to have the information you need. Whenever possible, that would be the person with the most intimate understanding of the patient and the most current information. For someone who is married or who still lives at home, a spouse or parent would be ideal. But it could also be a friend, a spiritual advisor, or even a coworker who knows the patient well.

Of course, you'll need the patient's agreement.* Obtaining this usually isn't a problem, but if you meet resistance, you can point out that the evaluation will stall and that resolution of the patient's problem will be delayed until you get the information. (According to the note from his boss, Brad is not supposed to return to work until his issues are sorted out.)

Ideally, the conversation with the informant will be private, so as to encourage complete candor, but sometimes the only way the patient will agree is to interview the informant while the patient sits in. Of course, then, if the informant is reluctant to speak candidly, you might have to draw inferences from body language and facial expressions. This is tricky. And it should be obvious that interviews conducted in person offer the greatest chance for meaningful information. However, through telephone calls or FaceTime, Skype, or some other form of video conferencing, even informants located in distant parts of the world can be accessible to inquiry.

Finally, what do you hope to learn? There are several types of information, including material that would help to resolve any previous conflicts of information; knowledge that would otherwise be inaccessible (such as the patient's own early childhood experiences and family history); and an objective view of whether—and how—the patient's behavior has changed over a period of time.

---

*Exceptions include people who are so medically ill that they cannot give informed consent, who are under conservatorship, or who are acutely suicidal or dangerous to other people.

Step 3

Brad's older sister, Lily, lives just outside town. She readily agrees to come in for an interview. At one point, she puts in a call to her aunt for perspective on some family history.

Lily remembers Brad as a pretty normal kid, much like their middle sibling, Jason. Brad got into the usual amount of trouble; he and Jason would tease her when she brought home a boyfriend. "Brad's always been very pleasant with people, a pretty good mixer, but perhaps a trifle shy," is Lily's assessment. He finished college, never served in the military, isn't religious, and has never had legal issues. She doesn't think he's been using drugs, and she's never seen him intoxicated. But some recent observations have troubled her.

During the time he's worked for Steve, Brad has lived in an apartment across town. A couple of months ago, he showed up on Lily's doorstep with the request to stay for a few days. He hadn't felt comfortable in his apartment, he said—his landlord had something against him and wanted him out. "Brad told me, 'It was probably so he could rent to a relative. Or something.' "

Lily and her husband have no children. "We have plenty of room, so of course I invited him to stay." That stay has now stretched into weeks, as Brad has shown no inclination to move out. Although he still goes to work, Lily has noticed in the last few weeks that he's become more and more distant. He has stopped eating meals with her and her husband; instead, he makes peanut butter sandwiches and takes these to his room. On weekends, he sleeps past noon, then slinks out the back door without so much as saying hello. Even on work nights, it appears that he stays up late. Once or twice, she's awakened to the sound of murmuring from his room. "It sounds as though he's talking to someone, but I'm certain there's no one else in the house." She has checked with other relatives, several of whom have reported that Brad has stopped emailing them; he doesn't even respond to text messages.

The call Lily makes to her aunt yields a surprise: Their family history isn't as spotless as Brad and Lily thought. When their mother's much older brother was a young adult, he became quiet and reclusive, refused to take baths, began to hallucinate, and was eventually hospitalized and treated with some sort of medication. Despite this care, he never left the hospital; after several years he died there, possibly by suicide. The family has never talked much about "Uncle Tad."

So, with this additional information, how would you assess—

Right, I've noted your virtual tap on my shoulder. I think I hear you saying, "Haven't we left something out?" It's big, so of course you've noticed it immediately. Right? If not, you can access a hint from the short list of interview sections we've created for Abby in Chapter 1's Step 2.

- ☐ Chief complaint
- ☐ History of the present illness
- ☐ Personal and social history
    - ☐ Early childhood relations
    - ☐ Family history

    - ☐ Schooling
    - ☐ Sexual and marital history
    - ☐ Employment history
    - ☐ Military experience
    - ☐ Legal issues
    - ☐ Religion
    - ☐ Leisure activities and interests
- ☐ Substance use
- ☐ Medical history and review of systems
- ☐ Mental status evaluation (MSE)
    - ☐ General appearance and behavior
    - ☐ Mood/affect
    - ☐ Flow of speech
    - ☐ Content of thought
    - ☐ Cognition (attention/concentration, orientation, language, executive functioning, memory, cultural information)
    - ☐ Insight and judgment

Rant

Handling complaints can be a chore for anyone, whether it's a personal issue or one related to work. Take a moment to reflect on any such stressful interactions you've had in the past. How did you respond? Would you—*should* you—have done anything differently?

Any type of "You did/No, I didn't" confrontation will probably generate more heat than light. Should the need arise, I like to draw from a small stock of responses that can encourage dialogue and defuse anger. You might want to see whether you can modify any of these to suit your own temperament:

> "You sound upset. Could you tell me more about what's wrong?"
> "I'm sorry to hear [whatever it might be]; what can I do to help you feel better?"
> "I don't think I've thought of it in quite that way. I'd like to hear more."

And if all else fails, you might consider using a quotation attributed to American writer H. L. Mencken. In response to any argumentative letter he might receive, he would send a note that read, in its entirety, "Dear Sir [or Madam]: You may be right."

Note C

The big issue we've left out is, of course, the *full* MSE, which I've expanded above. When you are sitting with a patient, it's easy to forget that your observations during a conversation net you only about half the material you need to complete all parts of the MSE. That is, you can notice how the patient dresses, sits, and moves, and whether there is eye contact. You can evaluate flow of speech (is it smooth, logical, coherent?), and you can probably make a stab at how the person is feeling (sad, happy, anxious, fearful, and so forth). Those are the parts of the MSE that you get "for free," so to speak—without having to ask a specific question.

But unless the patient voluntarily reveals it, you might not learn about such content of thought as hallucinations and delusions, obsessions and compulsions, phobias, and suicidal ideas. You might also be at a loss for an assessment of the patient's cognitive capabilities, including insight and judgment. For these functions, you will likely need to ask carefully tailored questions.

Step 4

In brief, here's how I'd describe Brad's MSE.

> Appearing a few years older (receding hairline and a few worry lines around his eyes) than his stated age of 25, Brad wears jeans and a dress shirt open at the neck. He carries a smartphone in a holster on his belt. He has no evident tattoos or piercings. He sits quietly; his activity level is neither excessive nor decreased. He says his mood is "OK," but his affect seems slightly depressed (slumped posture, hands motionless in his lap); it seems appropriate to his content of thought. Affective lability may be reduced a bit, but it does shift appropriately with changes in the topic of discussion. His speech is clear, coherent, and normal in rate and rhythm, except that he hesitates when asked to speak about what's on his mind.
>
> He begins with, "It's all rather puzzling, at least it is to me." He admits that a couple of months ago he began hearing "something, a voice—no, two voices. They are talking to me and about me." The voices tell Brad that his boss is trying to move him to another division in the company, so that Steve's nephew can take Brad's job. However, Brad denies having obsessions, compulsions, or phobias ("I don't care much for snakes, but I'm not afraid of them").
>
> He is fully oriented to date and day, place, and person; he can subtract sevens quickly and accurately, knows presidents, and appears fully aware of recent world events. Asked whether he is ill or needs treatment, he responds, "Well, I know I need to figure some stuff out about work. But it's not really my issue, it's Steve's." When asked whether he could be mistaken about his boss, Brad denies it, becoming quite animated as he does so.

And now, at last, considering Lily's information along with what we already know and the results of the formal MSE, what would you include in Brad's differential diagnosis? Yes, please, write it down. I've printed enough lines just below to accommodate each of the entries on my own differential diagnosis.

____

____

____

____

Rant

Let's pause and put into outline form the parts of a standard MSE. I've talked about it in Note C, but it'll be easier to comprehend if the outline is expanded a bit. We will make good use of it in future discussions.

- General appearance and behavior. Apparent age, race (if it bears on the diagnosis), posture, nutritional state, hygiene; clothing (neat? clean? type/fashion?); speech (clear? coherent?); activity level; mannerisms and stereotypies; eye contact; tremors; smiles.
- Mood/affect. Type of mood; lability; appropriateness (to content of thought).
- Flow of speech. Word associations (tight? loose?); rate and rhythm of speech.
- Content of thought. Phobias, obsessions–compulsions, suicidal ideas, delusions, hallucinations.
- Language. Comprehension, fluency, naming, repetition, reading, writing.
- Cognition. Orientation (person, place, time); memory (immediate, recent, remote); attention and concentration (serial sevens, counting backward); cultural information (for example, the five most recent presidents); abstract thinking (similarities, differences).
- Insight and judgment.

Note D

Now here's my differential diagnosis for Brad:

◊ Psychosis due to another medical condition ★
◊ Substance/medication-induced psychosis
◊ Mood disorder with psychosis
◊ Schizophreniform disorder
◊ Schizoaffective disorder
◊ Schizophrenia

Because I don't feel comfortable omitting anything, I've included all of the usual suspects here. That will be my default position when constructing a differential diagnosis.

Why have I arranged the list in this particular order? I always put medical disorders and substance use at the top of the possible causes for, well, just about anything. That's because I forever worry that one of these two etiologies *might* be the cause, and if that should turn out to be the case, I could miss a diagnosis that carries a potential of recovery, if identified and addressed quickly, and disaster if overlooked. If I put these possibilities on top, I *know* I'll consider them early.

Mood disorder comes next, not because I think it likely for Brad, but because it is found so frequently in the general population. Anything starting with *schizo-* will trail, because the relatively poor prognosis for these conditions in the sections on schizophrenia and psychotic disorders in most diagnostic manuals makes me very careful about being cavalier with these diagnoses.

This overall arrangement, from top to bottom, embodies what I call the *safety principle* of the differential diagnosis. At the top, I put the disorders that have immediate potential for serious harm or that offer a ready treatment approach. At the very bottom are those conditions that carry a frankly terrible prognosis, or for which treatment tends to be ineffective. In between goes everything else. This diagnostic principle is so important to keep in mind that I'll bring it up over and again.

Step 5

Wait a moment: I've included several diagnoses from the psychotic disorders category. Exactly what does the term *psychosis* mean, anyway, and what does it mean when a person has it? What I'd like from you is just a statement of definition; later, we'll get to the list of symptoms that can get a person into the psychosis ballpark. For the definition, as few as five words will do. (If you need a hint, unscramble the five words I've listed in the box below.)

To have a psychosis means that a person is

of out reality touch with

Note E

Stated simply, in one way or another, psychotic people are "out of touch with reality." That is, something about their thinking or behavior is radically different from an ordinary person's, and is at odds with the facts as others perceive them. Yet these patients may not realize just how different they are from other people. In fact, if their perceptions are pointed out to them as false, they are likely to deny that this could be the case. Someone with psychosis believes that other persons are the unusual ones, the ones who may need treatment. What we regard in psychotic people as abnormal, they experience as routine. In other words, they lack insight that there is something wrong, and that the problem lies within *them*.

Step 6

And now I'll give an example of each principal symptom of psychosis; you write in the term that describes the category. If you need a hint, I've listed the five choices in alphabetical order at the end of this Step.

- Arun lies flat on his back with his arm extended toward the ceiling in a sort of salute; when he is told that he can lower his hand, it remains elevated.

  This is an example of ______________________________

- Betty hears a voice just outside her head that encourages her to flee the country; no one else can hear it.

This is an example of ______________________________

- For the past 3 months, Charles has stayed in his room; when he does come out, he doesn't participate in family life or in any of the work around the house. It's been days since he's shown either joy or sorrow.

  These are examples of ______________________________

- Donald believes that his wife has been putting arsenic into his oatmeal. She tearfully denies it and eats the oatmeal herself without ill effects, but he clings to this belief.

  This is an example of ______________________________

- Ernestine's speech is so garbled with sentence fragments and made-up words that no one can follow her train of thought.

  This is an example of ______________________________

The hint: delusion, disorganized behavior, disorganized speech, hallucination, negative symptom.

Note F

In operational terms, a psychotic person will have at least one of the following five sorts of symptoms:

- *Delusions* (false ideas from which no one can dissuade the person). These ideas are commonly persecutory in nature (as with Donald), but sometimes they may instead be false ideas of poverty, guilt, infidelity (by a spouse or intimate partner), or mind reading/thought control.

- *Hallucinations.* These false sensory percepts are most commonly auditory (this was Betty's experience) or visual, but smells, tastes, and tactile sensations can also be hallucinated. Hallucinations must be distinguished from *illusions,* in which the person misidentifies an actual sensory input. For example, in the dead quiet of an empty room, the person hears a voice. If you ask whether there could be any other explanation, and the response is "Perhaps it was just a branch scraping against the window," then it's probably an illusion. However, if the response is that somebody (or something) is "actually talking—can't you hear it?", it is more likely that the person is experiencing a hallucination.

- *Disorganized speech.* Ernestine's speech output is garbled by puns, rhymes, and made-up words; the resulting output may not convey meaning to us as outside observers.

- *Disorganized behavior.* These are bits of behavior that do not appear to be goal-directed. Arun assumes unusual postures; others might maintain uncomfortable positions despite being told to "relax." Sometimes these behaviors are identified as *catatonic.*

- *Negative symptoms.* Charles seems to lack something that is normally present. That is, he shows very low variation in affect (sometimes it's termed *blunted* or *flattened affect*), and his lack of participation in family life we might interpret as the loss of will to accomplish something—called *avolition.* Paucity of speech in situations when more speech would be expected provides yet another example.

For a person to be diagnosed with a psychosis, at least one of the inclusion symptoms described above must be present. In DSM-5, these are the A criteria. For schizophrenia, schizoaffective disorder, and schizophreniform disorder, two of these symptoms must be present, and at least one of them must come from the first three types listed above. People whom we diagnose as suffering from delusional disorder have mainly—you guessed it—delusions, without any of the other symptoms. Well, maybe the odd hallucination, but only one that serves to support the delusions. For example, a patient with delusional disorder who believes that poison gas is being piped into the house claims to detect a characteristic odor when no one else can. Oh, yes, and someone whom we diagnose as having a psychosis caused by a medical condition or by substance use needs only one of the symptoms above.

By the way, I am not usually a fan of rote memorization; that's why we have computers and Wikipedia. But this is one set of definitions that you'll need time and again. Just learn it.

Step 7

Now, what best diagnosis would you choose for Brad? And why? What I'd actually like you to do is to go through the Note D list and put down reasons for including or excluding each one. That's what experienced diagnosticians do for each patient they see. (OK, they usually do it mentally, but I think you'll learn better if you commit your reasoning to paper.)

Psychosis due to another medical condition: ______________________

Substance/medication-induced psychosis: ______________________

Mood disorder with psychosis: ______________________

Schizophreniform disorder: ______________________

Schizoaffective disorder: ______________________

Schizophrenia: ______________________

Note G

And here is why I've ruled these diagnoses in or out. We'll use the safety principle and start at the top of our differential diagnosis for Brad.

- Just to be certain, Brad should have a complete physical examination, but there's nothing in the history, in the report from his sister, or in the MSE that would make us believe that a physical illness is causing his psychotic symptoms.
- His sister seems to agree that he doesn't currently use drugs or alcohol (nor has he ever) to any significant extent. But always, always, we try to keep these two potential diagnoses in mind, even after we've "ruled them out."
- Why do I include mood disorder at all? There are a couple of reasons. It is terribly common and highly treatable (so you'd hate to miss it), and some patients don't even recog-

nize that they feel depressed, so they don't report it. But with no evidence in the history to support a mood disorder diagnosis, we can pass it by—for Brad, for now.

Now let's move on to the *schizo*- diagnoses—schizoaffective disorder, schizophrenia, and schizophreniform disorder. We'll discuss them in alphabetical order, but note that each of these requires that the patient have at least two of the five symptoms of psychosis I've listed in Note F. Also note again the extra requirement, new in DSM-5, that at least one of these symptoms must be hallucinations, delusions, or disorganized speech/thinking. Brad appears to have both hallucinations *and* delusions.

- We can reject schizoaffective disorder for Brad, because by definition, it requires mood symptoms that meet criteria for a major depressive or manic episode throughout most of the patient's illness. We've already agreed that Brad has had no such mood symptoms.
- Schizophrenia is, unhappily, the first diagnosis some clinicians reach for when they encounter someone who has psychotic symptoms. I say *unhappily,* because when this diagnosis turns out not to be accurate, the patient may be stuck with an unwarranted label that's hard (if not impossible) to peel off. It's much better not to use the term in the first place, unless you can be truly certain. Of course, Brad does have the required number of inclusion symptoms (hallucinations and delusions), and he doesn't have evidence of a competing mood diagnosis. But he's apparently short on one factor: time. That is, as far as we can tell, he's been ill for just a few months, certainly less time than the minimum of 6 months required by DSM-5. That fact brings us to . . .
- Schizophreniform disorder. It's a concept that has been around much longer than half a century; yet, in my opinion, it still isn't used nearly often enough. Like its siblings above, it requires two or more of the psychotic symptoms, but you can diagnose it in patients who have been ill for as little as 1 month. It sets these "short-term" patients, some of whom will recover completely, off from those with true schizophrenia, who are far more likely to remain ill.

So schizophreniform disorder is the diagnosis I would assign to Brad, for now. If after another several months he were to recover, that would remain his diagnosis—unless another cause for psychotic symptoms were to become evident. However, after 6 months of continuous illness, we would then have to rediagnose him, probably as having schizophrenia.

Here's one more thought: The story of Brad's great-uncle might make us suspicious that there is a family history of schizophrenia, but I'd never place a high bet on a diagnosis beginning with *schizo*- based principally on family history.

Step 8

Just when we may have thought we were finished, uh-oh! A patient with schizophreniform disorder requires one further determination. That is, what is the likely prognosis for Brad? It's a simple good–poor dichotomy, so you could just offer your best guesstimate. But DSM-5 offers some guidelines. There are four criteria to consider. Can you intuit which of these is a feature that suggests a good outcome (that is, complete recovery), and which suggests a poor outcome? Underline your responses.

a. The appearance of confusion or perplexity (good/poor)
b. Good premorbid functioning (good/poor)
c. A normal range of affect (good/poor)
d. Onset of psychotic symptoms early (within the first month) in the overall course of the person's illness (good/poor)

Now, two further questions:

1. How many features, one way or another, are needed to predict a good outcome?
2. And what do we predict down the road for Brad?

Note H

If you underlined "good" for each of the features mentioned, you did goo—no, you did great! In excruciating detail, here they are again: (a) confusion or perplexity when psychosis is at its greatest; (b) good premorbid functioning with family, friends, and associates at work or school; (c) affect that has a normal range (I mean, it is not what we would call flat or blunted) when the patient is in the throes of illness; and (d) early onset of psychotic symptoms (within the first month that the patient appears ill in any way).

And having two or more of these four features suggests that this patient is more likely to recover completely and return to the previous level of functioning than is someone who has none or one of these features. How should we apply them in Brad's case? Is he likely to recover completely—that is, to return to his former, premorbid self—or remain ill? In other words, is he likely to meet criteria for a diagnosis of schizophrenia in the future?

Despite all the history we've given for Brad, it still isn't clear in my mind just how far into his illness the hallucinations and delusions began. But he definitely does have the first three of these features: He shows perplexity; by all accounts, he had good premorbid functioning; and his affect, as we've noted in Step 5, shows a range that is about normal and appropriate to the content of his thought. These three features are enough to suggest that in the next few weeks or months, he might recover.

The Takeaway

In our discussion of Brad, we've had to deal with conflict: two disparate chief complaints that must be evaluated and resolved, as well as two quite different versions of a patient's history. We haven't played favorites: We've valued them both. To make our evaluation, we've sought additional history from collateral sources—people who know the patient well. Along the way, we've discussed the sometimes delicate issue of obtaining the patient's agreement with acquiring this information.

We've learned this as well: Collateral history—in Brad's case, both from his boss and from his sister (yes, and from his aunt)—can sometimes trump history from the patient. We've also noted that though family history can be a useful pointer, it cannot supersede information about the patient's own behavior, emotions, and recent mental history.

Once we've established the basic symptoms of psychosis, we've noted that the diagnosis of schizophreniform disorder is a way of saying, "This patient is ill, but undiagnosed." (However, it is limited to a very few, highly specialized situations.) Then we've covered the guidelines for estimating prognosis for this rather peculiar, occasionally invaluable diagnosis.

Here are a few other important issues we've dealt with: how to confront, without going to war, a patient who presents discrepancies; the importance of the MSE; and the safety principle of diagnosis. Finally, we've revisited (not for the last time) the concept of best diagnosis.

Break Time

Let's talk about the movies. OK, that's too broad, so we'll focus it a bit. Let's discuss the mental health professions as they are depicted in films, on network and cable TV, and now in made-for-online-viewing videos and series. Sometimes the picture isn't all that rosy.

A film that comes immediately to mind—well, for those above a certain age—is *One Flew Over the Cuckoo's Nest.* This masterly portrayal of institutional neglect and malfeasance (filmed at an actual mental hospital in Oregon, my home state) shows Nurse Ratched running the place with little interference from the attending staff, to the detriment of the patients.

I'm also thinking of *Shock Treatment,* an even hoarier film from the 1960s in which Lauren Bacall plays a psychiatrist who gets off on administering electroconvulsive therapy to people who have no mental illness. (There is a moral: She ends up as a patient in her own facility.)

But wait. There's more! In fact, you can consult whole websites devoted to the theme of bad therapeutics in the popular media. Here's just a sample of what my informal search turned up:

- In *Running with Scissors,* Dr. Finch prescribes medications that aren't labeled and recommends behavior that isn't safe. He even suggests that his patient might avoid school by attempting suicide.
- In *Antichrist,* filmmaker Lars von Trier depicts a therapist who treats his own wife. A delicate assessment of the therapy would be "less than totally successful."
- Dr. Melvin Potts, the cigarette-smoking psychiatrist in *Girl, Interrupted,* diagnoses a patient as "borderline" because she has no goals in life other than to be sexually promiscuous.

- Dr. Brodsky, the doctor in *A Clockwork Orange,* prescribes experimental aversion therapy.
- In our first view of Dr. Jacoby, the psychiatrist in that (recently revived) television classic of another era, *Twin Peaks,* he is wearing glasses that have one red lens and one blue lens. He claims that they make the world appear three-dimensional. Generously described as "eccentric," in the original series, Jacoby ultimately had his license to practice revoked.
- Of course, Dr. Hannibal Lecter, the cannibalistic psychiatrist in *The Silence of the Lambs,* occupies a niche all his own.

On the other hand . . .

- *Good Will Hunting* presents an overall favorable portrayal (hey, it's Robin Williams!) of a clinician who, nonetheless, physically shakes a patient.
- In *Equus,* Dr. Dysart is basically a well-motivated psychiatrist who tries to help troubled kids, but questions his own profession.
- In the HBO classic *The Sopranos,* Dr. Jennifer Melfi is a pretty good therapist who, over the course of several seasons, helps Tony Soprano engage his demons. (On the other hand, the series' third season also features an older psychiatrist who, early in his first interview with Carmela, advises her to divorce Tony. Given what we know, that might not have been such a bad outcome—but as process, of course, it stinks.)
- *A Beautiful Mind* focuses on the patient, the actual mathematician John Nash; the psychiatrist appears competent, but remains a relatively minor figure.
- In *I Never Promised You a Rose Garden,* based on the novel of the same name, Dr. Clara Fried helps the patient (misdiagnosed with "borderline schizophrenia," we should note) to choose reality and fight her illness.

Positive and negative, there are many, many more examples out there; TV and the movies are chock-a-block with them. I'd love to know your favorites.

3

Past Is Prologue—Candice

Step 1

Candice is a farmer who has come in because of—well, at first, we're not sure just why she's sought care. She is accompanied by her wife, Sophie, with whom she's been arguing in the waiting room. When you invite Candice into the office, Sophie stands up, too. The two women resume their argument as Candice indicates clearly just how little she wants Sophie to join her in the interview room.

"This is my issue, and I'm going to have the first word!" Her yell morphs into a sob, and she resumes crying as Sophie tries to step ahead of her.

"Look, you need professional help, but first you need me." Sophie scowls and folds her arms across her chest.

Short of fisticuffs, how do you resolve the argument?

- ☐ Talk to Candice first?
- ☐ Start out with some background from Sophie? After all, at this point she sounds as though she's holding it together a little better.

And, can you formulate a principle on how to decide?

Note A

The question of whom to interview first isn't usually difficult; certainly that's the case for patients who are adults. With a young child, I take the accompanying adult first; with a patient in the teens or older, the patient almost always takes precedence. For ages in between, I play it by ear. But unless an adult patient requests you to speak first with the informant—or is obviously incapacitated by dementia or major problems with communication—the patient should be your first stop in the interview process. So Candice is the obvious candidate for first interview.

There's another question here: How do you smooth over what could be a rough patch at the beginning? And the answer is this: Hey! We're mental health clinicians; we're diagnosticians *and* we're therapists! Our stock in trade is persuading people to recognize that their own interests may lie on a path different from the one they have selected. And so we should be able to restructure nearly any situation so as to achieve more than one goal—in this case, to gather the material we need while keeping a lid on boiling emotions.

In such an instance, I'd say something like this:

> "Let's do what I normally do—hear first from the one who is the patient. But I am always interested in the viewpoints of people who know and care for each other. And so, Sophie, I'd like to speak first with Candice, privately. And then, with her permission, I'll listen to every bit of information you have to offer, too."

Coupled with your natural authority as the captain of the ship, that should settle the argument and give you the opportunity to speak with both partners.

Step 2

Making liberal use of the box of tissues on your desk, Candice tells this story.

> Until a couple of months ago, she and Sophie were happy and doing well with their farm, where they grow organic produce, mainly root vegetables. But there had been a fungus scare, and then they'd had a fight with a neighbor whom they suspected of using genetically modified seeds. "Those, plus a few other problems, were what started me downward," Candice says, reaching for yet another tissue.
>
> Gradually, she drifted into depression. Now she can admit that she had too easily become obsessed with the problems; perhaps that was why for several weeks she'd been unable to concentrate on her planting schedules. Sophie had had to take over many of Candice's responsibilities. And Candice had begun awakening even earlier than usual, sometimes even before the chickens were up. At your questioning glance, she adds, "Well, we're vegetarians, but we do need eggs."
>
> When her sex interest flagged, she'd considered trying flibanserin—"You know, 'the female Viagra?' "—but she hadn't felt motivated enough to make an appointment with her gynecologist. Sophie hadn't pressured her on this, "or much of anything else," Candice acknowledges. "She's been a peach—except that she keeps nagging me to eat more, my weight's fallen off so." Candice admits that most days she's been too tired even to eat dinner. "When I come in from the fields, all I want to do is go to bed. I'm just not interested in much of anything else."
>
> Had there ever been other episodes like this one? Yes, she'd had at least one other, when she was in college. Back then, it was a fractured relationship that had caused her to brood for several weeks; she couldn't study, and she "pretty much gave up eating and lost some weight. Hey, I looked terrific!" Her grades had begun to tumble when she "somehow dragged myself out of it. I realized I was actually lucky to be rid of my former 'significant other,' and for a couple of months, I was a ball of fire. I really burned through my courses and ended with all A's."
>
> During her interview, Candice repeatedly twists her fingers, and several times she gets up to pace to the window and back. Her speech is clear but rapid and, at times,

disjointed. Several times, she appears to lose her train of thought while she focuses on activities in the street outside the window.

When diagnosing anyone with depressive symptoms, perhaps the first thing we think about is this: Do the patient's symptoms qualify for a major depressive episode? DSM-5 requires that the patient have at least five of nine possible symptoms. (Yes, this is a reprise of the list we've encountered in Chapter 1 for Abby. Here it is again, as the lead-in to another important part of the diagnostic process. At least one of the first two symptoms is required.)

- ☐ Depressed mood (majority of the time)
- ☐ Decreased interest or pleasure (majority of the time)
- ☐ Loss or gain in weight or appetite
- ☐ Too little or too much sleep most days
- ☐ Activity level increased or decreased most days
- ☐ Fatigue or loss of energy
- ☐ Feeling worthless or inappropriately guilty
- ☐ Trouble concentrating or thinking
- ☐ Repeated thoughts about death or suicide

First, I'd like you to check off the symptoms that we know characterize Candice now. Then prepare to think about what else she would need to fulfill criteria for an episode of major depression. In addition to the inclusion symptoms, there are three requirements, and they are part of the boilerplate that we encounter in many (well, actually, most) mental health diagnoses.

Note B

The inclusion requirements for major depressive episode aren't onerous. You have probably already noted that Candice has depressed mood (you'd have to confirm that it lasts the majority of the day, most days, as indicated in the table on page 12). She is also experiencing loss of interest (low libido); she is agitated; she doesn't have much appetite; and she complains of fatigue. Even without digging further, she has five symptoms—enough to qualify.

Then there are those three boilerplate issues I've hinted at. But wait! Let's step back for a moment and talk a bit about the whole boiler, so to speak.

Before we can award our seal of approval to any diagnosis of major depressive disorder, or to many other mental or behavioral diagnoses, there is one further step: We must make sure to complete another diagnostic checklist that we should always keep in mind. I like to remember the four steps on this checklist with a mantra: "inclusion, exclusion, duration, distress." The mantra is in dactylic tetrameter; say it fast, and it sings.

And here it is, broken down for Candice's major depressive episode:

- *Inclusion.* We've done this part of the job, just above, and she's *in*.
- *Exclusion.* Most conditions carry with them a list of disorders that must first be

eliminated from consideration. For a major depressive episode, we must first rule out etiologies related to a physical health condition or to the use of substances. (This requirement is reflected in my obsessive placement of substance use and medical conditions at the top of every differential diagnosis I write.) Although we've been alerted, we haven't yet ruled out these other conditions that might apply to Candice's case.

• *Duration.* Most mental disorders have some sort of time requirement. For a major depressive episode or disorder, it's a minimum of 2 weeks. Candice has already passed that mark.

• *Distress.* And last on our list is a requirement that applies to most mental disorders in DSM-5: It must cause the patient to experience distress, often to the point of seeking clinical help. And if not distress, then there must be some sort of disability—impaired functioning at work or in some other aspect of the patient's personal or social life. (Of course, for a student, by "work" we also mean "school.") Many, perhaps most, patients experience *both* distress and disability. That's been the case for Candice, who is both suffering emotionally *and* having difficulties with her work and in her relationship with Sophie.

These four features—the mantra—form the bedrock of most mental disorder diagnoses. Quite frankly, I wish I could have introduced the idea even earlier, even in the Chapter 1 discussion of Abby. I haven't done it there because just too much else in Chapter 1 is new, but I promise to make up for my tardiness by coming back to the mantra again and again.

Step 3

Now what would you include in Candice's differential diagnosis? Jot down a couple of words of justification concerning each one. We've already done this exercise a couple of times; for some hints about the sorts of choices you can make, review Note E for Abby (page 13) or Note D for Brad (page 24).

____

____

____

____

____

____

Note C

Here's my back-of-the-envelope first pass at Candice's differential diagnosis, along with justifications for my choices.

◊ Depressive disorder due to another medical condition. Of course, we must *always* consider this possibility. But I don't see it as any real likelihood at this point. Still, a trip to the family doctor wouldn't be amiss.
◊ Substance/medication-induced depressive disorder. There's probably nothing here to worry a lot over, either. But wouldn't it be a good idea to take a complete substance use history, and to verify with Sophie what you learn?
◊ Major depressive disorder. Candice definitely qualifies for this one—assuming that we don't find information to support the next entry on the list.
◊ A bipolar disorder. With nothing said to the contrary, "something bipolar" definitely still belongs in the running—pending further information.
◊ Adjustment disorder with depressed mood. This one is a rather hard sell. DSM-5 and other diagnostic manuals make it clear that just about every other type of disorder must be eliminated first. Somehow, I don't think we're going to accomplish that. But it's often a good idea to consider adjustment disorder at least briefly, assuming that the history will yield a suitable stimulus.
◊ Unspecified personality disorder. Of course, this might feature in just about any differential diagnosis, but is it likely to cause a sudden change such as Candice has described? Highly unlikely. Note that personality disorder should languish at or pretty near the bottom of the possible diagnoses for any given individual's symptoms.

Step 4

Now it's Sophie's turn. She says she's happy to speak with Candice present in the room, though to encourage candor, I usually prefer to interview each person privately. In this case, you yield to the importance of preventing any further rupture of their relationship.

"So did she tell you about her past episodes?" Sophie wants to know.

Of course, you nod *yes*.

"I'll bet anything—anything!—that she didn't say 'boo!' about her hyper periods."

Candice interrupts: "I wasn't hyper—I'm *never* hyper. Sometimes I'm just normal, that's all." She bursts into tears. With more tissues and time, Candice calms down, and Sophie continues.

At least twice since they've been together, Candice has experienced episodes where her activity level and her outlook on the world in general have changed in synchrony. "It's as though she's become—perhaps not a different person; it's just as if she's put on makeup and clothing that render her nearly unrecognizable. At least by me."

Candice tries again to object, but Sophie ignores her and continues.

"For maybe a month, she'll seem to move faster than normal. It isn't, like, warp speed, but she even talks noticeably faster than usual. And there isn't the normal delay between thought and action; it all seems to happen at once. Here's a typical example: I might say something, and where she'll usually pause and reflect for a moment or two, instead she'll start to answer, even before I've finished."

"Oh, for Pete's sake, that's never—"

But Sophie waves her off and continues. "Look, she can actually be a lot of fun then. She chatters, she has lots of suggestions for activities—once we just left the tractor right in the middle of the field, packed up, and drove to the beach!

"At these times she doesn't sleep much, doesn't seem to need it. Normally, we go to bed at the same time. When she's, um, hyper [another scowl from Candice], she comes to bed late and wakes me up, wanting sex. And then next morning, there she is, up first, making breakfast, as alert as if she'd slept 8 hours." These "up" episodes tend to last several weeks. In response to questions, Sophie says that they didn't seem related to any particular time of year, or to Candice's menstrual cycle.

During one "up" episode, Candice thought that it might be a good thing to grow marijuana. Legalization was coming, and they could get in on the ground floor—never mind that their climate might require special, hard-to-grow cultivars. So, without discussing it further, she had ordered lights and other equipment for *indoor* cultivation. "Where, exactly? In the basement? We could just take out the furnace? Luckily, I was able to cancel the order; no harm done. But her judgment simply isn't up to the mark when she's hyper like that."

"I'm only normal. It's when I feel *well,*" Candice puts in. "I'm not high, just *normal.*"

"You *are* high! For several weeks, you are witty and laugh at stuff and seem to feel that the world is just one big joke. But you can also become quite irritable!" exclaims Sophie. "Like now, but more so—*really* pissed off! I walk on eggshells the whole time, so as not to set you off."

"I'm never irritable!" Candice almost screams it out.

So, with this information, we can mention two diagnostic principles: (1) History sometimes beats the patient's cross-sectional appearance, and (2) collateral history sometimes beats the patient's own viewpoint. In the course of a clinical practice, each of these will get a heavy workout; each is important to keep in mind.

The information from Sophie leaves us now obviously needing to discuss manic symptoms a bit further. In fact, we need to consider four separate conditions: bipolar I, bipolar II, and cyclothymic disorders; and the *with mixed features* specifier for manic or hypomanic symptoms during a depressive episode. Can you *very* briefly outline the features that differentiate them? This is a free-form question of the sort I won't ask very often, but you may be itching to express your creativity. In defining the differences, it might help if you consider these things:

a. The severity of any manic-like symptoms
b. How long they last
c. Their relationship to any depressive symptoms
d. How noticeable an effect they have had

Bipolar I: ______________________________

Bipolar II: ______________________________

Cyclothymia: ______________________________

Mixed features specifier: ______________________________

Note D

First, I'll give my own very brief take on what differentiates these four conditions. Then I'll toss in a couple of tables to provide guidelines that are a bit more detailed.

The extremely short version is this: Bipolar I disorder has manic episodes, and bipolar II has hypomanic episodes. Each of these episode types is a pure "up" phase, and activity level is increased in each. Although the symptoms are similar in the two types, they are more extreme with manic than with hypomanic episodes. Episodes with mixed features have aspects of both highs and lows at the same time. And cyclothymic disorder has comparatively mild, rather brief ups and downs that alternate.

Now let's go through it again, with more detail. Patients with bipolar I or bipolar II disorder have high periods when they have heightened mood and feel good about themselves. They tend to talk a lot and to be more active than usual; they don't seem to need much sleep; and they show poor judgment. The major difference between the two is that the symptoms of bipolar II (that is, during a hypomanic episode) are not as extreme as those in a full-blown manic episode of bipolar I. Specifically, patients with bipolar II are *not* psychotic and *do not* require hospitalization; also, they can be diagnosed if they have symptoms for a time as brief as 4 days. For a manic episode, symptoms must be present for at least a week. Note that if a patient with bipolar II ever requires hospitalization for a high episode, that's mania, and that patient will have to be reclassified as having bipolar I.

In cyclothymic disorder, a patient's moods vary with considerable frequency—perhaps every few days or weeks. And the highs and lows are *never* severe enough to qualify as a major depressive, manic, or hypomanic episode.

And, finally, there's the specifier *with mixed features.* For this specifier, as you can see from the tables on the facing page, DSM-5 requires that a patient who meets full criteria for an episode of either mania (or hypomania) or major depression must have several features of the "opposite" episode type—on most of the days that the patient has symptoms at all. The requirements, as DSM-5 prints them, are complicated; I hope that a little time with the tables I've provided will help.

By the way, have you noticed how vehemently Candice denies being irritable? That sort of self-justifying statement is termed a *defense mechanism.* Hers is of a type called, you won't be surprised to learn, *denial.* There are many, many others. We'll have more to say about defense mechanisms much later in the book.

Step 5

And now we have to apply all of this information about diagnostic criteria to Candice's case history. Applying the information in Steps 2 and 4 and Notes C and D to the six contenders, what would you finally determine to be her diagnosis? And why?

Best diagnosis for Candice: ____

And the reason(s): ____

Comparing Manic and Hypomanic Episodes with Mixed Features during a Major Depressive Episode

<table>
<tr><th>Manic episode</th><th>Hypomanic episode</th><th>Mixed features—manic during depressive episode</th></tr>
<tr><td>Duration: 7 consecutive days</td><td>Duration: 4 consecutive days</td><td>Duration: Most days of a major depressive episode</td></tr>
<tr><td colspan="2">↑ energy or activity level plus mood that is elevated, expansive, or irritable</td><td>—</td></tr>
<tr><td colspan="2">3+ (4+ if mood is only irritable) of the following:
↑ self-esteem/grandiosity
↓ need for sleep
↑ talking or pressured speech
Flight of ideas or racing thoughts
Distractibility
Agitation or ↑ goal-directed activity
Excess activity showing poor judgment
—</td><td>3+ of the following:
↑ self-esteem/grandiosity
↓ need for sleep
↑ talking or pressured speech
Flight of ideas or racing thoughts
—
↑ goal-directed activity or ↑ energy
Excess activity showing poor judgment
Elevated or expansive mood</td></tr>
<tr><td>Markedly impaired functioning or psychosis, or need for hospitalization</td><td>Never psychotic or hospitalized</td><td>—</td></tr>
</table>

Comparing Major Depressive Episode with Mixed Features during a Manic or Hypomanic Episode

Major depressive episode	Mixed features—depressed during manic or hypomanic episode
Duration: 2 weeks	Duration: Most days of a manic or hypomanic episode
5+ of (must include at least 1 of first 2):	3+ of:
Depressed mood	Depressed mood (felt or observed)
Loss of interest or pleasure in most activities	Loss of interest or pleasure in most activities
Marked change (↑ or ↓) in weight or appetite	—
Sleep change (↑ or ↓)	—
Psychomotor activity change (↑ or ↓)	Psychomotor retardation
Tired or ↓ energy	Tired or ↓ energy
Feelings of worthlessness or inappropriate guilt	Feelings of worthlessness or inappropriate guilt
↓ ability to think or concentrate	—
Recurring thoughts of death, suicide	Recurring thoughts of death, suicide

Note E

Let's quickly dispose of one possibility: cyclothymic disorder. People with this diagnosis have relatively mild ups and downs of mood, with many of the hypomanic symptoms we've already discussed. However, in cyclothymia, the symptoms must never qualify for any of the three types of mood episodes—manic, hypomanic, or major depressive. We've already agreed (Note B) that Candice has a major depressive episode, and this rules out cyclothymic disorder.

Some variety of bipolar disorder is beginning to look like a winner, but we need to validate it by carefully scrutinizing Candice's symptoms and the diagnostic requirements.

In Step 4, Sophie describes Candice's symptoms of mania/hypomania during a previous "hyper" episode (you can compare them to the requirements in the table on page 39): increased talkativeness, decreased need for sleep, and involvement in activities that show poor judgment—such as buying way too much material for growing pot indoors. (In DSM-5 language, *poor judgment* is referred to as "activities that have a high potential of painful consequences . . .")

As for mood, Sophie describes Candice as being higher than usual during an "up" episode, but most notably, she's just irritable. *Really* irritable, as we have seen during their conversation in Step 4. And, as required by the DSM-5 definition, her noticeable change in mood is coupled with increased activity level—Sophie's noted that Candice typically has quite a lot of energy during these times. These symptoms last several weeks; in all, Candice has more than enough for either a manic or a hypomanic episode. A diagnostic principle at work here is that collateral information sometimes beats the patient's own history.

Now how do we decide between bipolar I and bipolar II? Again, let's construct a table (see page 41) that uses DSM-5's requirements for all the relevant mood episodes and disorders.

Differentiating between bipolar I and II depends heavily on the degree of distress or impairment from symptoms during the "up" episode. Note that the features of Candice's current depression don't help at all (though a depressive episode in bipolar II must be serious enough to cause distress or impairment—which Candice's surely is—or the frequent, unpredictable switch between highs and lows must cause distress or impairment). The episode duration doesn't help, either: each of Candice's "up" episodes has lasted longer than 7 days. She is definitely ill (others can notice her symptoms), but is she severely incapacitated? Probably not—Sophie, of course, notices a change, but Candice has never been psychotic, and she has certainly never required treatment in a hospital. Not yet, anyway.

In summary, Candice has relatively mild symptoms that, relying on our excellent clinical judgment, we regard as insufficiently severe to regard as an episode of mania—but are perfectly congruent with the symptoms of hypomania. We can point to at least one episode of major depression (the current one), and that's the final piece of the puzzle that allows us to diagnose bipolar II disorder. Note that in getting here, we've used all four parts of our diagnostic mantra: inclusion, exclusion, duration, and distress.

Just for the sake of argument, suppose we had encountered Candice during her first-ever hypomanic episode? Then we'd have had to defer diagnosis, because she wouldn't yet have had an episode of major depression. Unlikely, you say? But that's what the differential

Comparing Bipolar I and Bipolar II Disorders

	Bipolar I disorder	Bipolar II disorder
Duration of episode	7+ days	4+ days
Symptoms	3+ of the 7 listed in the table on page 39	
Mood ("up" phase)	Expansive, elevated, or irritable *plus* ↑ activity or energy	
Major depressive episode	Can have, but not required	1+ prior episode required
Psychotic features	Can have, but not required	Cannot have
Manic episode	Required	None ever
Hypomanic episode	Can have, but not required	Required
Substance use	Must be ruled out as cause	
Another medical condition	Must be ruled out as cause	
Other mental disorders	Psychotic disorder doesn't explain symptoms better	
Distress/impairment	Marked impairment, psychosis, or need for hospitalization	"Up" episode → definite change (others can recognize mood and changed functioning), but impairment is not marked; does *not* require hospitalization; depressive episodes and/or mood shifts also distress or impairment

diagnosis is all about—sorting out the likely from the unlikely. And the unlikely sometimes turns out to be the case.

Step 6

One last thought: Because Candice has also been agitated and distractible during her current major depressive episode, we wonder whether she might warrant the *with mixed features* specifier (see the table on page 39). Yes? No? And why?

Note F

Taking another look at the "Mixed features—manic during depressive episode" column, we find that the mania-like criteria include increased talking, decreased sleep, and so forth. But agitation and distractibility, which seem sort of mania-like, don't even make the cut. Candice has exactly zero of the three or more listed symptoms. The bottom line, then, is *no*: We wouldn't invoke the specifier for Candice's episode of major depression.

The Takeaway

We've started out with two people—patient and informant—vying for our attention. In such a situation, we most often should allow the patient to take precedence. Candice claims that her past upswings of mood were "normal," but the diagnostic principle that collateral information sometimes beats the patient's own history prevails here. Using all our clinical skills, we have developed information that qualifies Candice for a current major depressive episode, but Sophie makes it clear that Candice also has a history of mood swings going "above the line"—in other words, toward the "up" end of the mood spectrum. At this, we can invoke another diagnostic principle: History beats the patient's current appearance.

We've also discussed the intricacies of diagnosis of manic and hypomanic symptoms, to the point that we can sort out Candice's ultimate diagnosis (bipolar II disorder) from the competition—bipolar I disorder, cyclothymic disorder, and major depressive disorder with mixed features. And along the way, we've considered the importance of the consequences of illness (distress/disability). We've even mentioned the use of denial, and promised more about defense mechanisms—later. Finally, we've introduced the elements required for making any mental health diagnosis, which we've referred to as a mantra: "inclusion, exclusion, duration, distress." All things considered, it's been a pretty good outing.

Rant

Patients' clinical presentations can be devilishly hard to unravel. Histories are often convoluted, and the diagnostic requirements are sometimes confusing as written. That's why I recommend you do what I did in the case of Candice as I wrote this chapter: In separate columns, I wrote down her symptoms during her current episode and her symptoms during her prior "hyper" episodes. Then I compared each of these against the DSM-5 diagnostic criteria for each of the conditions in my differential diagnosis. Only then could I be sure that I'd given her the full, careful evaluation that she (and every patient) deserves.

Break Time

Perhaps the best-ever book depicting bipolar disorder was written over 100 years ago. It is *A Mind That Found Itself*, by Clifford W. Beers, who in 1900 at the age of 24 was hospitalized for severe depression. His book, published in 1908, details the treatment he received (nothing that was especially helpful for his condition) and the switch he experienced into mania.

OK, this book is sort of a busman's holiday—but it is a terrific read, and will imprint on you forever the experience of a bipolar disorder in the era of no effective treatment. It is still in print if you want a hard copy, but you can download it free of charge as a PDF from Project Gutenberg. Imagine that: A Break Time that gives your budget a break!

4

Decision Tree—Douglas

Step 1

Douglas enters the office and sits down. Wordlessly, he lays a tiny recorder on the table and turns it on. Here is what you hear.

VOICE: Hello, my name is Alex Harper. And you are . . .

DOUGLAS: Douglas.

VOICE: Why are you here?

DOUGLAS: Well, I've had this anxiety . . . (*Pauses.*)

VOICE: How long have you had it?

DOUGLAS: I think it started when I was 16.

VOICE: How old are you now?

DOUGLAS: I'm 23.

VOICE: Are you married?

DOUGLAS: No.

VOICE: Where were you born?

DOUGLAS: Right here, in town.

VOICE: How far have you gone in school?

DOUGLAS: (*Voice rising*) Listen, do you even care about my problem?

VOICE: What could you mean by that?

Douglas turns off the recorder and scowls. "I'm sure that clinician was able to tick off every box on the intake form. That wasn't all that got ticked off."

I think you're going to recognize right away what's wrong in this snippet. But I'd like to focus on the effect of such an interview. There are two main goals of an initial clinical interview; which one of them has probably been ruined?

- ☒ Rapport with the patient
- ☐ Obtaining a complete database

Note A

Of course, the answer is the first choice. The clinician on the recording left no opportunity for free speech right at the beginning, setting the stage for a yawning gap in rapport. And to form a solid clinical relationship is one of the two principal reasons why I like to give my patients plenty of time to express themselves freely, right at the beginning of our clinical interaction. (The other reason is to identify as many as possible of the problems the patient brings to the first session.)

I don't think I've exaggerated the importance of early interactions to the therapeutic relationship. As the clinician, you are, in effect, selling yourself. Ordinarily, that sales job should be pretty easy: Most patients enter the office expecting to like you. You'd have to work hard—or be careless in the extreme—to challenge that expectation. Although I've long maintained that there is hardly any interviewer gaffe from which recovery is not possible, patients do form initial impressions that can be hard to shake. Responding to provocation, whether real or imagined, some patients have been known to bolt from the room during an initial interview. And so, right from the beginning, you must be deeply invested in forming the strongest alliance possible. If nothing else, it helps ensure that you will obtain the most accurate and complete dataset possible.

Right: If you want to be picky, the opportunity to obtain the clinical information was also seriously damaged in Douglas's recorded interview. But that's a downstream consequence of the devastated working relationship.

Step 2

So let's begin anew, once again asking Douglas some variation of "Why did you come in today?"

> DOUGLAS: Well, I've had this anxiety . . . (*Pauses.*)
>
> YOU: —

And isn't that exactly the problem? How do you decide what to say to encourage a patient to respond with more speech? Just below, I've listed several possibilities. Check each one that you think has a chance of success. Then put an asterisk after the one you prefer.

- ☒ Say nothing and wait some more.
- ☒ Use a verbal or nonverbal encouragement to further speech.*
- ☒ Use Douglas's own words to help him regain the thread of his thought.
- ☐ Ask the question again, perhaps slightly rephrased.

Note B

If you've checked any of the first three methods, we're on the same page. Each could encourage further speech on the patient's part without specifying content.

In Douglas's case (in most cases, actually), I'd be tempted simply to remain quiet and give him a little more time to think. Some people have problems organizing their thoughts, and need the freedom of a bit more time to pull themselves together. Saying nothing—for a few seconds, not forever—would be a way of telling Douglas, "I'm interested in what you have to say. In fact, I'm interested enough that I'm going to give you some space to express it."

A little further on, assuming that he still hasn't made much progress, you could encourage further speech by using his own words: "You were saying you had some anxiety . . . ?" Or simply use a slight variation on the interviewer's favorite traditional verbal encouragement (yes, these are all called *encouragements*): "Tell me more about that." Even a smile, assuming that Douglas is looking right at you, could say in effect, "It's fine to just proceed at your own pace." (I would probably have offered a smile right at the beginning, too.) In effect, any of these three responses is likely to produce better results than the rat-a-tat assault caught on the Step 1 recording.

I'm not quite so enamored of the fourth choice, which is to ask a variation of the same question. Of course, it might prompt more speech (so if you've checked this box, don't beat yourself up), but to me it sounds a little too much like criticism—a nagging sort of "C'mon, let's get this thing moving." It also carries with it the whiff of the intolerant pedagogue who's talking down to a not-very-bright pupil. For those reasons, I'd probably steer clear of that final option.

Step 3

In his own words, related almost completely without further prompting or direction (though lightly edited for continuity and concision), here's the story Douglas tells:

> "I've had this anxiety, where I can be sitting quietly, minding my own business, thinking about nothing in particular, and wham!—Down it comes, and I'm practically on the floor, quivering and shaking with fear.
>
> "Now I'm not an especially timid person. I've worked as an arborist all my adult life; it was the job I could get when I left college. So I'm used to climbing trees, working high up in the branches. That doesn't intimidate me at all; of course, I do wear a safety harness. Really, I love my job—keeps me out in the (mostly) fresh air, gives me exercise. I'm fit and trim.
>
> "So why do I have these attacks of horrible anxiety? They come on me once or twice a day and leave me wiped out for minutes and minutes afterwards. If I'm at work, I'll have to take a break. The other guys—our team has been together for several years—are terrific about it. They just say, 'Douglas's having a little down time; let's all take a break.' I mean, who gets *that* kind of consideration from

coworkers? One day last week I was sitting high up in a fir tree when the anxiety hit again, and I'd finally had enough. I decided, 'Whatever else, I'm gonna make an appointment and try to fix this.'

"Um, I guess that right now, I'd like to hear *how* to fix it. I've read some stuff on the 'Net about panic and fear, so I know that there are a number of different steps we could take . . . "

And with that, Douglas finally pauses.

That's a pretty good dollop of information, gained by simply encouraging Douglas to talk freely. Perhaps we can take advantage of his current pause and try for some specifics. Of course, there's a lot of stuff we need to know, but at the moment we especially want to learn details pertaining to his present illness. So, next, please, a two-parter:

1. Right near the end of the Step 3 vignette, Douglas says something suggesting that your efforts at building rapport are paying off. What is it?
2. And then how would you deal with his request to consider treatment?

- ☐ Just ignore it—it's too soon.
- ☐ Take a short break from the information-gathering process and discuss the options.
- ☐ Explain why you need to delay that discussion.

Note C

1. The clue I've been fishing for is Douglas's use of the first-person plural (" . . . steps *we* could take . . . "). To me, it suggests that he's getting past the ire provoked by the first interviewer. Another indicator of a gathering rapprochement is his apparent willingness to speak freely about his issues. Clearly, you've advanced the therapeutic alliance.
2. As to his request about treatment options, I wouldn't ignore it. (Apologies if I lured you off the scent.) But neither would I drop everything to have a conversation that would be, quite frankly, premature. Rather, you'll contribute still further to the mutual good feeling if you begin by acknowledging the request, and then explain why you need to put it off. You can probably do the job with something as simple as this: "I want to discuss treatment as soon as possible, but to do a good job of that, first we need to gather a few more facts and establish a diagnosis."

Step 4

Before moving on, we'd like more information about some facts that Douglas has already divulged. Of course, we could just let him talk until he spontaneously says everything we need, but that could take a very long time. What we need instead is a series of probes that can increase our understanding of his situation.

Let me be clear: Probing doesn't mean being unacceptably intrusive (like aliens with an abducted earthling in a Grade B science fiction movie). We can obtain most of the details while maintaining a conversational tone that won't cause patients to feel we are muscling into their personal space. But it does mean trying to learn all about every aspect of the history of the present illness: Usually, this will be the *who, what, where, when, why,* and *how*—questions that are bread and butter, both for journalists and for clinicians. We'll also want to learn the consequences of certain symptoms, previous attempts at remedy, and (possibly) attempts at prevention.

In the history from Douglas that follows, the underlined passages followed by superscript numbers refer to some questions I'll pose afterward (and answer in Note D).

Douglas's episodes of anxiety, which he readily identifies as "panic,"[1] can come on at almost any time.[2] He rarely has any forewarning;[3] they seem to arise "out of a blue sky." The attacks can happen as often as two or three times in a day; however, he's occasionally gone a week or more without having one.[4]

At first the attack feels mild, perhaps only a hint of apprehension.[5] But it rapidly builds[6] to engulf him in terror so severe that he feels virtually paralyzed. His heart beats rapidly;[7] he has the sensation of being unable to catch his breath.[8] His legs feel like jelly,[9] and he must stop what he is doing, lest he collapse.[10] He sometimes tries to tell himself to "chill,"[11] but that doesn't usually make much difference.

With prompting ("I haven't thought about it in years"), Douglas recalls his earliest experience with anxiety.[12] It occurred during his first year of college.[13] He and some of his new classmates had gone to stay at the lodge their school maintained in the mountains. "The accommodations were somewhat spartan," Douglas reports. "We brought a camp stove and had to carry in water from town. The loo wasn't working, either, so we had to use a privy located outside the back door. The first evening, I was in there minding my own business when my friends sneaked up and put a stick through the latch, so I couldn't open the door. Then they went off down the mountain to party with some women we'd met."

Douglas shifts uneasily in his chair and sneezes. "I was there for hours. At first, I tried to laugh about it, but the smell, the dark, and—most of all—the closeness of those four walls pretty much killed my sense of humor. After a few minutes of beating on the door and yelling, I realized no one was going to come. So I crouched in a corner and tried to contemplate the big questions in life—such as the meaning of friendship and the value of trust. But all I could really focus on was my heartbeat, which seemed to be getting faster, and the cold sweat that was pouring off me into the stinky air. As the evening wore on, they seemed to be squeezing in on me, like in that Poe story about the Inquisition."

Since then, Douglas has had repeated episodes[14] of severe anxiety, where "I basically succumb to terror." Several times a week,[15] he says, without any provocation or warning,[16] his anxiety level begins to build.[17] Over the next few minutes, he'll become "too aware" of the beating of his heart,[18] which he sometimes worries will "accelerate to one huge, final thump before it stops completely." He feels acutely short of breath;[19] his chest hurts;[20] and he's so weak[21] that his legs will not support him and he has to sit down. During some of these episodes, he's also experienced dizziness ("It's more of a lightheaded feeling"),[22] hands trembling,[23] numbness[24] of his fingers, and the feeling that he is about to vomit.[25] "If I'm up in a tree, God forbid, I'll come down[26] as fast as I can. If I'm really high up, I may just have to sit down on a limb until it passes.[27] That can take half an hour,[28] though sometimes it's shorter than that." Douglas has never sought treatment before.[29] Although this appointment was his own idea, his boss has hinted that unless he gets his problem sorted out, "he might have to let me go."

Douglas still hates being closed in.[30] He won't crawl into any tightly confined space, even the time it meant that he had to hire someone to check for gas leaks in the crawl space under his house. "Just the thought of squeezing in there makes me feel literally sick with dread." However, he claims he has no other specific fears.[31] Other than concern about having further attacks, he doesn't think he worries more than anyone else.[32] He denies feeling depressed, says that his appetite and sleep are "just fine," and maintains that he enjoys his leisure-time activities[33] as much as ever.

Further questioning reveals that he regards his childhood as "normal." He has two sisters (one older, one younger); there's no family history of mental illness at all. His MSE is completely normal.

Once or twice, Douglas has tried to "attack the attacks with chemistry,[34] but I've never gotten much past opening a beer before the symptoms fade." After doing a complete physical exam ("normal, normal, normal"),[35] his primary care physician once offered him Valium,[36] but he never even filled the prescription. "Don't you think I have enough problems without adding an addiction?"

Below are the questions that elicited the further history Douglas has just given us. Just mark the number(s) of the underlined passage(s) corresponding to each question. (At the end, you'll find that most questions refer to several underlined passages.)

"Will you describe what you feel during an attack?" ____________
"Under what circumstances do the attacks occur?" ____________
"When did you first experience an attack?" ____________
"How often do they occur?" ____________
"What seems to precipitate an attack?" ____________
"How quickly does the attack develop?" ____________
"How do you respond when these attacks occur?" ____________
"How long do they last?" ____________
"What treatment have you sought before?" ____________
"Have you had any other experiences with fear or anxiety?" ____________
"Any problems with your mood? Or sleep? Or appetite?" ____________
"Have you had any physical or substance use problems?" ____________

These are the sorts of probing questions you'll need to ask just about any patient concerning just about any set of symptoms.

Note D

And here's how I'd match up Douglas's underlined statements to the questions listed above.

"Will you describe what you feel during an attack?" 1, 5, 7–9, 17–25
"Under what circumstances do the attacks occur?" 2

"When did you first experience an attack?" 12, 13
"How often do they occur?" 4, 14, 15
"What seems to precipitate an attack?" 3, 16
"How quickly does the attack develop?" 6
"How do you respond when these attacks occur?" 10, 11, 26, 27
"How long do they last?" 28
"What treatment have you sought before?" 29, 34
"Have you had any other experiences with fear or anxiety?" 30, 31, 32
"Any problems with your mood? Or sleep? Or appetite?" 33
"Have you had any physical or substance use problems?" 35, 36

Let me reiterate that with time and experience, these are the sorts of questions that you'll be able to rattle off (almost without thinking) about most of the complaints your patients will bring to you for evaluation. But there will probably always be a few that will, from time to time, have you returning to a textbook to obtain more information or refresh your memory.

Step 5

Well, we may have glossed over one or two items that a complete evaluation should include, but I think we now have enough information that you can formulate a reasonably thorough differential diagnosis. I hope that you'll write it down.

____
____
____
____
____
____
____
____

Note E

Here's my differential diagnosis for Douglas:

◊ Anxiety disorder due to another medical condition
◊ Substance/medication-induced anxiety disorder
◊ Panic disorder

◊ Agoraphobia
◊ Specific phobia
◊ Generalized anxiety disorder (GAD)
◊ Social anxiety disorder
◊ Obsessive–compulsive disorder (OCD)

There are several diagnoses that I'll almost always include in the differential diagnosis for someone with anxiety or panic symptoms—in fact, all of those on the list above (just as you suspected). As you also may have noticed, I tend not to be too creative in the differential lists I write. I include just about anything that seems remotely possible—sometimes, even beyond remotely. It helps keep my own anxiety level at a minimum.

Rant

Why not posttraumatic stress disorder (PTSD)? In the past, I've received emails from readers asking why I haven't included PTSD in the differential diagnoses of some of my other case histories. This time, I'll get ahead of the issue.

For Douglas, the reason is that although his experience in the outhouse was undeniably distressing, it simply does not rise to the standard of seriousness established by the diagnostic guidelines. That is, he was not exposed to death, serious injury (except perhaps to his pride), or sexual assault—either as an actual occurrence or as a threat. Furthermore, he stated explicitly that for many years he hadn't relived, or even recalled, the outhouse experience. Although the clinical history doesn't further explore the criteria for PTSD, these two omissions by themselves are enough to disqualify the diagnosis from our further consideration.

Step 6

By now, you know the drill. Which of the possibilities in Note E should we choose for Douglas (best diagnosis)? And why? Yes, you need to jot down any reasons you have for eliminating the other possible disorders from your consideration.

Best diagnosis for Douglas: ______________________________

And the reason(s): ______________________________

Note F

It's the "reason(s)" part of Step 6 that causes confusion, which in turn sometimes leads us into temptation—to omit disorders in a differential list that really ought to be there.

For example, in Step 4 we've made a big deal of presenting material that speaks against both medical issues and substance use as prospective causes for Douglas's symptoms. It is true that the risk for these etiologies is very small indeed. And, quite frankly, even though I reject them for Douglas—his diagnosis is based on a pretty good history, but a physical exam and lab studies would help confirm this conclusion—I'll still keep them in mind as possibilities. If the course of treatment doesn't run smoothly, or if further symptoms develop, I might want to reconsider. Substance use and medical issues are just too important to dismiss beyond reach of recall.

GAD is there because Douglas worries a lot; we can now discount the diagnosis because his worry focuses on a single issue (having more attacks), rather than on many different issues, as is typical of GAD. People with social anxiety disorder have anxiety symptoms that stem from being observed while participating in such activities as writing, having a drink, performing, speaking, or even using a public toilet. OCD involves having, well, obsessions or compulsions, neither of which is the case for Douglas. OK, we're closing in on closure.

Panic disorder is a good bet. In fact, it's extraordinarily good, inasmuch as we've seen in Steps 3 and 4 that Douglas has many symptoms typical of a panic attack—rapid heartbeat, shortness of breath, chest pain, weakness, a feeling of dread, dizziness, tremor, numbness of extremities, and nausea. I therefore invoke one of my diagnostic principles, which is that having many symptoms of a disorder makes the diagnosis more likely than if there are barely enough for diagnosis. The duration Douglas reports (about half an hour) is also typical for a panic attack. Agoraphobia (fear of being alone or away from home) often accompanies panic disorder, but either disorder can exist independently of the other. I've included agoraphobia in the Note E differential diagnosis, but it obviously doesn't apply to Douglas.

Finally, there's specific phobia, which is where Douglas's story started (with the episode in the outhouse). It is fortunate, isn't it, that he fears being closed in, and not heights, which in his line of work he experiences daily? But the claustrophobia has lasted longer than 6 months, causes distress or disability, and is reliably stressful to Douglas. It is often comorbid with panic disorder. We would classify his specific phobia as a situational type; another example of this type would be fear of air travel.

Step 7

And now, in what order would you list these two diagnoses—specific phobia and panic disorder—when you write up Douglas's history? And why? Here are some possibilities.

- ☐ Alphabetical. This is clear and simple.
- ☐ Chronological. This tells you which started first.
- ☐ Most in need of treatment. This could help you determine what to recommend by way of therapy.

Note G

The good news is that there isn't any wrong way to list these diagnoses. Even if you just opt for the alphabetical, you've listed each diagnosis to remind you (and subsequent clinicians) what's important to pay attention to for a given patient.

However, if one disorder is causing a lot of misery or suggests a potentially dire outcome—a mood disorder with suicidal ideas, for example—then obviously that's what deserves pride of place in your list.

As often as possible, I also like to put diagnoses in chronological order. Not only does this tell you what has been around the longest, but it sometimes also suggests causative links in the chain of a person's illness history.

Sometimes it works out so that different strategies yield the same order of listing. However, in Douglas's case, I'd list panic disorder first: Its symptoms, by their severity, demand prompt attention. Only after dealing with it would I want to address the far less problematic, though chronologically earlier, specific phobia.

Rant

Speaking of trees, if you haven't already been introduced, let me acquaint you with *decision trees.* These are devices that can help you sort through symptoms and other material to arrive at logical choices for a person's diagnosis. For example, the decision tree for anxiety symptoms would allow you to conclude that Douglas has—surprise!—panic disorder and specific phobia. I've reprinted the one for anxiety and fears from one of my other books (see the figure on the facing page). *Diagnosis Made Easier* contains quite a number of other decision trees, for disorders as varied as mood disorders, psychoses, and cognitive problems.

The Takeaway

In Douglas, we've met a patient whose history encourages a discussion of the differential diagnosis of anxiety disorders. His story also demonstrates the importance of the first interview in establishing rapport, and the use of verbal encouragements. We've been introduced to the issue of probing for details of the history of the present episode of illness. In a Rant, we've read about using decision trees as an adjunct to diagnosis. Oh, yes, and we've started out with a clear example of an opening question: "Why did you come in today?"

Douglas has a *lot* of symptoms of panic attack and panic disorder; together, they illustrate the use of this diagnostic principle: More symptoms of a given illness increase the likelihood that it is the correct diagnosis. We've also talked about how to prioritize a list of diagnoses, when the final diagnosis includes more than one disorder. And once again, we've emphasized (or overemphasized!) the need to write down a complete differential diagnosis every time we evaluate a new patient. At some point, we'll start to take that bit of advice for granted, and stop saying it every time. But not yet.

Break Time

Think about fear and anxiety as we see it portrayed in the movies and on TV. Sometimes it's fear of an actual threat (*Nightmare on Elm Street,* for example); or it may be played for laughs, as in *High Anxiety,* the 1977 Mel Brooks film that

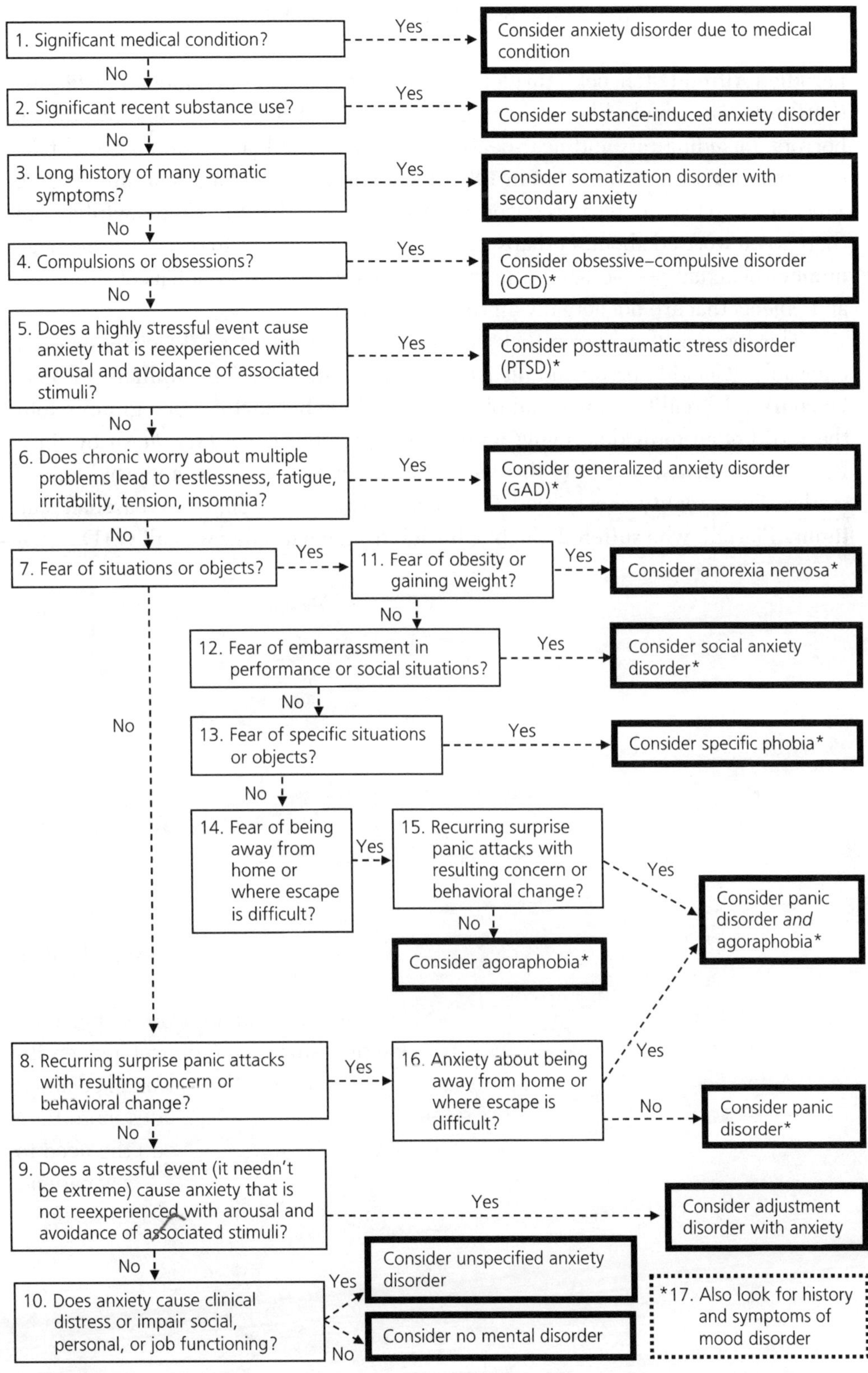

Decision tree for a patient who has fear, anxiety, panic, obsessions, or continuing worry.

parodied Alfred Hitchcock's thrillers. (Douglas, our patient, mentions *The Pit and the Pendulum,* which, like so many of Edgar Allan Poe's stories, features actual horrors, including rats and near-death from a swinging blade. Poe's original tale, of course, was a short story, but in 1961 Roger Corman made it into a film starring Vincent Price.) Such offerings encourage us to believe that there's an awful lot out there to be worried about. Perhaps this subtly encourages us to disregard the huge number of actual people who suffer from panic disorder and phobias of situations and objects that are not actually all that threatening.

The tension of a horror flick is sometimes described as delicious or even enjoyable. (Google *horror* and *pleasure* together, and you'll get millions of hits.) Of course, the reality of an actual phobia is anything but joyful. For a glimpse into the world of an individual living with phobias, try the novel *Live Flesh* by Ruth Rendell, the British writer of thrillers. It's about a man who has a morbid fear of turtles. For a reality check, read *Fear Strikes Out,* the memoir by baseball star Jimmy Piersall, who suffered much of his life from what today we call GAD.

5

Transitions—Elinor

Step 1

Elinor works as a medical records clerk just across the hall. As arranged a couple of days ago, she drops by during her lunch hour. She glances warily around as she closes the door. "It has to do with a miscarriage last year," she volunteers, then sits quietly, waiting.

After a few seconds' pause, you respond, "Could you tell me some more about that?"

Except for bereavement and a few panic attacks after the loss of her first baby to sudden infant death syndrome (SIDS) several years ago, Elinor has always been emotionally well. She wasn't even seriously troubled a few months back when a supervisor told her that something in the environment at work could have caused her, and three other employees, to have miscarriages. But in the past 2 weeks, since discovering that she is again pregnant, she has been by turns fretful and anxious. Although an environmental survey was completed for part of the clinic, it did not include her own work area. So she worries that the environment could harm the fetus she is carrying, even though she has been assured that all is well. Now she has requested either a full investigation or time off work until the end of her first trimester.

Elinor pauses again and looks at you. After you respond, "Uh-huh?," she continues with her story.

Whenever she recalls her first pregnancy, the memory of those troubles comes tumbling back upon her. Then she will feel "scared and depressed. In fact, a couple of times I was a little frantic."

Now, she says, she often feels depressed and anxious, especially during the week, when just being at her work station reminds her of her previous losses and current worries. It's enough to cause her to "sometimes blank out when I'm trying to work." She says that she's made some careless filing errors that are not typical of her usual meticulous work habits. She's also felt irritable, with a decrease in her energy and in her interest for her usual activities. The panic attacks, however, have not come back. The worst episode occurred last week on her way to work, when, at a stop sign, her attention drifted for a moment and she rear-ended the car ahead of her. It caused no injuries and only dented the bumper of her own car. "But, still, it made me feel I was losing it."

For a few days Elinor's appetite was down, but her weight has been steady, her sleep is approximately normal, and she has had no death wishes or suicidal ideas. On the weekends, she feels "pretty much my normal self."

Again, she pauses. This time, you only nod and smile. After a moment, she resumes talking.

So far, we've experienced three separate pauses in Elinor's story, which you have instinctively met with *encouragements*. These are ways of moving the conversation along, and they can be . . .

- Verbal or nonverbal
- Directive or nondirective (the latter does not specify the type of information you are seeking)
- Open-ended or closed-ended (the latter can be answered in a word or two, such as yes/no)

Underline the characteristics of each of the three encouragements you've used here:

" . . . tell me some more . . . ": verbal/nonverbal, directive/nondirective, open-ended/closed-ended
"Uh-huh?": verbal/nonverbal, directive/nondirective, open-ended/closed-ended
[Nod and smile]: verbal/nonverbal, directive/nondirective, open-ended/closed-ended

The answers will help define why such responses should be used more often.

Note A

" . . . tell me some more . . . ": **verbal**/nonverbal, **directive**/nondirective, **open-ended**/closed-ended
"Uh-huh?": **verbal**/nonverbal, directive/**nondirective,** **open-ended**/closed-ended
[Nod and smile]: verbal/**nonverbal,** directive/**nondirective,** **open-ended**/closed-ended

Each of these encouragements prompts Elinor to keep talking and tell us more. The first one is verbal and directive, so that she knows just what area you want her to address. Because it requires an answer of more than a word or two , this encouragement is also open-ended.

The second one is verbal, though just barely. It is also open-ended and nondirective. And the third one is just a facial expression and a head nod of approval, which accomplish the same end as the second does.

Nonverbal encouragements are great because they don't intrude into the patient's stream of consciousness; clinicians should use nonverbal (and barely verbal) encouragements almost without thinking, throughout the interview process. And open-ended questions are very important to use, especially early in the interview process. They encourage patients to speak candidly about what they are thinking; they promote free exchange of ideas; and they help to forge the bonds of rapport so necessary to the interview—and therapeutic—process.

On the other hand, "Tell me more about that," though directive, is one of the most useful phrases in the clinician's toolbox. I use this open-ended request a lot.

Do take notice of the fact that in every case, we've opted for an encouragement that is open-ended: It allows Elinor scope to choose how she will express her answer. That would be quite usual this early in the interview. In a later chapter, we'll explore the merits of closed-ended questions.

Rant

Note that *nondirective* and *nonverbal* aren't the same thing. You can make several combinations of these two techniques. I concede, however, that it would be pretty hard to make a nonverbal *directive* request without waving your arms a lot and looking pretty silly.

Step 2

With encouragement, Elinor continues with her story.

> Elinor and Brian, her husband, now both 26 years of age, have been married for 4 years. Their marital problems have been so serious that for the past year they have been living apart. Elinor has been staying with her father and stepmother (she gets along well with both) while she and Brian have been "working on getting back together." Working with some effect, it would seem: He is the father of her unborn child.
>
> "Brian isn't as worried as I am about the clinic environment," she says. "Of course, we're both in the middle of some big personal issues, but they especially affect me." Again, she mentions the possible environmental condition at work, and how unhappy she felt after her earlier miscarriage.

At this point, you realize that Elinor has begun to recycle some of her earlier statements; she needs redirection. There are several verbal devices, sometimes called *bridges,* to turn the conversation in a new direction that will yield fresh information. You could:

- Use something the patient has just said as a pivot to turn the conversation in a different direction.
- Pick up on something the patient said *earlier* to use as a springboard to a new topic.
- Flag your change of direction by pointing out that you are, well, changing directions.

With what's already presented in Steps 1 and 2, construct (in your mind, if nowhere else!) an example of each method.

Note B

When shifting topics in a mental health interview, you don't actually *have* to do anything special; you could just ask a different question. After all, you're directing this conversation, right?

Well, yes and no. Of course, you are the one who's gathering the data. But it is the two of you, clinician and patient, who need to form a relationship. That means paying attention not only to what you ask, but to how you ask it. If you are changing directions, you want to do it in a way that doesn't cause the patient to feel interrogated, herded, or bullied.

Moving from one topic to another with a transition (or *bridge*) that's both graceful and productive is something of an art form. I think of it as trying to make the interview as much as possible resemble a normal conversation. This means that you should try to create an understandable connection between subjects, just as you would do in conversing with a friend.

1. One way to do that is by taking something that the patient has just said, and keying off it with a twist. Let's say you'd like to know about Elinor's current mood.

   "That unhappiness you felt with the miscarriage—have you been feeling anything like it recently?"

2. A second method would be to refer back to an earlier statement the patient has made.

   "A bit ago, you mentioned the death of your baby. How does the way you felt then compare with how you have been feeling in the last few days?" Notice that the question is directive, but still open-ended. If instead you were to ask a closed-ended, "Does the way you felt then seem a lot like you feel now?", you'd be limiting Elinor to a yes/no response that might not allow enough scope for the fullest expression of her feelings.

Each of these two methods almost seamlessly eases the patient from one topic to another.

3. But sometimes you will need to make a more abrupt transition to an unrelated topic. Then it's a good idea to note the fact that you are changing directions. This gives the patient an opportunity to move with you, rather than feeling jerked around like a puppy on a leash. For instance, you might say to Elinor, "I think I understand about your concerns regarding the workplace. So for a moment I'd like to change direction and ask this: Has anyone in your family had similar problems with depression?" The phrase "understand about your concerns" provides additional reassurance that you aren't ignoring the patient's other issue, but have in fact noted it.

I prefer to use one of the first two methods, but of course that depends on whether my patient has actually said something (that I can remember) that provides a useful bridge.

Step 3

Responding well to your encouragements and bridges, Elinor continues to elaborate her story, yielding this information.

> She was born in Texas, where her father was stationed while in the Air Force. She was the oldest of four children (two brothers and one sister). When she was 11, her parents divorced, and her mother began working as a nurse's aide. Through her father, she has a much-younger half-sister. Her father has had a severe alcohol use disorder, but has now been "dry" for 5 years; his example has given her such a horror of substance use that only infrequently will she even sip a glass of wine. During a "nervous breakdown" years ago, her mother was depressed and suicidal. One brother has had serious alcohol problems (divorce and a ruined career).
>
> To help with her siblings when her mother went to work, Elinor dropped out of school in the 12th grade, before graduation; subsequently she obtained a GED. She has worked steadily in clerical positions since then, sticking with each job for several years before moving up to a better one. She has worked at this clinic for nearly 2 years.
>
> Other than an allergy to sulfa drugs, her physical health has "always been terrific"; her obstetrician did a complete exam recently and said that her health was excellent. Other than a multivitamin, she takes no medications; she's had no major illnesses and seldom needs to see her doctor. A Caesarian section has been her only operation.
>
> Elinor's clothing is appropriate to the workplace environment, and she shows no behavioral abnormalities. She has a pleasant demeanor and is clearly in command of herself. Although her eyes redden when discussing the SIDS death of her baby, she accepts a tissue and is able to smile and continue speaking. Her affect, if a bit labile, is thus appropriate to her content of thought . . .

We interrupt Elinor's narrative for this bulletin. Well, it's actually a quick question, with three answers: What are the qualities (there are broad hints just above) we must always look for and describe in a patient's affect? This is one of those issues that clinicians really need to have at their fingertips, so, without apology, I ask you to answer without prompts.

1. ____________ of affect
2. ____________ of affect
3. ____________ of affect

Note C

You need to keep firmly in mind the three aspects to the assessment of affect. (Remember that the terms *affect* and *mood* are often used interchangeably. But careful clinicians do make this distinction: Mood is what the patient feels, and affect is what the patient *appears* to be feeling.)

1. *Quality* of affect. Does the patient's emotional state seem to be one of anger, anxiety, contempt, disgust, fear, guilt, joy, love, sadness, shame, or surprise?
2. *Lability* of affect. Is the person's emotional state pretty stable, or does it move around

a lot? When it swings wildly from one extreme to another (joy to sadness and back within moments), we say that affect is *excessively labile.* On the other hand, little or no variation at all in the way the patient appears to be feeling (when we would expect at least some) we call *affective blunting* or *flattening.*

3. *Appropriateness* of affect. How well does the affect (mood) seem to fit with this person's content of thought? For example, laughing at something sad, like the death of a friend or relative, we would usually describe as affect that is inappropriate.

If you needed help in conjuring up these three fundamental aspects, I'd recommend that you spend a few moments right now committing them firmly to memory.

Step 4

. . . her content of thought, which reveals no delusions, hallucinations, phobias, obsessions, compulsions, or other abnormalities. She acknowledges that her miscarriage could have been "completely natural." There is no evidence that she thinks there is some sort of a conspiracy. However, she does point out, logically enough, that her concern could be justified: She didn't go to her supervisor looking for information about her miscarriage; he came to her. Her intelligence appears above average, her insight and judgment excellent. She is fully oriented, and she can relate recent events (she briefly rants about the outcome of a recent election). She subtracts serial sevens quickly and accurately.

Wait a minute: Why do we always ask our patients to subtract sevens? Is it to judge:

- ☐ Mathematical ability?
- ☐ Ability to comply with an instruction?
- ☐ Comprehension of the spoken word?
- ☐ Attention span?

And what if someone cannot subtract sevens? Is there anything we can substitute?

Note D

Of course, the purpose of serial sevens isn't to judge the patient's facility with math—or any of those first three choices. We actually use it as a formal test of attention span. (Trouble keeping her mind on the interview—remember those pauses in her narrative in Step 1?—has already figured in Elinor's story, heightening our interest in this aspect of her evaluation.)

With good attention span, defined as the ability to focus well on a task, a person will continue to subtract another seven from each successive remainder: 93 – 86 – 79 – 72 – 65 – 58 . . . and so on (and on, should the clinician neglect to call a merciful halt). There may be a mistake or two, but the test is "passed" if the subtractions are continued below 60 with mostly correct answers. It isn't a great test, but as Tevye says, it's tradition, so we continue to use it.

Someone who cannot do sevens (whose math skills are hopelessly deficient) can be asked instead to count backward by ones from 50, with the instruction to stop at, perhaps, 27. This introduces an instruction that the person must hold in mind and implement a bit later; in other words, it's another test of attention, just one that packs a bit less tradition.

And finally, based on how well the patient focuses on the interview overall, you can also make a reasonably accurate judgment of attention.

Step 5

Now, no surprise: Determine the differential diagnosis for Elinor. It'll be wide-ranging, so I've included lots of blank lines. Feel free to add more if you wish. For now, don't bother with arranging them; just try to get all your thoughts onto the page.

____

____

____

____

____

____

____

____

____

____

____

____

____

____

Note E

Here is my differential list for Elinor, arranged alphabetically. I've warned you, it's a long one.

- ◊ Adjustment disorder with mixed anxiety and depressed mood
- ◊ Anxiety disorder due to another medical condition

◊ Uncomplicated bereavement
◊ Depressive disorder due to another medical condition
◊ Generalized anxiety disorder (GAD)
◊ Major depressive disorder
◊ Panic disorder
◊ Personality disorder
◊ Posttraumatic stress disorder (PTSD)
◊ Relationship distress with spouse
◊ Somatic symptom disorder
◊ Specific phobia
◊ Substance/medication-induced anxiety disorder
◊ Substance/medication-induced depressive disorder

As I've indicated, you may even want to add some other disorders. For example, some people might specifically mention a depressed episode of a bipolar disorder, on the theory that in the future, Elinor *could* have an episode of mania or hypomania. I won't argue the point, though I consider the possibility is pretty far downstream from our current evidence, so I didn't include it on my list. In general, though, when it comes to the differential diagnosis, the more the merrier.

Step 6

However, we don't (or shouldn't) just stick disorders onto a list without some principle of organization. Of course, the alphabet *is* an organizing principle of sorts, but it doesn't really accomplish much other than to help us find our place. What I prefer, and will ask you to do, is to impose order based on these factors:

- How urgent is it to treat the condition?
- How readily can it be treated?
- How much harm can be averted by treating it?
- How complete a recovery can we expect, assuming adequate treatment?

That's quite a lot to sort through, but the end product is important. I call this organizing principle the *safety principle* or *safety hierarchy,* and I've mentioned it before. Yep, you'll probably hear about it again.

In the Note E list of differential diagnoses, which I've printed again just below, circle or underline the T (top), M (middle), or B (bottom) after each choice to indicate where you'd place it in your safety hierarchy. And here again is a brief definition of what those positions mean.

Those at the Top are conditions that, even if rarely encountered, would require immediate treatment and could represent a serious threat to the individual's overall health. At the Bottom, I place conditions that may not respond well to treatment—or, treatments may not even be available. Everything else goes into the Middle group; you and I could argue forever about the exact order.

◊ Adjustment disorder with mixed anxiety and depressed mood (T/M/B)
◊ Anxiety disorder due to another medical condition (T/M/B)
◊ Uncomplicated bereavement (T/M/B)
◊ Depressive disorder due to another medical condition (T/M/B)
◊ GAD (T/M/B)
◊ Major depressive disorder (T/M/B)
◊ Panic disorder (T/M/B)
◊ Personality disorder (T/M/B)
◊ PTSD (T/M/B)
◊ Relationship distress with spouse (T/M/B)
◊ Somatic symptom disorder (T/M/B)
◊ Specific phobia (T/M/B)
◊ Substance/medication-induced anxiety disorder (T/M/B)
◊ Substance/medication-induced depressive disorder (T/M/B)

Note F

And here is my differential list again, this time arranged according to the safety hierarchy.

Top

◊ Depressive disorder due to another medical condition
◊ Anxiety disorder due to another medical condition
◊ Substance/medication-induced depressive disorder
◊ Substance/medication-induced anxiety disorder
◊ Major depressive disorder

Middle

◊ Uncomplicated bereavement
◊ Panic disorder
◊ PTSD
◊ GAD
◊ Specific phobia
◊ Adjustment disorder with mixed anxiety and depressed mood
◊ Relationship distress with spouse

Bottom

◊ Somatic symptom disorder
◊ Personality disorder

Major depressive disorder belongs in the top/"most urgent" category because it usually responds well to treatment, and because it can yield dire consequences—suicide comes to mind—if it is left untreated. For the same reasons, medical condition and substance use etiologies always belong high on the list. The two disorders in the bottom category are conditions that are relatively hard to treat or respond slowly to treatment, so we consider them only once we've eliminated everything else. If disorders such as dementia (major neurocognitive disorder) or schizophrenia were in the running for Elinor, they'd go at the bottom, too.

Step 7

And now for the *pièce de résistance,* your best diagnosis for Elinor. Once again, include a few notes justifying your selection. Then in Note G, you can compare your efforts with what I've written.

Best diagnosis for Elinor: ____

And the reason(s): ____

Note G

Let's take it from the top, then. The first four disorders I'd eliminate at one stroke: Even without following her around to see whether she frequents pubs and taverns, from her reliable history we can state that Elinor's symptoms of depression or anxiety aren't due to alcohol or drug use. Furthermore, her physical health seems excellent. (So why did we even put these possibilities on our list, let alone at the top? It's because we *always* include them, as a reminder to ourselves.)

Let's move on, a bit more slowly. For any patient who complains of depression, major depressive disorder comes trippingly to the word processor. And so it should, because it is one of the most frequently encountered emotional disorders in the world. However, this diagnosis requires certain features that Elinor just plain lacks. Especially, episodes of major depression must last more or less all day nearly every day, for at least a couple of weeks, whereas Elinor's symptoms abate on weekends. There may also be too few inclusion symptoms—insomnia, significant anorexia, and the like—to qualify, but the sole issue of duration is enough for us to reject a major depressive episode (or depressive disorder).

Now we've moved through the top layer of our list to the midlevel possibilities. Although Elinor complains of anxiety, there simply aren't enough inclusion symptoms of any anxiety disorder to persuade me that one of them should be Elinor's best diagnosis. In particular, she doesn't have panic attacks (she did several years ago, after her baby died). And her worries are confined to the possibility of having another miscarriage, rather than a wide-ranging concern about all manner of problems; multiple worries would be the case with generalized anxiety disorder. Although she was bereaved after the SIDS death, that death happened several years ago, and she apparently recovered fully.

Of course, any time there is a stressor, we should think about PTSD and its sibling, acute stress disorder. However, we must reject them here because Elinor's situation doesn't involve anything truly awful, such as death, grave injury, or an act of violence or sexual attack. We can rule out specific phobia because the condition has been present for far less time than the required 6 months.

I'll rule out relationship distress in part because it isn't really a diagnosis at all; rather, it is used when the focus of treatment is on a problematic interpersonal relationship. Of course, Elinor and her husband are going through a rough patch, but that's been going on for a long time, and her symptoms have come up more recently. We might want to consider it as an adjunct to another diagnosis, but for now, let's move on.

From near the bottom of the pile, somatic symptom disorder? A diagnostic principle asks us to consider it often, but for Elinor it's not so likely, considering that she has very few somatic symptoms (and even those she does have aren't the focus of her concern). Although she could have a coexisting personality disorder, we haven't seen evidence of marked personality issues that have persisted throughout her adult life. Besides, I am always very careful about diagnosing a personality disorder in the face of a major mental disorder.

That leaves only adjustment disorder, which should be regarded as a condition of "almost last resort." That's because other disorders are defined better and have more specific available treatments. Nonetheless, Elinor does meet the basic requirement: A specific stressor has apparently caused a symptom response greater than you'd expect for most people in similar circumstances. Of course, we could argue about what an expected response to a possible environmental threat might be, but for me (and, I think, for DSM-5), the temporal contiguity of stressor and response, coupled with the importance the patient lays on these factors, is enough to substantiate the diagnosis. The subtype is dictated by the presence of both anxiety and mood symptoms.

Elinor has only one diagnosis, so we needn't worry about what to list first. But there are a couple of other issues—pregnancy and marital problems—that we'll include as we sign out her case:

◊ Adjustment disorder with mixed anxiety and depressed mood
◊ Early pregnancy
◊ Separated from husband

We've included the line concerning the separation from her husband as a reminder to ourselves, and to any future clinicians who work with Elinor, that a relationship problem could complicate the future need for or provision of services. To keep things tidy, the record room will slap on a code number* (this and similar codes are known as *Z-codes,* since in DSM-5 they each begin with a Z). The fact that she is now pregnant also gets a code number, but we'll leave it alone: We're clinicians, not bean counters.

---

*It's Z63.0, Relationship Distress With Spouse or Intimate Partner. Alternatively, we could have used Z63.5, Disruption of family by separation or divorce. I chose the former, to focus on the relationship, which is ongoing, rather than the separation.

The Takeaway

In the evaluation of Elinor, we have appreciated the importance of moving through an interview in a way that provides a good experience for the patient (it permits bonding with the interviewer) *and* that obtains good diagnostic information. The techniques include the use of encouragements, both verbal and nonverbal, which can either shift the interview in a different direction or simply provide space for the patient to express content of thought more fully. Another technique we've discussed is the use of bridges to change topics without unduly distorting the flow of conversation. Along the way, we've discussed the three qualities we use to describe mood/affect; the assessment of attention span with serial sevens and other tests; and the diagnostic safety principle to help us arrange our differential diagnosis. We've mentioned relationship (spousal) distress, which is not really a mental health diagnosis at all, but rather a condition to be considered as possibly influencing our treatment of a patient who has another disorder. I've cautioned about overuse of adjustment disorder, which is a perfectly good diagnosis in its place. And that place comes after just about everything else under the sun has been eliminated.

Rant

Adjustment disorder is a diagnosis often made in the context of general health care. I suspect this is because health care providers too often attribute a mood disorder to whatever is going on in the patient's life, without paying enough attention to other possible diagnoses—especially depressive disorders. The rule for making a diagnosis of adjustment disorder is, or should be, that you use it only when you've ruled out just about everything else in the universe of mental health care. Adjustment disorder is one of those diagnoses that may be used far too often—along with borderline personality disorder and perhaps major depressive disorder (though major depression is probably also used too little).

Break Time

Elinor's story has been about techniques we can use to facilitate interviews with patients. But what about our interactions with friends and with family members? How effective are we in casual conversation? Do we even realize we are *using* techniques in talking with friends? Do we ask open-ended questions? Do we respond to the answers by listening actively?

I suspect most of us would respond, "Hey, no problem here!" But how can we know? Do we indeed formulate questions that give plenty of time for free speech, employ active listening, and avoid telegraphing answers we might want to hear? And do we fairly divide the time, so that our friends and loved ones get what they want—especially time to hold the stage themselves?

The poet Robert Burns famously wrote (I'm cleaning up the spelling and omitting the Scottish dialect), "O would some Power give us the gift to see ourselves as others see us." In the 21st century, the Power is Apple (and Samsung and Google)—the gods among us that produce devices bearing apps with which we can record speech in virtually any situation. I'd recommend an experiment with recording some of your own casual conversations, to assess your effectiveness in these. Of course, first obtain permission, lest your current friends become former ones.

6

Safety First—Fritz

Step 1

"Oh, criminy! It's back. And I'm feeling just awful."

The voice on the phone is anguished—and familiar. The call comes in midafternoon, squeezed between office patients; you look at your bulging schedule and say, "Try to outline it for me, please."

As Fritz begins to speak, an image shimmers into focus: There was a previous history of major depressive disorder (successfully treated with cognitive-behavioral therapy and a selective serotonin reuptake inhibitor [SSRI] antidepressant); a divorce; the loss of a job. Then serenity and calm, and a resumption of Fritz's climb up the greasy pole of employment in his competitive workplace. But now, in a few short hours, it had all come crashing down again. "When I was depressed the first time, it started just this way. I was fine the day before and foul the next. Now I'm having trouble keeping my mind on work, and I'm so cranky I could strangle anyone who comes through the door. I don't think I can stand to go through this again!"

As your next scheduled patient sits down in the waiting room, you consider how to respond.

What should you say? Hint: it's an overriding duty of clinicians.

Here's what you'd say: ______________________________

And here's what you'd do: ______________________________

Note A

Fritz sounds distraught, and there's no telling what impulsive act a frantic person might embrace—perhaps even some desperate act of self-harm. Of course, the overarching principle with someone who may be suicidal is that you must first ensure the patient's safety.

How you accomplish this will depend on the situation: Call 911? Pursue hospital admission? Persuade a trusted relative or close friend to confiscate firearms? Conduct a more extended interview with the patient? I could go on.

In the present situation, where self-harm has been implied ("I don't think I can stand to go through this again!") but not expressly threatened, more information seems critical to the mission. Regardless of how many others you keep waiting, your duty is to stick with this patient until you've obtained enough information to enable action that is informed and effective. So here's what I'd say to Fritz:

> "Thank you so much! You did exactly the right thing, calling me when you did! The most important thing is this: Let's keep you safe. I'd like you to come to the office right away. If at all possible, get a friend to bring you and stay with you. Once you're here, I'll see you just as soon as I possibly can. Will you do that? Good! See you in a bit."

Once Fritz arrives, you see him immediately. Even if that means you have to postpone another appointment. Even if it means you have to *cancel* another appointment! Patients understand these things, and most people won't take offense at being moved aside for the sake of a true emergency. After all, by and large, our patients realize that one day they could be in exactly the same position. Safety—our patients' and our own—must be a core value for every one of us as health care practitioners.

Step 2

As your previous patient departs, Fritz sinks into a chair. In the waiting room, his partner types away on an iPad.

Fritz seems composed, though a couple of times he launches himself to his feet and walks around the room. He even laughs once or twice as he describes his mood: "Midway between twitchy and bitchy—I nearly bit the head off someone at work today, and all she did was say she thought I looked nervous. Talk about shooting the messenger!"

He admits that every so often, a wave of depression sweeps over him: "Just like a couple of years ago, before I started the SSRI." Although he's "pretty distraught" right now, he denies any active thoughts of harming himself. He's oriented, and he waves his hand dismissively when you ask about delusions and hallucinations.

Until recently, Fritz has been doing well. "Even off the antidepressant for months now, my mood has been good and steady, until today." His job has been going well, he thinks—at any rate, his supervisor seems to like him, and he's made friends with some of his new coworkers.

Fritz's physical health has also been good, he says, and that takes into account his preemployment physical for his new job. But last night he was unable to sleep, and he worried into the wee hours about "well, just everything."

From his earlier evaluation, you recall that Fritz had been the assistant purser and safety officer on a cruise ship. There he was responsible for lifeboat drills, accident prevention, inspection of the ship's stores for proper labeling and storage, and checks of generators and lights. But that job had disappeared in the aftermath of his previous depressive episode. At his present job, he's persuaded his boss to create a safety committee, "to ensure well-being in the workplace and draft an evacuation plan, in the event of a 9/11-type crisis."

Fritz was adopted at birth and knows nothing of his biological parents. He's been in his current stable relationship for about 10 years; Allan supported him through the treatment for his previous episode. "Today, too," Fritz volunteers. "He's been a rock."

Before deciding on a plan of action, we need to review what we know. Below is that pesky short-form listing of the parts of an initial mental health interview. Sure, there's a lot missing, but what *vital* piece of history do we need?

- ☐ Chief complaint
- ☐ History of the present illness
- ☐ Personal and social history
  - ☐ Early childhood relations
  - ☐ Family history
  - ☐ Schooling
  - ☐ Sexual and marital history
  - ☐ Employment history
  - ☐ Military experience
  - ☐ Legal issues
  - ☐ Religion
  - ☐ Leisure activities and interests
- ☐ Substance use
- ☐ Medical history and review of systems
- ☐ Mental status evaluation (MSE)

Note B

Yep, substance use is the bit of history that we need to cover. I'm making a big deal of this, not because we often gloss over it (though that's easy to do—a history of serious mood disorder tends to outshine everything else), but because it can be truly dangerous to omit. So let's dig into Fritz's substance use history.

Step 3

Fritz reminds you that during his episode several years ago, he'd begun showing up for work intoxicated; finally, after repeated warnings, he was let go. He hadn't been able to return to that job—"they're a little skittish; I can't say I blame them." But he's continued to attend Alcoholics Anonymous meetings four times a week; for over a year, he's been clean and sober.

"No drinking," he says, "no illicit drugs. Period!"

Now what? Do we need to retake every part of the history, as we've outlined it above? Or is there something else we could ask as a shortcut?

Note C

There are a couple of ways to approach the problem. As suggested, one would be to move systematically through the entirety of a typical mental health evaluation. I have mentioned most of it in Step 2 above. That's a lot of stuff, but thorough reviews are, well, thorough, and I wouldn't for a moment discourage this approach. However, shortcuts are often useful, and not only when you are short on time.

Even when I'm pretty sure I have all the facts needed for my evaluation, I will still sometimes ask a patient for a bit of help: "What's happened just recently that we haven't yet discussed?" Phrasing it that way may encourage the patient to think just a little more deeply about anything we might have overlooked. In any event, I'd want to take every step possible before deciding that Fritz's *very* recent onset of symptoms marks the onset of yet another major depressive episode.

Step 4

So you take the shortcut and ask, "Has anything else happened, even a *little* event, that could have upset you here?"

Fritz pauses to consider. "No, everything was fine until yesterday," he says. "I've been really stable. Doing so well, in fact, that I decided I could finally stop my pack-a-day smoking habit. Threw away my cigarettes yesterday morning."

You ask, "Have you ever tried that before?"

He replies, "Sure. I've tried and tried. This time, I decided I was just gonna *do* it!"

In a couple of words, what diagnosis does this new information suggest?

Note D

Of course, the two words are *tobacco withdrawal.*

I wish it were otherwise, but it's really easy to miss something as commonplace as smoking cessation. I've done it myself, I'm embarrassed to say. Also, it's easy to overlook something that's gone missing in action, such as a habit that the patient has abandoned and would like to forget all about.

Let's think a bit broadly about substance use. There are quite a few different substance use conditions that can lead to anxiety or depression. The table on page 78 shows a summary of some effects on mood.

The number of substances that can be responsible for psychological symptoms, and the range of emotional states, are pretty broad; together, they generate a table that would be hard to remember. Perhaps we should keep this one handy, to use whenever we consider the effects of substance use on mood.

	Substance intoxication								Substance withdrawal					
	Alcohol/sedatives	Cannabis	Stimulants	Caffeine	Hallucinogens	Inhalants	Opioids	Phencyclidine (PCP)	Alcohol/sedatives	Cannabis	Stimulants	Caffeine	Tobacco	Opioids
Labile mood	×													
Anxiety		×	×		×				×	×			×	
Euphoria		×	×			×	×							
Blunted affect, apathy			×			×	×							
Anger			×							×			×	
Dysphoria, depression					×		×			×	×	×	×	×
Irritability										×		×	×	

Rant

Wouldn't you think that Fritz might have figured this cause-and-effect relationship out for himself? It's a thought that's crossed my mind, as it has for other readers. But the variety of events people can experience without recognizing their importance is astonishing, as a partly fictionalized example of a monarch's physical health problem illustrates. The first two episodes of *The Crown,* a Netflix miniseries about Queen Elizabeth II, portray a long period during which her father, King George VI, who had a long-time habit of heavy smoking, was coughing up blood from lung cancer. Even after he'd had a lung resected, he seemed happy to believe that his problem was only "structural changes" and that he'd soon be on the mend. In the event, he died within months of the surgery.

We humans are predisposed to think the best—for ourselves and for those we love—and to ignore or misinterpret warning signs that, if we were to observe them in someone removed from us, would be immediately obvious. The underlying motivations are probably varied, with fear and anxiety (and hope) prominent among them. Our duty as health care professionals is to view our patients objectively and to help them break through their defenses—or perhaps only to live with them—whatever they might be.

Step 5

By this time, you might think it unnecessary to construct a differential diagnosis for Fritz's mood symptoms, but humor me: It's what I do—and so should you. And while we're at it, let's decide on the best diagnosis (as if it weren't already set in stone).

Note E

For his mood symptoms alone, Fritz's differential diagnosis *is* pretty straightforward; under the circumstances, I think we can keep this relatively brief.

- ◊ Depressive disorder due to another medical condition
- ◊ Substance/medication-induced depressive disorder
- ◊ Major depressive disorder (and other primary mood disorders)
- ◊ Generalized anxiety disorder (GAD)
- ◊ Adjustment disorder with depressed mood
- ◊ Personality disorder

Now let's run through the possibilities to arrive at our best diagnosis. Of course, we always need to think of the many physical disorders that can cause depressed mood. Prominent among them are AIDS, brain tumors, cerebrovascular disease, thyroid and parathyroid disorders, Lyme disease, and premenstrual syndrome. None of them seems a good fit for Fritz, whose depression has started up again abruptly and in the context of other issues.

Fritz's mood has only been down for a day, which is far too brief to allow a diagnosis of major depressive disorder—or of a depressed episode of a bipolar disorder, or of dysthymia. I suppose someone, somewhere will make a case for adjustment disorder with depressed mood, but exactly what would Fritz be adjusting to—other than the loss of his cigarettes, of course? There really needs to be an identifiable stressor, and he seems to be adjusting well to his new job and his domestic relationship. As for a personality disorder, well, I often include that category for the sake of completeness, but we have no information that would support, say, borderline personality disorder, which often features unstable mood.

That leaves substance/medication-induced depressive disorder, and we have finally stumbled onto the fact that Fritz has just stopped smoking. His symptoms—depressed mood, irritability, anxiety, restlessness, insomnia, and trouble concentrating—are absolutely classical for nicotine withdrawal (called *tobacco withdrawal* by DSM-5, which has reverted to the terminology used in DSM-III and abandoned in DSM-IV; go figure). If we were to speak with him just a little longer, we might also learn that his appetite is on the upswing. In addition, the time frame for tobacco withdrawal (his symptoms began within

24 hours of when he gave up smoking) is perfect. I really don't think we need to look any further.

The diagnostic principle here is crystal-clear: Recent history beats ancient history. That is, we give greater weight to what's happened recently than we do to what happened some time ago.

Step 6

Your own anxiety is almost palpable as you ask, "Well, what about his tobacco use? Shouldn't we consider *that* as a disorder for Fritz, too?"

The answer is "Yes, of course we should consider it." Using the official DSM-5 criteria for any substance use disorder, how would you evaluate it?

Just below, I've written down the 11 classic characteristics of substance use disorder. For any substance, a use disorder can be diagnosed in someone who, within a 12-month period, fulfills as few as 2 of these criteria, *if* the person is distressed or clinically impaired. For Fritz, I'd like you to rate each potential symptom as Yes (Y), No (N), or Requires further evaluation (R). Circle your answer in each case.

- Using more. Many patients use more of their substance of choice than they intend. Y/N/R
- Control issues. The person wants to control use or repeatedly fails in attempts at control. Y/N/R
- Time investment. Many people, especially those who use drugs other than alcohol, spend much of their time in ensuring their supply or just in using the substances. Y/N/R
- Craving. A lasting desire for the substance has been linked to dopamine release in chemical dependence and other addictive behaviors such as gambling. Y/N/R
- Shirking obligations. Patients may abandon their roles at home, in the community, or at work in favor of substance use. Y/N/R
- Worsening social or interpersonal relations. Use continues, despite the fact that it leads to fights or arguments with close associates. Y/N/R
- Reduction of other activities. Patients ignore work and social interests. Y/N/R
- Ignoring physical dangers. Principal examples are driving a vehicle and operating heavy machinery when intoxicated. Y/N/R
- Ignoring health warnings. These can include ulcers; liver disease; the well-known risks of HIV/AIDS and hepatitis; and suicidal ideas, mood disorders, and psychoses. Y/N/R
- Tolerance. Tolerance has developed when prolonged use causes the body to become accustomed to the chemical effects (especially those of alcohol, opioids, and sedatives). The patient either requires more of the substance to obtain the same effect or feels less effect from the same dose. Y/N/R
- Withdrawal. Sudden discontinuation of use causes a symptom picture that is charac-

teristic for the specific class of substance. For tobacco withdrawal, symptoms must include four or more of the following.) Y/N/R for each:

- Irritability, anger, feelings of frustration
- Anxiety
- Poor concentration
- Feelings of hunger
- Restlessness or fidgeting
- Depressed mood
- Trouble sleeping

Note F

You've probably rated the items on this list exactly the way I did: mostly with a whole flock of R's, indicating that we haven't done such a swell job of evaluation—yet. But do we have enough for *any* statement about Fritz's tobacco use?

Well, we know from his own statements that he has repeatedly failed in his attempts to stop using, so that's the control issue we've marked with a Y. And what about tobacco withdrawal? Based on the information from Steps 1 and 2, I'd give these a Y rating:

- Irritability, anger, feelings of frustration
- Poor concentration
- Restlessness or fidgeting
- Depressed mood
- Trouble sleeping

That's plenty to identify a tobacco withdrawal syndrome.

A diagnosis of mild tobacco use disorder requires only two symptoms. With a more robust history, we'd probably score at least one or two more. (Surely Fritz has been exposed to, and ignored, health warnings—they're everywhere, even on cigarette packages.)

The bottom line is that, even with this limited information, we can note these diagnoses in Fritz's record:

◊ Tobacco withdrawal
◊ Tobacco use disorder

Rant

One way never to overlook an element of history is to use a checklist every time you interview a patient. Then you won't ever fall victim to your own lapses of memory. This approach, as we've seen in Chapter 4 in the case of Douglas, is also fraught with the concern that you might intrude on the conversational feel of your interview. That risks possible loss of rapport, and it potentially reduces all of your professional relationships to a series of interchanges that could as well be generated by Dr. Microsoft.

The Takeaway

Fritz's story is something of a cautionary tale (to be sure, that's the intent of every case in this book). The principal lesson is the importance of obtaining a *complete* history every time; the corollary for someone we've seen before is to update the history with each renewed evaluation. Any stone we leave unturned could end up as a stumbling block on the road to treatment nirvana. His story also illustrates the virtue of always considering substance use disorders, even when there's a previous history of a different behavioral or emotional syndrome.

Along the way, we've discussed patient safety in the context of an interview—not the last time this issue will arise, by the way. And we've seen the importance of exploring all aspects of a patient's medical history, including reviewing medical issues and any changes in habits such as tobacco use. Finally, we've encountered in action this diagnostic principle: Recent history beats ancient history.

The follow-up: Fritz slaps on a nicotine patch; within a few hours, his mood is back to normal, and his other symptoms have begun to dissipate.

Break Time

The mention just above of the change in terminology from *nicotine-* to *tobacco-*related disorders reminds me of a spreadsheet I once constructed that shows all the changes in terminology, all the additions and subtractions to and from the various DSM editions over my professional lifetime, and even before. You can view it—heck, you can download the PDF for free from a website of mine (*www.jamesmorrisonmd.org*). Click on the "DSM History Spreadsheet" link, and use your Control and + keys (Option and + keys for Mac) to enlarge the spreadsheet enough to read. It's not recommended for smartphone viewing.

This Break Time does focus rather exactly on diagnosis and classification—topics that are pretty closely allied to our usual workaday world. But it's also an interesting take (OK, it interested me) on changes in the tools we use every day.

7

Central Casting—Gloria

Step 1

"I'm not really sure why I'm here," Gloria begins. "I don't think this is the sort of problem you can help me with."

At 47, Gloria is a slender woman with greying hair. She glances warily around; then, with a grace that borders on stealth, she glides to the indicated seat. There she sits, perched far forward on her chair, looking as though she were about to fly. She has carried in a small stack of books and papers; rather than set them down, she holds them against her chest and abdomen, like a shield against the world.

It's an emergency evaluation; you have no information, other than the referring clinician's evident concern. What should be your response (and why?) to someone who shows so little faith in the system? Here are a few possibilities:

- ☐ "Well, why did you make the appointment?"
- ☐ "What *would* you like to talk about?"
- ☑ "Perhaps you could tell me about it anyway."

Note A

Of course, your follow-up question should be some variant on "Please tell me about it anyway." I'm only a little sorry to keep harping on this sort of open-ended invitation. My purposeful nagging is with the intent of instilling this overwhelmingly important concept: A major goal of any evaluation is to encourage the patient to reveal the information you need to make a diagnosis. You are hoping, in other words, to encourage enough speech that you can identify these concerns. The second purpose, as I've also noted before (also well worth repeating), is to establish the groundwork for a relationship with the person. And nothing works better for building bridges than a clinician's evident interest that spans the full range of what that person has to say.

Step 2

Little by little, with repeated verbal and nonverbal (smiles and head nods) encouragements, Gloria reveals that she is a professional actor whose new play opens in just over a month. The theater is small, the play is experimental, and no one expects it to make any money. Gloria actually has three roles to perform, frequently changing costumes during the action as she assumes different characters. And that troubles her.

"Every time I change characters, I know that everyone is watching me. I mean, more than any audience ever would. After we started rehearsals, the lighting designer was replaced by a person who is there just to keep an eye on me."

She opens one of her notebooks and displays what she has jotted down—page after page of dates that begin over a year ago, time of day, the exact locations (diagrams!) where she was standing, where the "observer" was standing, what was being said. "And he's recruited others in the show to watch me. Last night, two people followed me home. I don't feel safe now, anywhere."

So how do you respond to someone who seems so suspicious? (Note that I didn't say, ". . . who is psychotic?" There are lots of reasons to explain suspiciousness, and being delusional is only one of them. It is terribly important not to foreclose your evaluation before all the evidence is in.) Here are some choices:

- ☐ Perhaps you feel like arguing the point(s) with her, but is that wise?
- ☐ Perhaps you should just roll over and agree that she could be under surveillance?
- ☐ You could simply decline to comment.
- ☐ You could direct attention away from the content, and instead focus on her feelings about the situation.
- ☐ Or you could ask her to tell you more about it.

I'd like you to check the box you prefer, and then write down a few words defending your choice.

Note B

I'll admit that it can be hard to ignore clear violations of logic; the impetus to stand up for what's right and reasonable can feel overwhelming. However, arguing about something a new patient passionately believes in is just about the worst response you could make. It puts you on opposite sides on an issue that doesn't demand confrontation, whereas without penalty, you could instead let just about any inaccuracy slip past without refuting it. If you offer a rebuttal, the likely upshot will be to reduce the amount of information you obtain, and perhaps to harm your developing relationship. Remember that you are searching not to determine a scientific truth, but to understand how this patient experiences the world.

On the other hand, neither should you agree with something that's patently wrong. If what you've been told is false, to suggest otherwise would only reinforce thinking that could be delusional. And *that* could eventually undermine trust.

Simply passing over the questionable material is probably better than some of the other choices, but it's not what I'd prefer, either: It ignores something that is important to the patient and must eventually be addressed. Rather, I'd approach the dilemma from another direction—some variation on an open-ended "Tell me more about that." More details may help give you a handle on the genesis of the patient's beliefs, and might even suggest an approach to countering them.

Another approach is the often effective tactic of moving away from the content to focus instead on the accompanying emotional issues: "Tell me how that makes you feel." Regardless of substance, the feelings about any issue are undeniably the patient's property, something that no one can question or quarrel with. This response also demonstrates empathy for the patient while you are gradually moving away from potentially conflicted territory. Of course, the battleground will have to be revisited sometime in the future—but only after you have had the chance to build solid rapport.

Rant

Decades ago, in a popular book called *The Fifty-Minute Hour,* psychoanalyst Robert Lindner described how he had persuaded a patient to give up his delusional system by participating in the psychosis. In the chapter titled "The Jet-Propelled Couch," he wrote that the outcome of the case was predicated on "a commonplace: it is impossible for two objects to occupy the same place at the same time. It is as if a delusion . . . has room in it only for one person at a time." Unsurprisingly, the technique hasn't caught on in a big way. Few clinicians today would argue that agreeing with a person's delusions is a good idea.

Step 3

Accordingly, you continue: "I can understand that this sort of experience would make anyone uncomfortable—perhaps especially an actress who is trying to get into a part. Could you tell me more?"

Gloria responds, "OK, but that term, *actress,* offends me. I'm an *actor.*"

Uh-oh. How did this bump in the road happen, and how do you deal with it?

- ☐ Ignore it.
- ☐ Ask her to tell you more about this issue.
- ☐ Briefly apologize and move on.
- ☐ Do you have a better idea?

Note C

Wow! This interview seems to be an unending series of false starts and diversions. What you've stumbled into this time is a minor example of something that can affect a developing therapeutic relationship. At issue is learning to speak the patient's own language, in the sense of using words, expressions, and (sometimes) emotions in a way that the patient finds familiar and comfortable.

As it happens, many people in the world of theater do not want to be identified by a label that divides professionals according to gender. Hence both men and women are commonly referred to as *actors.* Similarly, many deaf people bridle at the notion that they are *handicapped,* whereas parents of children with dyslexia may reject the label of *learning disability.* Any time we health care professionals encounter one of these issues, we should seize the opportunity to learn something and, at no cost to anyone, make another deposit in a patient's trust account.

Of course, talking the patient's language extends way beyond metaphor. It is always appropriate (indeed, necessary) to use words and concepts the patient understands. You may need to adjust your own expressions and choice of words to fit the education, cognitive abilities, and cultural background of individual patients.

So what response should you make to Gloria? If this were other than an initial interview, I'd ask her to tell me more about the issue. Patients love educating their clinicians about any area of their expertise. However, whereas of course you want to protect rapport, your objective right now is to gain diagnostic information. I might say, "I'm sorry, I didn't think. I'd like to hear more about that from you later on."

Step 4

You thank Gloria for her correction and again request further information about her recent experiences as an actor.

She reveals that her concern has been growing for several months. She has begun to wonder whether her whole life is part of a giant theatrical script, in which she plays the central role. "When I came into your office, there was a guy outside who looked like he might be dressing the set for a scene. Also, the lighting in the hallway—it looked, well, staged. You know what I mean?"

You point out that the "set dresser" was only washing the windows; Gloria ignores your comment, instead saying, "And that person playing the receptionist seemed to be running her lines."

Unmarried, Gloria has had no lovers or intimate relationships for 2 or 3 years. She used to share her apartment with a cat, but she recently decided that she didn't like the responsibility. ("I don't even have houseplants anymore.") She emphatically denies having any hallucinations, either auditory or visual. When talking about the play that features her own story, she becomes animated and even grows visibly angry when she mentions the people who are "working on the set of my life." The only other person in whom she has confided is her director, who thought she should discuss her concerns with a clinician. Although she didn't think it would help, she wants to please the director, and so she has come for this evaluation.

Gloria has spent much of her adult life auditioning for roles on the stage, most of which have gone to other actors. She supports herself with the free-lance designing of websites, which she does for people who want to have a hassle-free online presence.

"I'm good with a computer. It's work I like to do, though maybe it interferes with getting the roles I deserve," she says. Although her town is "pretty good for theater, very few people here can afford to live on what they make from acting. We mostly need day jobs."

In response to further questioning, Gloria denies any family history of mental disorder; her physical health, she says, is excellent. She admits that she drinks some, but "wine only"; she doesn't "care to disclose just how much. If anything ever gets out, no matter how little, it might harm my career," she says, with a nervous glance toward the door. "You can't be too careful."

Throughout your time together, Gloria's speech is clear, coherent, and relevant to the questions she is being asked. Her affect is about normal in intensity and quality, certainly appropriate to her thought content. To your direct questioning, she denies feeling depressed or anxious; she says she takes a lot of pleasure in reading. She's never wished she were dead or had suicidal ideas. What about the experiences of hearing voices or seeing things others cannot hear or see? She answers, "No, never—I'm not crazy, you know." She briefly scowls, but then appears to lighten up: For just a moment, she smiles.

Now what should your differential diagnosis include for this patient? Please write your choices down in some sort of safety order, as we've discussed for Brad in Chapter 2 (page 24).

____

____

____

____

____

____

____

Note D

Here's my differential diagnosis for Gloria:

- ◊ Substance/medication-induced psychotic disorder
- ◊ Psychotic disorder due to another medical condition
- ◊ No mental illness
- ◊ Schizophrenia
- ◊ Schizoaffective disorder
- ◊ Schizophreniform disorder

◊ Delusional disorder
◊ Paranoid personality disorder

The first two are potentially more treatable than the others, and they would certainly need urgent attention, which is why they (as usual) occupy the top positions. I haven't tried to put the fourth through sixth choices (the ones beginning with *schizo-*) into any safety order. In the presence of major psychopathology, if I think personality disorder is a possibility, I'll always place it toward the bottom—to consider only after I've accounted for the major mental disorders.

As for the third choice, no mental illness, I promised myself that I'd include it somewhere in this book. Of course, it seems highly unlikely in Gloria's case, but we do have to keep in mind that, of all the patients we encounter in the course of our busy professional lives, there will inevitably be some for whom no formal diagnosis of a mental disorder is warranted. Although Gloria is not likely to be one of these patients, keep thinking about the possibility in the cases to come.

I can almost hear you whisper, "Haven't you forgotten mood disorders?" I did think about including some form of depressive disorder in the list, which would be in accord with one of my own diagnostic principles, but even my wide-reaching differential diagnosis has its limits: In response to direct questions, Gloria has denied having depression or loss of pleasure in her activities. However, if you've included it, do not deduct points. Points?

Step 5

And now the step we've all been waiting for: the denouement vis-à-vis Gloria's diagnosis. Please jot down arguments for and against each of the possibilities outlined in Note D. What you should end up with is your best diagnosis. Let's see if it's the same as mine.

Best diagnosis for Gloria: ____

And the reason(s): ____

Note E

Here's my discussion, which meanders through the Note D differential diagnosis.

No actual mental illness? I've mentioned this one first, because it is the null hypothesis we must negotiate to justify any of the remaining choices. Gloria has simply ignored the suggestion that the "set dresser" was only washing windows; in fact, she's doubled down on her paranoid ideas, claiming that the receptionist was practicing a speaking part. Of course, we should have asked her directly whether any other interpretation is possible, but for now her false ideas do seem fixed, and hence delusional.

Substance/medication-induced psychotic disorder? Whoa, at the first crack of the bat, we've hit a foul ball. Because, although you pitched the question, Gloria hasn't swung quite hard enough. In fact, whereas she's sort of rejected the idea that she might be misusing alcohol, she's definitely pushed back against giving a full, frank answer. We'll have to leave this one "unproven." Perhaps a later interview and/or collateral information will give us the information we need. For now, let's put this one on the bench.

Gloria's physical health is good. That doesn't absolutely rule out psychotic disorder due to another medical condition, but it shoves the possibility far down on the list.

To earn a diagnosis of schizophrenia, Gloria would have to have psychotic symptoms other than delusions. However, she has emphatically denied having any hallucinations, and we've seen evidence that she does *not* have negative symptoms: Her affect is quite appropriate, even forceful (she becomes angry when she thinks it's implied that she is psychotic), and in her determination to succeed in her career, she seems to be anything but apathetic. We have seen nothing to indicate that she has catatonia or other evidence of disorganized behavior; we have experienced enough of her speech to determine that it's pretty well organized. Therefore, by virtue of the fact that she has only one of the *A* criteria/inclusion symptoms—which are all listed in the Chapter 2 discussion of Brad (page 26)—she cannot have schizophrenia.

Schizoaffective disorder is ruled out because, in addition to the A-list schizophrenia requirements, Gloria would have to meet inclusion criteria for a mood episode. Evidence for that is entirely lacking. Schizophreniform disorder is also ruled out both by lack of the requisite A-list symptoms and by the fact that her symptoms have lasted longer than 6 months.

Paranoid personality disorder? Sure, as an add-on, it's a possibility, but it cannot explain the presence of actual delusions. For that, you need to invoke a psychotic disorder. Besides, one of our diagnostic principles is that we try to avoid making a personality disorder diagnosis in the face of a probable acute, major mental health diagnosis.

Unless more evidence turns up regarding Gloria's substance use, our best diagnosis will likely turn out to be delusional disorder. In this condition, the patient is out of touch with reality (the definition of being psychotic) all right, but with a lone symptom type: delusions. (Well, some patients with delusional disorder may have hallucinations, but these will be subsidiary and only serve to reinforce the delusions.) Though the delusions have lasted a month or more, Gloria's functioning remains relatively unimpaired. And that definition seems to fit Gloria perfectly—like a part that was written for her.

Rant

What is a *disease?* The word comes from, no surprise, the combination of *dis* (a negation) + *ease,* and the *Oxford English Dictionary* (OED) dates it as early as the mid-1300s. The authorities I've consulted all point out the word's implication that some part of the body has been structurally changed, and that this physical state is serious, prolonged, and active. The cause is usually something we can identify.

Sickness is a more common word we trot out for everyday use ("sleeping sickness"), and it's often pretty nonspecific ("We've had so much sickness this winter"). *Illness,* on the other hand, just sounds more formal (we speak of people who are "mentally ill," not "mentally diseased"). *Ailment* describes something of lesser magnitude, perhaps of unclear type or origin—something even as mild as a common cold. *Indisposition* is a stuffy way of saying much the same thing, with just a hint that the patient might be more unwilling than unwell.

Complaint completely takes the patient's point of view of whatever issue might be causing distress; it also places emphasis on that person's initial contact with a health care provider. *Syndrome* is sometimes used interchangeably with *disease,* but its specific meaning is a group of symptoms that go together to form an identifiable pattern. For those with really long memories (OK, back to the mid-1300s again, according to the OED), *distemper* once referred to human ills; to use it that way now would invite derision and lots of dog videos. A *malady* is a disease of longer standing, perhaps chronic, with the implication that it is mysterious and often fatal, like tuberculosis. (And for you in the back of the room, No! It's *nothing* like a pretty girl!)

Under the influence of the American psychiatrist Adolph Meyer, *reaction* found favor in the original DSM (1952) as the preferred term for many mental ills. It emphasized the theory that many mental disorders result from the response of individuals to their psychobiological life situations. By the time DSM-II appeared (1968), the term, with its implications for etiology, was history.

Even with all this, we still haven't come to the end. *Condition* is now used with no implication of cause or severity. *Affection* can apply to states of body or mind, but it's now pretty much obsolete in this sense. But what about *affliction? Infirmity? Disability? Scourge? Plague?* Most, if not all, of these you can probably figure out for yourself.

Rather, let's focus for a bit on *disorder*—the term currently preferred for mental health, and the one that's attached to nearly every condition included in DSM-5 (which uses several of the terms we've just discussed, while defining none). The OED says that *disorder* is a weaker term than *disease,* and that it doesn't necessarily imply change in physical structure. Philosopher John Locke may have been the first (1704) to use *disorder* in anything that approaches its modern sense—a disturbance of physical or mental functioning. However, if we reach even further back in time, Shakespeare used it (in *King John*) to mean a "disturbance or agitation of mind." Nowadays, *disorder* doesn't usually imply a cause, which is probably one reason that it has been seized upon by each of the famously atheoretical DSMs since 1980. As far back as 1883, *disorder* implied a functional disturbance; of course, that relationship is changing as we grow ever closer to unearthing the biological roots of each of the conditions (ailments?) we encounter.

By the way, did you notice how the word *disturbance* has wormed its way into the previous paragraph? It is the term of art DSM-5 reaches for when it wants to avoid saying *disease* or *disorder*—or any of the other words we've talked about above. As *destourbaunce,* it too goes back to the (late) 14th century, when living was hard and spelling was easy (in that it operated largely without rules). The OED says that disturbance then indicated "an interruption of mental tranquillity or equanimity," and it gives *mental agitation, excitement,* and *discomposure* as alternatives. *Discomposure?*

In the end, the terms we use matter only to the degree that they enable us to convey meaning with a degree of precision. From the evidence, we're still a long way from lexicographic nirvana.

The Takeaway

Gloria's story reminds us how important it is to work at developing rapport, even when the patient tries to stand aloof. Along the way, we have discussed using the patient's own language and open-ended questions to foster communication: We've focused on responding to statements that may be delusional. We've also reviewed the A-class symptoms of schizophrenia, but have come to the conclusion that delusional disorder best fits her symptoms. We've mentioned, to disparagement in her case, the possibilities of no mental disorder and of a personality disorder. And in an extended Rant, we have discussed some of the many terms used to denote ill health.

Break Time

We've talked about mental health issues, and mental health professionals, as they are depicted in motion pictures. But clinicians as the stars of TV and cable series? Seems improbable! Have there been any? Well, yes, and here's a sample:

- *Cracker.* This police procedural drama from the United Kingdom featured Robbie Coltrane as Edward Fitzgerald, a psychologist who assists the Manchester police in solving serious crimes. "Fitz" overeats, chain-smokes, gambles addictively—and always gets his man (or woman). The award-winning show was remade in the late 1990s with an American cast and locales.
- *The Bob Newhart Show.* If you remember this one, you've been around for a while! It was wildly popular in its time, but that was years before many mental health professionals practicing today were even born. Bob Newhart played the group therapist Bob Hartley, a psychologist whose relationships with patients and family members (mainly his wife, played by Suzanne Pleshette) are fodder for laughs, not drama or intrigue. Its 141 episodes spanned five seasons.
- *Web Therapy.* In another comedy show, this one much more contemporary, a female therapist named Fiona Wallice (played by Lisa Kudrow) offers her help via Internet sessions. With a stellar cast, it ran for four seasons on Showtime.
- *Wire in the Blood.* This British crime series, based on books by novelist Val McDermid, featured psychologist Tony Hill (portrayed by Robson Green). Using a variety of methods (intuition, role playing, and vivid visions of murder victims), Hill profiles repeat offenders to solve crimes too complex for the police. His personal history awash in childhood trauma, Hill himself has considerable psychological baggage, including Asperger's disorder, symptoms of developmental coordination disorder, and feelings of inadequacy.
- *In Treatment.* This series ran five nights a week for three seasons on HBO. It featured Gabriel Byrne as Paul Weston, a psychologist who treats a series of patients, with each of four evenings devoted to a different patient. As a result, we got to know these people pretty well as each season developed. In the episodes that aired on Fridays, Weston sees his own therapist (Diane Wiest). Much of the material was based on *BeTipul,* a series that originated on Israeli TV in the mid-2000s.
- *The Mentalist.* Patrick Jane (played by Simon Baker) works as a "mental health professional" of a different sort—a celebrated con-man psychic who later uses his insight into human behavior and motivations to consult for the California

Bureau of Investigation. His initial goal in changing sides is to locate the madman serial killer who murdered his wife and daughter, but the plot branches out from there. The show went on to 150 episodes across seven seasons.

- *Perception.* In this 2012 TV series, Daniel Pierce (portrayed by Eric McCormack) is a neuropsychiatrist touched with the unusual: He has paranoid schizophrenia, and one of his hallucinations serves as an assistant who helps him detect clues that have eluded the FBI in criminal cases. Wow!
- *Hannibal.* Perhaps the *ne plus ultra* of the genre, *Hannibal* was a prequel to *The Silence of the Lambs,* which I've mentioned in an earlier Break Time. The action of the TV series takes place before the apprehension and imprisonment of the antihero—psychiatrist Hannibal Lecter (played on TV by Mads Mikkelsen)—as he develops a relationship with a young female FBI profiler.

Can you think of others? I'd love to hear.

8

Self-Defense—Hank

Step 1

You're trying to take a history from the new patient who limped into the emergency room a few minutes earlier. He's young: He appears to be in his early 20s, though he's so tall and husky that you might be wrong about his age. So far, about all you've learned is his name.

Hank nervously taps the chair arm with the fingers of his left hand; his right lies quietly in his lap. His expression is a bit lopsided; one corner of his mouth droops. You've just asked, "Why are you here?" when he shifts suddenly in his chair, leans forward, and suggests that you can "go fuck yourself." He clenches his left fist, glowers, and shifts his feet to place them squarely under him. Is he preparing to pounce?

You know that sooner or later I'm bound to ask, "Now what do you do?" But first, because your actions could depend in part on your immediate surroundings, let's back up a bit and consider this: What should your seating arrangement be for any patient? Refer to the diagram on page 88, and then circle or check the arrangement listed below that you'd prefer.

a. [You and the patient facing each other across the desk or table, with your back to the door]
b. [You and the patient facing each other across the corner of the desk/table, with your back to the door]
c. [You and the patient sitting side by side, with the desk or table between you both and the door, and with both of you facing the door]
d. [You and the patient facing each other across the desk or table, with the patient's back to the door]
e. [You and the patient facing each other across the corner of the desk or table, with the patient's back to the door]
f. [You and the patient sitting side by side, each with your back to the door]

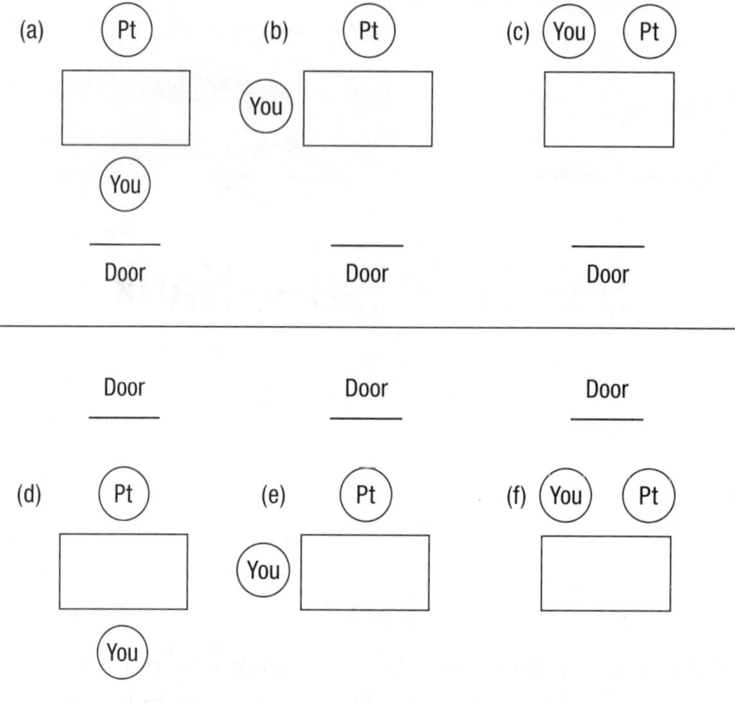

Six possible seating arrangements for a patient (Pt) and you as the clinician (You), in a room with a desk or table.

Note A

Right off the bat, we can discard choices d and e: You don't want anyone or anything in a position to interfere with your potential escape route. Indeed, I've only included them for completeness—and because some interviewing rooms are (unfortunately) set up that way. Choice f is only marginally better; perhaps it could be justified for an office where you see ongoing patients, but even then it sets you up for a possible frantic dash to control the door (which we hope swings outward).

The arguments for and against the other arrangements are a little more nuanced. It's pretty easy to understand why you might choose not to sit across the desk or table from the patient with your back to the door (choice a). Despite the fact that the across-the-desk positioning is the arrangement shown in every film and TV drama ever made about clinicians and their patients, it sets up a barrier between you and the patient.* And this is contrary to one of the two principal goals of the initial interview—to establish rapport with the patient that will provide strength for your future working relationship.

Sitting across the corner of the desk/table from the patient, with your back to the door (choice b), would be my preference—now for more reasons than ever. I like it mainly

*So why do filmmakers and cartoonists show it that way? I suspect it has a lot to do with emphasizing the authority of the clinician, who sits behind a big desk that might as well sport a sign saying "BOSS." Drama is all about symbolism, to which realism and true therapeutic relationship take a back seat. I do hope that I'll get a flood of emails with counterexamples, but I don't think it likely.

because it allows you to vary your distance from the patient according to the content of the discussion and your perception of the patient's demeanor. You can retreat if you detect anger or the need for space, and you can lean in when support is indicated—for instance, perhaps when the patient's affect suggests anxiety or depression. And now, with note taking on a computer so prevalent, you can position your screen so that it appears almost next to the patient in your field of vision. If you must take notes while speaking with the patient, you can minimize loss of the all-important eye contact.

Of course, you might be able to accomplish the same goals with choice c, the first side-by-side arrangement. But then you forgo the ability to use the furniture to form a tiny bit of added psychological barrier between the two of you when you need it. At least it offers you a sporting chance, in the event you'd ever have to race a patient to the door.

And by the way, I hope there's an emergency alarm built into the underside of the desk/table where you're sitting; if not, advocate for its installation. Also, does your clinic hold drills for practicing what to do if anyone should ever sound the alarm? It is a first principle of mental health care that providers take care of one another, and here is an excellent opportunity to do just that.

Step 2

Now for a quick quiz. Which of these behaviors should warn you that a patient is showing potential aggression? Check all that apply:

- ☐ Restlessness or pacing
- ☐ Increased amount of speech
- ☐ Mumbling, yelling, quarreling; abusive, rude language
- ☐ Clenching of fists
- ☐ Irritability
- ☐ Shifting gaze
- ☐ Glaring

Note B

That wasn't hard, was it? Of course, it's all of them, and I suspect that you've issued a flurry of checkmarks. In that case, we are clearly thinking as one.

Each of those behaviors is associated with the risk of aggression, even violence. The first three are more frequently observed in inpatients. Of course, close observation to learn all you can about a patient's state of mind is always important. Here, however, your own safety (and that of others around you) provides an added incentive for remaining alert to any hints of danger a patient throws off. Let's try to boil the list down into a single phrase: "Be alert for anything that suggests increasing agitation." That will cover most patient behaviors you need to watch for.

But there's one more situation to be aware of, and unfortunately it isn't something you can easily defend against: the patient with psychosis. The affect of someone who is high on a street drug or in the throes of an endogenous psychosis may not faithfully reveal that person's emotional state. When that's the case, aggressive behavior may appear without warning.

> With chagrin I remember Tina, a petite teenager who was experiencing the early stages of what turned out to be a chronic psychotic disorder. As we sat together in the hospital dayroom, she was calm and focused, and she smiled pleasantly as we chatted amiably together. It was a bit noisy there, what with other patients and staff members conducting their own business all around us, so I leaned forward to hear and be heard. With no warning, in a flash she had raked the nails of one hand across my face, barely missing my eye. Astonished, I fell back, but Tina only continued to nod and speak and smile—as though nothing untoward had happened.

Patients like Tina will be in the small minority, however, and the overwhelming majority of people with mental health disorders will never commit a violent offense. (In fact, they are at increased risk for being the victims of violence themselves.) With that said, it remains vitally important to be alert to the signs we've discussed, which can guide you to take appropriate precautions.

Step 3

OK, now your seating arrangement is sorted out, and you're alert to signs of potential violence. Hank is still sitting there, clenching his fist and staring fixedly; your heart is in your mouth. There are all sorts of responses you could make, many of which we can list as alternatives. For each pair, underline your choice of either A or B. Would you:

A	*B*
Speak quietly?	Raise your voice to be heard?
Ignore the insult?	Reject it ("You can't talk like that")?
Use open-ended questions to try to engage the patient in conversation?	Maintain control with closed-ended questions?
Intervene early?	Wait to see how it plays out?
Announce your intentions before getting up or taking other measures?	Act quickly (so the patient cannot forestall you)?
Maintain a neutral expression?	Frown to show disapproval?
Try to name the patient's feelings?	Focus on the behavior, not the emotion?

Note C

If in each of these seven instances you chose the response from column A, we are again fishing from the same stream. These are the actions likely to help deescalate aggressive, potentially violent situations. Based on respect for and maintenance of the patient's dignity and autonomy, deescalation depends on showing empathy and forming an alliance, as opposed to confrontation and dominance. Speaking softly is one of the clinician behaviors that can advance this agenda. (It might also help restrain you from escalating a situation right along with the patient.)

I'll also particularly note that false statements and inappropriate requests of the sort Hank makes are best handled by ignoring them; the patient probably doesn't need anything additional (such as your retorts) to fight about. You can also promote comity by identifying the patient's feelings; you might even validate them. ("I don't blame you for being upset; anyone who felt forced to come to the hospital would be.")

Don't frown, but don't smile, either. Smiles can be misinterpreted as amusement, or even mockery, which is especially problematic for someone who might already be suspicious of your intentions. You should also try not to show fear, contempt, anger, anxiety, or a judgmental attitude. And here's a verbal tic that I've heard many clinicians use with patients when they shouldn't: Saying "OK?" after you've made a statement shuts down a patient's ability to choose a response other than "Yes" (or "No way"). Using it repeatedly only compounds the patient's frustration. So don't use it. OK?

Listen and paraphrase, to show you've heard what's been said. And asking your questions in an open-ended manner will permit more options for response, which could reduce your patient's feeling of being closed in.

Here are some other points that don't as neatly fit the A–B forced-choice format in Step 3:

- Approach any patient with caution, moving with a pace that is slow and steady. You might clear your throat or softly say "Hello," so as not to startle someone who's already jittery.
- At all times, be patient and deliberate; don't try to hurry things.
- Try to project self-confidence without being bossy.
- Don't try to BS the patient; it can backfire.
- Make yourself appear nonthreatening, perhaps by leaning back or crossing your ankles. Of course, crossing your arms on your chest or balling your fists are signs of confrontation; monitor your own behavior so as to avoid them.
- When you do need to set limits, provide choices. ("Would you prefer to sit down and talk here, or should we find someplace quieter? Or should I call someone else to help us with this?")
- Don't argue unnecessarily. Rude requests like Hank's don't require a response, and you'll never persuade an acutely psychotic person that weird pronouncements such as "I am the Messiah!" are false.
- Keep facing the patient; it only invites attack if you turn your back (perhaps to show you are not afraid—when you should be!).
- Try to distract the patient, perhaps with the offer of food or a beverage (not, of course, one that's hot or served in a hard container).
- You can be firm, yet show compassion. ("I realize you are feeling upset, but I need you to try to stop shouting. Maybe you could do some stretches.")
- When you are about to engage with a potentially aggressive patient, remember to leave behind any objects that could serve as a weapon against you—or be used as a garrote.

I well remember the time I confronted someone creating a disturbance in a hospital waiting room. I was the senior clinician at the facility, so when the patient became unruly and refused a social worker's request to sit down, the staff had called me. Our dress code for men was shirt and tie, with or without a jacket. It should have been without the tie, for upon seeing me, the patient stepped forward, grabbed mine, and hoisted me upward into his snarling face. Fortunately, the throng of witnesses quickly rescued me, but the incident calls into question the wisdom of ties and scarves of any description—and of name tags worn on lanyards, a means of identification nearly universal in health care facilities.*

Rant

Besides causing anxiety (and potential hostility) in all who associate with an acting-out patient, disruptive behavior has another decided disadvantage: It can cause clinicians to diagnose patients incorrectly. That was the conclusion of a 2016 study done in The Netherlands, whose authors reported that the misdiagnoses were not simply an effect of clinicians' spending insufficient time in their evaluations.

And the issue of rudeness cuts both ways. Recent experimental studies in Israel have reported that rude remarks from either clients or clinicians disrupt team processes (such as sharing of information and workload) that are vital in providing high-quality care.

Step 4

You've survived the emergency, and now, at last, you're ready for Hank's history. It's obtained mainly from an interview with his clearly worried mother, who has been waiting in the corridor.

A quiet, studious child, Hank had never played much with the other kids in the neighborhood—or even with his two siblings, an older brother and a younger sister. But he walked and talked at the usual ages, and he'd shown an early talent for athletics. His mother had been a tennis pro before she'd married at the relatively advanced age of 39. Then she'd borne her three children in rapid succession.

When he was 13, just a few months after first stepping onto a tennis court, Hank had come close to beating his mother in singles. But in his first year—in the first *month*—of high school, he'd hung up his racket ("too tame") in favor of football. He went on to become the first freshman ever to make the varsity team at his school. "He was a pretty big kid," his mother says, "easily a match for anybody, even for seniors on the team."

Hank was simply a spectacular athlete. Playing middle linebacker that year, he not only earned his varsity letter, but finished a close second in the school's annual Most Valuable Player competition. After that, he only improved; by the beginning of his junior year, he seemed a certain choice for the honorary state all-star team. But in early November, his performance slackened.

*The two personal anecdotes I've related in this chapter may give the impression that my professional life has been one of nonstop combat. In my entire career, I've only been assaulted three times, with no serious injuries ever. If I'd had the same good advice I've been dispensing, I might have avoided those embarrassments.

For several months, Hank had seemed quieter than usual. Although he attended classes, his participation dwindled; his literature teacher phoned his parents to express her worries that Hank hadn't turned in assignments and seemed barely to pay attention in class. Then he stopped returning phone calls from friends.

But on the football field, Hank stepped up his game. Whereas he had never participated much in locker room horseplay, now he remained completely silent, even in the huddles. But during scrimmages he hit hard and often, to the point that some of his teammates complained of excessive roughness. Then in a game with their crosstown rivals, he hit the opposing quarterback with a tackle so vicious that it sidelined him for the rest of the season. When the coach tried to speak to Hank, he just walked away.

"That was the last game he ever played," his mother said. "Actually, it was the last time he went to school. At first, he'd get up each morning and head out, as though he were walking to school as always. But we found out later that he usually just went to the park, sometimes the bowling alley. Once he learned we were on to him, he'd mostly stay home. He'd just sit at his desk and play video games."

From time to time, she would enter his room, or try to; he usually asked her to leave. Once when he was in the shower, she'd gone in to try to straighten up, and saw some notes on his computer screen that she thought might refer to satanic rituals. In the end, his father forced his way into Hank's room and demanded to discuss Hank's behavior.

"Now my Jerome is a big man," Hank's mother explained, "but Hank is bigger. First he tried to push Jerry out, and when that didn't work, he hit him in the face. I never thought I'd see my husband crumple like that, but all he could do afterward was remain seated. That's when we called for police assistance to bring Hank here."

After the first 10 minutes, Hank refused to cooperate with the initial interview. But the few sentences he did speak suggested that for some weeks he had been hearing voices that advised him not to go to school. If he did, they seemed to say, he might be locked up, tortured, or killed.

Now, as you muster your thoughts for the differential diagnosis, have we forgotten to ask anything? What I really mean is this: What vital part of the traditional mental health evaluation have we neglected? Have you dog-eared the place in Chapter 1 where that brief outline is given? It's in Step 2 of the evaluation of Abby, on page 8. Turn back to it if you need a reminder.

Note D

That's right—we've hardly breathed a word about Hank's physical health. It's especially easy to forget that vital step for someone who has been playing varsity football, but in Hank's case, it turns out to be truly crucial. Because every once in a while the information about physical health is decisive, we must consider it every time. That often entails running through a *review of systems* for the patient, asking about symptoms from each of the body's functional areas—vision, hearing, heartbeat, breathing, digestions, urination, neurological functioning, and so on—to ensure that nothing gets overlooked. For Hank, here is the relevant information.

Step 5

Say, didn't you notice something just a little off about Hank's gait when he entered the room? Didn't he limp just a little, perhaps dragging his right foot? Come to think of it, didn't his right hand lie in his lap a bit unnaturally? And there was that lopsided facial expression. It would be understandable if you disregarded those signs in the initial efforts at assuring your own safety while obtaining a mental health history.

Prompted by your questioning, his mother remembers that once or twice, she'd noticed Hank making hand gestures that she thought peculiar. "Like he might be practicing sign language? Only he isn't hard of hearing!" she explains. And last week, while ordering her from his room, he suddenly stopped speaking "and just stood there, staring blankly—his jaw working, his lips moving, but nothing coming out. I wondered if he could be having a seizure, but then, after a few seconds, his eyes refocused and he turned away. I assumed he'd just forgotten what he'd wanted to say."

In retrospect, don't you wish you'd obtained this information much earlier? Actually, it's pretty terrific to have it during the initial evaluation—so often, it gets glossed over completely.

Now let's condense a few steps of the differential diagnosis process we've been following to this point. First, use the blanks below to write down a differential diagnosis for Hank, and mention the pros and cons of each diagnosis. Then mark your best diagnosis with your choice of a star, an arrow, or heck, a smiley face! Emojis are taking over the world, anyway. I'll do the same in my own differential list in Note E.

____

____

____

____

____

____

____

____

____

Note E

Here is my differential diagnosis for Hank, now as complete as I can make it, and with my best diagnosis marked as indicated above. Let's begin by noting once again that a differential diagnosis is supposed to include all possibilities, even if we think we've already sorted out the best diagnosis. With that as the goal, some entries are likely to seem pretty fantastical, and that's what we see here.

- ◊ Psychosis due to another medical condition ☺
- ◊ Substance/medication-induced psychotic disorder
- ◊ Stimulant intoxication
- ◊ Bipolar disorders
- ◊ Intermittent explosive disorder (IED)
- ◊ Schizophreniform disorder
- ◊ Schizophrenia
- ◊ Delusional disorder
- ◊ Antisocial personality disorder (ASPD)

Let's start the discussion from the bottom of the list, to eliminate the least likely possibilities. Here is my thinking about each of these disorders in regard to Hank.

A diagnosis of ASPD could be sustained only with a lot of additional information indicating that Hank's earlier childhood behavior was consistent with conduct disorder. Such a finding would be at odds with the history from his mother, which doesn't even hint at childhood or early adolescent misbehavior. According to DSM-5's rules, we'd also have to wait until Hank turned 18 to diagnose ASPD. Indeed, *any* diagnosis of personality disorder would be hard to sustain in a teenager, even one who has progressed fairly far through adolescence.

Next (moving up the list), we come to three psychotic disorders. In general, schizophrenia and its cousins carry a poor prognosis; that's why we honor the safety principle by placing these conditions toward the bottom of the differential diagnosis. Hank's delusions could indicate a delusional disorder, but he's also reported having some hallucinations. As we've noted in discussing Brad (Chapter 2) and Gloria (Chapter 7), people with delusional disorder don't usually have hallucinations, unless they are closely related to the content of the delusion. And a diagnosis of schizophrenia is unsustainable until we've eliminated everything else that could explain the symptoms. The same argument goes for schizophreniform disorder, which has symptoms similar to schizophrenia but a relatively brief (under 6 months) duration of illness. Each of these for now belongs on the sidelines, although they might be back in play, should we eliminate the possibilities higher up on the list.

IED, in which people fly off the handle with little or no provocation, has some of the trappings of a personality disorder: onset in childhood or teens, long-term persistence, impulsivity, and comorbidity with other personality disorders. But with treatment difficult and nonspecific, and prognosis uncertain, IED deserves to dwell in the nether regions of the safety hierarchy; it too should be diagnosed only after just about everything else has been ruled out. And we're still a long way from meeting that standard.

People with bipolar disorders often have emotional outbursts; sometimes these are accompanied by physical threats, or even actual violence. Whenever psychosis is involved, I prefer to consider bipolar disorders (or sometimes major depression) over schizophrenia and its cousins; mood disorders are more common, more readily treatable, and have a better prognosis, and so appear much further up the safety hierarchy. So far, not much information about Hank's mood has been revealed. That would be the work of the next interview session, because mood disorders are my go-to diagnoses of choice. Here is where I'd next focus my attention in the case of Hank, were it not for issues still higher on the differential diagnosis.

There's no information to persuade us that substance use has entered the picture, but then we cannot absolutely rule it out, either. It's safest to keep thinking about it as a possibility—always.

Finally, we arrive at psychosis due to another medical condition. Its top-level position might seem, in a sense, *pro forma*: after all, I *always* put it at or near the top of my differentials. But in this case, the practice has more than custom to recommend it. The symptoms (as described by Hank's mother) of delusions and sudden violent outbursts alternating with retreats into silence can be caused by brain tumors or other space-occupying lesions. Hank has also shown a couple of signs: the foot-dragging and the stillness with which he holds one hand—oh, yes, and the asymmetry of his mouth, and that incident where his mom wondered whether he was having a seizure. Indeed, it should be imbedded deep within our professional DNA first to rule out physical causes of emotional and behavioral pathology.

Usually, when I discuss with students a physical cause for mental symptoms, the likelihood I have in mind is in the low single digits. In the case of Hank, I would regard this possibility as an order of magnitude greater. And the relevant diagnostic principle is this one, of course: Physical disorders can cause or worsen mental symptoms.

Rant

Schizophrenia is in a funny position: a condition with careful, specific inclusion criteria that we nonetheless save as a diagnosis of exclusion—indeed, of almost last resort. Its close relative, schizophreniform disorder (when symptoms have been present for less than 6 months), occupies a perch just a notch higher in a differential diagnosis. This is a good example of the safety principle of differential diagnosis, which means putting those diagnoses with a good prognosis, relatively easy treatment, and symptoms that bode ill for the patient if not treated, higher on the list. Have I said this before? Good. I plan to mention it again.

The Takeaway

Hank's story is all about safety—safety for the patient, safety for the clinician, and safety for the diagnostic process. For the clinician, it involves preparation (thoughtful arrangement of office furniture; knowing what procedures to follow when confronting a hostile, potentially violent patient). For the patient, we have discussed the principle of the diagnostic safety hierarchy. We've also discussed some of the possible signs that a patient may be on the verge of aggression, or worse.

As for Hank's diagnosis, the one toward which the data appear to point is a mental disorder due to another medical condition. We don't often encounter someone who bears this diagnosis, but it is terribly important to include it in every differential list. The relevant diagnostic principle is this: "Physical disorders can cause or worsen mental symptoms."

The follow-up: Hank has been diagnosed with a slow-growing astrocytoma, which has been treated with surgery and radiation therapy. At his 2-year follow-up, he still walks with a limp. Without using psychotropic medications, he now has no psychotic symptoms. But he has never again played football.

Break Time

Do an online search for "patient attacks on [type of clinicians]" (you can fill in your own professional identifier here), and be prepared to be appalled at what you find. Every few months, there's another story about some clinician—a physician, a nurse, a psychologist—who in the line of duty has been assaulted, or worse. That should help put you into a safety-oriented frame of mind for—

Uh-oh. I think I heard someone say, "I'm on break, and this isn't relaxing me one bit!"

So, instead, let's turn the question on its head and Google "[type of clinicians] who kill patients." You'll find a shocking number of medical personnel who have turned into serial killers. Especially doctors and nurses—they've been on police radar as far back as the 19th century. (Right: Radar wasn't invented until just before World War II.)

Some of these deadly clinicians have been motivated by greed—they sought through inheritance to profit from murdering their patients. At least one, the notorious Josef Mengele, was enabled by the Nazi regime for which he worked. But a few may have been mentally deranged (or brainwashed), taking perverse pleasure in taking life.

I was deriving some solace from the notion that none of the documented helpers-turned-killers was a psychiatrist or mental health care worker of any profession—until I remembered Nidal Hasan, the U.S. Army psychiatrist who at Fort Hood, Texas, murdered 13 people and wounded 32 others in a shooting rampage that may have been in part motivated by ideology. And then there's Radovan Karadzic, the "Butcher of Bosnia," who got his start as a psychiatrist. He was ultimately sentenced to 40 years in prison for genocide. His story isn't all that restful, either.

9

A Mystery and an Enigma—Inez

Step 1

The police have brought a young woman to the emergency room. She carries no identification, and you know only that she has just been pulled from a car that was involved in a single-vehicle traffic accident. She wasn't driving; in fact, the driver is dead. No one else was in the car—a loaner from a car dealership.

You have only a few minutes to interview her: She must be moved to the operating room to stabilize her fractured pelvis. She speaks slowly, deliberately, in simple sentences; her pronunciation is clear. Her speech is coherent, but it conveys remarkably little information: She responds to most questions with "I don't know," or, occasionally, she simply doesn't respond at all. Her only spontaneous request is "I want my mom." During the interview, such as it is, she keeps her gaze firmly fixed on you. Her speech is a bit circumstantial; should we call it tangential? There's a bruise on the side of her head. Her pupils are equal. Her affect is uniformly flat.

Inez has a nearly empty pill bottle in her pocket; it bears no label, and no one in the emergency room recognizes the remaining tablets. No purse or wallet accompanies her from the scene of the accident. From her demeanor and speech, you can't determine enough to decide whether she needs further evaluation before she goes into surgery. Time is of the essence; besides surgery for her fractured pelvis, she needs to be evaluated for possible internal bleeding.

Right from the opening seconds of the interview, experienced clinicians start to compile a list of possible causes for what they observe. Based on what we've observed in Inez so far—slow speech, a paucity of information in her thought content, dull affect—what would be on your list of conditions to rule out? Write them down, and then compare them with mine in Note A. I'm betting that at least one of mine will surprise you.

Note A

Here's my list of disorders in which we could expect to encounter a combination of dull affect, limited content of thought, and slow speech.

- Traumatic brain injury with delirium
- Substance/medication-induced depressive disorder
- Substance intoxication
- Schizophrenia (and other psychotic disorders, such as schizophreniform disorder)
- Major depressive disorder (and other mood disorders)
- Autism spectrum disorder
- Intellectual disability (ID)

I wouldn't call this list a differential diagnosis. Rather, it's a game plan for how to approach someone with Inez's special requirements. It will inform your interview with the patient over the next 30 minutes, or whatever time you have before they haul her off to surgery.

I thought that the inclusion of ID might surprise you. That's because, though it is one of the most common mental conditions on the face of the earth (to one degree or another, it affects 3% of the overall population), the majority of people affected by it look no different from anyone else. That allows this diagnosis sometimes to fly undetected beneath our diagnostic radar.

Of course, Inez's final diagnosis may not even be on our initial list. Perhaps we haven't yet observed the behaviors that would lead us to the correct diagnosis. But the conditions listed are the ones that should guide us as we pursue our interview with her.

Rant

Intellectual disability (ID) is the current term of choice for what was once called *mental retardation.* For a little over 100 years, that term (or the single word *retardation*) was used as a description of intellect. As such, it once comprised a number of other, even less desirable terms: *idiot, imbecile, moron*—each of which was supposed to denote a specific IQ range. These pejoratives are well behind us now, for which we can be grateful, but the "R word" is still with us—recently as an epithet of abuse in popular film and literature, and, way too often, in personal discourse. Rosa's Law was named for then 9-year-old Rosa Marcellino, who has Down syndrome and with her family worked to replace *mental retardation* in law with *intellectual disability*. They succeeded, first in their own state of Maryland, then nationally; President Barack Obama signed it into law in 2010.

However, even beyond semantics, there remains the problem of precision. The strict meaning of the term *retarded*—"slowed down"—suggests a person who is intellectually running behind now, but who might catch up later. Of course, the vast majority of affected people will never truly catch up, though they may, with education, coaching, and accommodation, come to compensate in part for their condition. ID is currently defined not on the basis of raw intelligence alone, but also on the degree to which the individual's adaptive functioning is impaired. A rival term, *intellectual developmental disorder* (IDD), currently used in the 11th revision of the *International Classification of Diseases* (ICD-11), and as an alternative term to ID in DSM-5, further underscores the fact that the cognitive deficits begin early in the developmental period. With their emphasis on the degree to which affected persons can compensate for their disability, either of these terms is a vast improvement on the old definition of mental retardation.

Whichever of these two terms we use, we are engaged in an effort that goes beyond a simple, though laudable, effort to achieve political correctness. Even well into the 21st century, we are still in the process of learning to describe mental disorder in general, and ID in particular, in ways that are both accurate and useful.

Step 2

Inez is still lying on a gurney in the emergency room, awaiting transport to the operating room. You stand at her side, armed with your tentative list of the mental problems she might have. Now you must rapidly work your way through them, selecting open-ended and closed-ended questions to complete the task.

Time management means that you will need to consider the advantages of closed-ended questions as opposed to open-ended ones. We've talked a bit about this earlier in Step 1 and Note A of Elinor's story (Chapter 5, page 56). Now let's identify the characteristics of each type of question. I've tried to make it easy by listing many of the features of each type. After each question, just circle the O or the C for open-ended or closed-ended, respectively.

- You can spend more time listening. O/C
- Answers take just a few words. O/C
- You can obtain a broader scope of information. O/C
- It discourages evasiveness. O/C
- It facilitates expression of feelings. O/C
- It's generally used early in an interview. O/C
- It's generally used later in an interview. O/C
- It helps establish rapport. O/C
- It can elicit significant negatives. O/C
- It helps pin down a diagnosis. O/C
- It may suggest an answer the patient thinks you want to hear. O/C
- It requires longer answers. O/C
- It's useful for clarifying an earlier response. O/C

- It helps obtain details about an event or emotion. O/C
- The information it yields tends to be valid. O/C
- It can yield a broad range of concerns from the patient. O/C
- It may help you cut to the chase when time is of the essence. O/C
- You may want to shift to this type when the other type hasn't been very successful. O/C

After you've tagged each characteristic, which type of question points the way for your further evaluation of Inez?

Note B

Here are my answers to the features of open-ended (O) and closed-ended (C) questions:

- You can spend more time listening. O
- Answers take just a few words. C
- You can obtain a broader scope of information. O
- It discourages evasiveness. C
- It facilitates expression of feelings. O
- It's generally used early in an interview. O
- It's generally used later in an interview. C
- It helps establish rapport. O
- It can elicit significant negatives. C
- It helps pin down a diagnosis. C
- It may suggest an answer the patient thinks you want to hear. C
- It requires longer answers. O
- It's useful for clarifying an earlier response. C
- It helps obtain details about an event or emotion. C
- The information it yields tends to be valid. O
- It can yield a broad range of concerns from the patient. O
- It may help you cut to the chase when time is of the essence. C
- You may want to shift to this type when the other type hasn't been very successful. C

Adding up the O's and C's yields many features in favor of each type. Considering what we've encountered so far in Inez, who doesn't show a lot of spontaneity anyway, the last item in the list is the clincher: it suggests that, for the present, you will be more successful with questions that are generally closed-ended. And that judgment is reinforced by the strictures of time, as noted in the next-to-last item in the list.

By the way, time management is one of two main uses of the closed-ended question. Keep reading; before too long, we'll encounter another use.

Step 3

Considering our tentative list of conditions to explore and the fact that our time with Inez is limited, what closed-ended question should we choose to start off in the right direction? I'll offer some alternatives:

- ☐ "How are you feeling right now—happy, sad, something else?"
- ☐ "Have you had any experiences such as hearing voices when no one was talking, or seeing things that other people couldn't see?"
- ☐ "Will you tell me your name?"

Note C

My answer (no, my *question*) would be the third choice. Of course, we already know her name—but the question serves as a proxy for the entirety of the formal mental status evaluation (MSE). Here's why I think we should focus on it with Inez:

We already have some indication that Inez's brain may not be working as well as it should, and we know that she has very recently been in an accident. Furthermore, we don't have a baseline against which to assess change in mental functioning. Outside information from a friend or relative would probably help us with some of these issues, but we don't have the luxury of that resource. Instead, I'd move right away to a careful appraisal of her current cognitive functioning.

Step 4

Just below is the outline of *cognitive* features we usually include in an MSE. We'll use the check boxes once we get to the end of this Step.

Orientation
- ☐ Person
- ☐ Place
- ☐ Time

Memory
- ☐ Immediate
- ☐ Recent
- ☐ Remote

Attention and concentration
- ☐ Serial sevens
- ☐ Counting backward

Cultural information
- ☐ Examples: recent presidents/prime ministers, state governors or provincial prime ministers

Abstract thinking
- ☐ Similarities
- ☐ Differences

Insight and judgment
- ☐ Insight
- ☐ Judgment

And here, with Inez's responses, are the MSE questions that pertain to cognition. To give the flavor of the whole interview, I've written out the exchange verbatim, adding in the occasional comment. At the end, I'm going to ask you to evaluate her cognitive status.

Q: I'd like to ask you some routine questions to help me understand what sort of problem you might be having.

A: (*No answer*)

Q: Will you tell me your name?

A: (*After a few moments' pause*) It's Inez.

Q: Great! And your last name?

A: Inez Paisley.

Q: Super! My name is (*you give it*). Will you please repeat it back right now?

A: (*She accurately repeats your name.*)

Q: Excellent! And can you tell me what the date is today?

A: I don't know.

Q: Well, how about just the month?

A: Um, maybe October?

Q: That's right. Very good! Now how about the date?

A: I don't know.

Q: OK, is it early in the month?

A: Halloween's coming.

Q: You are right about that! Is Halloween coming soon?

A: I think so. Day after tomorrow. I've bought candy.

Q: So what would be the day of the month today?

A: (*Long pause*) October 29th.

Q: And the year?

A: (*After one false start, she corrects herself and then states it correctly.*)

Q: Perfect! And do you know where you are right now?

A: I don't know—a hospital?

Q: Yes, this is a hospital emergency room. Do you know the name of this hospital?

A: No.

Q: What city are we in?

A: (*After a pause, she gives the correct answer.*)

Q: Excellent! Now I'm wondering: Do you feel up for a little math? We clinicians are always asking people to do math problems. It's just part of the routine.

A: I don't know. I'm not very good at math.

Q: Well, let's just give it a try. Can you subtract 7 from 100?

A: I can with a pencil. And paper. (*Long pause*)

Q: OK, instead, can you just count backward from 30 and stop when you get to 15?

A: Um, 30, 29 . . . ?

Q: Great! Keep going to 15.

A: 30, 29, 28 . . . (*She keeps counting until she gets to 15, then stops.*)

Q: Excellent! Now let's try something different. Would you multiply 2 times 3?

A: That's 6.

Q. Great. Now 2 times 6?

A: Um . . . 12.

Q: Good. Can you keep going?

A: Going where?

Q: Well, 2 times 12.

A: (*Pause*) 24?

Q: Good. And 2 times 24?

A: (*Long pause*) No, that's too hard.

Q: OK. Let's try something that isn't math. What does it mean when I say, "Don't cry over spilt milk"?

A: Well, if you spill the milk, you shouldn't cry about it.

Q: Right. But does it have any other meaning?

A: Just, don't spill the milk.

Q: OK, and what did I tell you my name is?

A: (*After a pause, Inez states it correctly.*)

Q: Do you know what's happened to you? I mean, why you are here?

A: Well, I was riding in the car.

Q: Yes, and what happened?

A: I think I hit my head. And my leg hurts, up here. (*She points to her hip.*)

Q: That's right; it got broken in an accident. Do you want the doctors to fix it? It means an operation.

A: I want it well again.

Q: Do you think you should have the operation?

A: If that will fix it, sure.

Given the information we have so far, please go back and make a checkmark beside each indicator of cognitive status in the list at the beginning of this Step for which we have at least a modest amount of information.

Note D

With only a start on the MSE, and hardly any history at all, we've actually accomplished quite a lot. Perhaps in response to encouragements and overt praise, Inez is now talking more than she did at first, and she's demonstrated that she's fully oriented to person, place, and time. Furthermore, she can focus pretty well—she's paid attention through several minutes (12 by actual count) of formal testing, and throughout a countdown to stop at a specific number. She has also retained a name and repeated it after more than 5 minutes, so her short-term memory is intact. However, she doesn't appear able to abstract a general principle from a proverb. Even though we haven't evaluated her store of cultural information or her insight and judgment, what Inez has demonstrated is a far better cognitive performance overall than we might expect from someone with, for example, delirium from head trauma.

Step 5

How would you evaluate Inez's differential diagnosis against the choices listed in Note A now? It would be a good thing, using those choices, to make a few notes here as to why you would favor or reject each one.

____

____

____

____

____

____

____

Note E

Brace yourself: I'm going to take my usual methodical stroll through the suggestions we have so far. Right now, the differential diagnosis stands as the temporary list we've formulated in Note A.

We've already mentioned the fact that Inez's cognitive status is more nearly intact than we'd expect from someone with a delirium. The criteria for delirium require problems with attention *and* orientation, and Inez appears to have neither. Reduced affective lability can of course be encountered in schizophrenia and other psychotic disorders, but we have so far turned up no evidence of hallucinations or delusions. Furthermore, Inez's thinking, when she does speak, is pretty much linear and responsive to the line of questioning. In other words, we find no evidence that she has the sort of A criteria (we've discussed them for Brad in Chapter 2, page 26) that would be needed to diagnose a psychosis.

Both affect and content of thought can be restricted in mood conditions, such as a major depressive episode. We would have to dig for a lot more information—especially an expression of feeling depressed!—before we could diagnose a depressive disorder. Autism spectrum disorder can cause patients to have limited affect and difficulty relating to other people, but Inez appears to warm to the interview situation; we'd need a lot of historical information to sustain this diagnosis. People who are under the influence of alcohol or other substances sometimes have flattened affect and may offer limited responses to questions, but again, substance use in this case would require history that I don't think will be forthcoming.

So what about ID? It certainly fits with her presentation, and I'm betting that it will appear when we settle on her final diagnosis—but that'll be somewhat later. Right now, we cannot affirm ID, either: It requires information that her symptoms began in early childhood and that they have limited her ability to be socially and personally independent. What we do have so far is consistent with mild ID, but this is a diagnosis for which there is no effective treatment, so we must be certain of our ground before lumbering Inez with the label. We simply cannot justify making this diagnosis without more information.

Uh-oh: For one reason or another, we've rejected every potential diagnosis on our list. Where does this leave us? Without enough material to make any solid diagnosis, her formal diagnosis at this point would have to be *undiagnosed.*

And we would tell anyone with a need to know—especially the surgeons—that with the present information, her diagnosis is most consistent with mild ID. Period.

Rant

Let's stipulate, for the sake of discussion, that Inez has mild ID. Obviously, it began when she was an infant—probably even before she was born. Hers is only one of the disorders that we sometimes forget to consider, because we tend to think of them as "kids' diseases." Yet diagnoses such as ID and certain others that are usually made in childhood continue to follow affected patients throughout their lives. These conditions include autism spectrum disorder, Tourette's disorder, and learning disorders, which are generally first diagnosed in childhood (or sometimes the teen years) but persist into adulthood. Others, such as separation anxiety disorder, reactive attachment disorder, and pica, were once included in the section of the diagnostic manuals devoted to what are now called *neurodevelopmental disorders.* Still other disorders are clearly intended to be applied to children, but are listed in sections of the manuals specific to behavior rather than to age (the brand-new DSM-5 diagnosis of disruptive mood dysregulation disorder is the obvious example).

When determining a differential diagnosis, we need to keep in mind so-called "childhood disorders" that persist. In the second edition of *Interviewing Children and Adolescents,* Kathryn Flegel and I have included an appendix that lists every major mental disorder (omitting the paraphilias), with our estimation of the earliest age at which each one might be reported to occur, as well as the period of life that it might most often be found. Of 110 disorders, we've reckoned that only 5 would never occur for the first time in children: 4 neurocognitive disorders (still commonly called dementias when they are major), plus rapid eye movement sleep behavior disorder. To be sure, 70 are most often encountered in adults (or, in some cases, youth in their late adolescence). But the bottom line is this: Very few of the conditions we discuss in our differential diagnoses are exclusive either to adults or to children/teenagers. Clinicians who work with patients of any age range need to be aware of the full spectrum of mental disorders, regardless of the typical age at which the disorders are first encountered.

Step 6

Inez is about to have a further diagnostic workup, followed by surgical care. Don't we need to consider whether she has the ability to give informed consent?

Let's review the traditional guidelines for judging whether a patient's consent to a medical procedure is appropriately informed:

1. Sufficient maturity. Children are too young to have the perspective and judgment required for the evaluation of health care issues; by the time they are in their mid- to late teens, this capacity has usually developed sufficiently, but the determination must be made case by case.
2. Ability to appreciate the consequences of the procedure and the possible outcome if it is not performed. Adults are presumed to have this capacity, in the absence of marked ID or other mental or emotional disorder.
3. Consent freely given. This means that there must be (a) no coercion employed and (b) adequate time for considered reflection, if possible. However, some situations are emergent and must be rapidly evaluated and decided upon.
4. Clinician candor. Especially in circumstances such as research studies, it is also important that the patient be apprised of any possible conflict of interest the clinician might have.

On the basis of these guidelines, and considering what we know about Inez, how would you evaluate her capacity to consent to an operation on her hip? If we need more information to make this determination, what would that be?

Note F

Of course, Inez is old enough to make this sort of decision, and there is no evidence to suggest that she is in any way being coerced. Rather, the issue has to do with her ability to understand the fact that she requires surgery. Quite frankly, I'd feel a little more secure if we'd taken the time to ask, "Do you understand that sometimes surgery can go wrong and people can get even sicker?" But, given her absolute need for the procedure and the fact that there's no one available to act as her proxy, I believe we should allow her to sign for her own care.

The Takeaway

In Inez, we've encountered a time-limited situation with a patient who doesn't spontaneously offer much information; this has forced us to rely heavily on closed-answer questions. We've discussed her likely diagnosis of mild ID; despite its ubiquity, it is easy to overlook. However, lacking the necessary collateral information, we must ultimately fall back on the diagnostic principle that advises us to use the term *undiagnosed* when we are unsure of the diagnosis. We have also discussed what steps we should take to ensure that a patient is competent to give informed consent for a medical procedure.

Break Time

Who doesn't like free stuff? As I've noted in an earlier Break Time, there are a lot of great reads you can download just for the asking from Project Gutenberg and other free sites. Some of these books feature characters with mental health issues, and some of *them* make for interesting diagnostic problems.

One such is the central character of Herman Melville's classic short story "Bartleby, the Scrivener." First published in 1853 and subtitled "A Story of Wall-Street," it concerns the new clerk (Melville gives him no first name) hired by the narrator, a Wall Street lawyer (who remains totally nameless throughout). Bartleby is initially hard-working and productive, but he later comes to answer every request with the refrain "I would prefer not to." And indeed, as time goes by, he accomplishes less and less, eventually spending his days staring at the brick wall visible from his office window. Ultimately he prefers not even to eat and dies of starvation. I'm not going to tell you more. But I will say this: At the end, there is considerable doubt as to just what is the matter with Bartleby.

You can approach this Break Time in a manner that's about as quick, or perhaps as slow, as you wish. (OK, the absolute speediest method is to stop reading now and skip to Chapter 10. Absent this back-of-your-hand dismissal, you can just read "Bartleby" as an interesting story that you may not have encountered before.)

But if you do engage in this experiment, the story itself will be a quick read (at 14,000 words, you can probably knock it off in an hour). Go ahead and download it from the Project Gutenberg website, and then—as so many clinicians find themselves compelled to do when they read the classics of literature—try to figure out just what ails Bartleby. You can even construct a differential diagnosis. And if your interest has been truly piqued, you can visit my website to see what I think about Bartleby's condition, and what lessons his story might hold for us today. You may end up agreeing with the narrator, who in the last line of the story sighs, "Ah Bartleby! Ah humanity!"

10

Now and Then—Julio

Step 1

"Oh my God, am I ever glad to be out of that car! I thought I'd go crazy, cooped up with those two for 500 miles. I don't think that I've—"

At his college, the first place Julio goes (or, strictly speaking, is taken) is the infirmary, and that's where you find yourself interviewing him in a cubicle barely large enough for the gurney. You have to step over some of his stuff, which has been dumped all over the floor.

"How are you doing now?" you ask. "Sorry to butt in."

Julio takes a tighter grip on the rails of the gurney and forges ahead. "That was the trip from hell. I don't think I've ever experienced anything quite like it. I half thought those guys were going to kill me. For the last 50 miles or so, Billy sat on me. I guess he thought I was going to jump out of the car, or something insane like that. Actually sat on me! What the *hell* kind of treatment is *that,* I'd like to know?"

At this point, with time and the patient *both* flying, how would you proceed? OK, maybe this is too hard as a fill-in-the-blank question, so let's make it multiple-choice. You could:

- ☐ Tolerate the rambling and keep on listening.
- ☐ Put your finger to your lips to suggest the need for quiet.
- ☐ Ask some yes–no, closed-ended questions.
- ☐ Interrupt the patient and repeat your question—over and over again, if necessary.

Now make your choice(s), but I'd like you to write down a note or two to justify each one that you choose, as well as each that you reject. If you favor more than one choice, in what order would you try them out?

Note A

Of course, any of the four approaches listed above might yield results, but some have greater potential than others for providing the information you need. As it happens, I've listed them in the order in which I'd probably try them—with most patients.

So let's start with the first. Actually, isn't this pretty much the same thing as the free speech that I intermittently advocate throughout this workbook (everywhere, actually)? There's a lot to be said for listening to the top concerns of any patient you're interviewing for the first time. As I've pointed out before, encouraging free speech not only gives you a window into the immediate issue that prompted the evaluation; it also promotes the understanding that you are an alert, caring provider who is interested in learning the full extent of the patient's current concerns.

But do we know anything that might suggest how hopeless further free speech would be for Julio? Look again at how he responds to your question "How are you doing now?" It's with further ranting and rambling, threatening to drive your interview into the tall grass. Sure, we want to give every patient scope for expression—but the direction this interview has taken leads, in my opinion, exactly nowhere.

So I might instead try a symbolic finger to the lips. If I do it right, my slightly humorous demeanor will indicate to most patients the need for restraint, without provoking them further. It is similar to the raised finger you might sometimes use to signal that you want to interrupt a patient. (Hey! Index finger!)

Next, I may well switch to closed-ended questions that can be answered with a "yes" or "no." Although the message ("I'd appreciate succinct answers") could be a bit subtle for this patient, it is one worth trying to get across. Along with this message, I might well add something even more explicit, saying in so many words: "I think we'll get places more quickly if you will respond with a word or two. We can explore each of your issues later, after you've given me the broad picture."

But Julio has such a death grip on the interview that even this directive approach might not yield the material needed for diagnosis. So if his loquacity continues, I wouldn't hesitate to put in my oar repeatedly—asking the same question with each interruption—until either I get a usable answer, or I determine that this patient simply hasn't enough control to give the needed information.

Step 2

Let's say we've run through the above-described steps to little avail. Where do we go next? What can we do to get the data we need? We've discussed it before, so I'm not giving any hints. Your thoughts? ____

____

Note B

The answer is, of course, that with little crucial information likely to come from the patient, we need an alternative source. That could mean obtaining a history from a previous health care provider (medical records), but we're likely to get more help from talking with informants who have known the patient well, for a long time, and recently. Collateral information is the most efficient way forward; considering Julio's current mental state, perhaps it's the only way. The obvious next step is to talk to Julio's buddies.

Step 3

First, let's take a bit of a detour: When, if ever, should we *not* interview relatives or other informants? Make a short list. Please.

Note C

Actually, a list of the conditions under which you wouldn't speak with potential informants *is* a pretty short one.

First, obviously, you won't speak with informants if there are none available. That will only rarely be the case; perhaps the classic example is a homeless person or someone who has appeared in your emergency room, having just drifted into town, carrying no identification—and who is unwilling or unable to give you the sort of contact information you'd need to telephone friends and relatives. (We've just encountered such an example in the case of Inez in Chapter 9.) A little investigative work on a smartphone will usually render this sort of situation relatively infrequent.

Occasionally, however, a patient will say "no" to your request to speak with Mom and Dad or with a former spouse or partner. The reasons will be varied—concern about a soured relationship; worries (perhaps even based in psychotic thinking) that your contact will feed into a plot against the patient; a desire to conceal current whereabouts; or fear that a secret might be revealed. On occasions when I've been refused permission, I've sometimes found that a warm demeanor and repeated explanations will convey the understanding that accurate information can work to the patient's advantage—that it might help achieve relief from symptoms such as depression or fear, or even lead to release from the hospital or from detention.

In any event, when you do speak with informants, be sure that you are careful only to receive information, and not to give it out against the patient's wishes. To do otherwise would be a violation of your duty to maintain the patient's confidentiality. We'll talk more about clinician ethics in Chapter 26, when we encounter Zander.

Step 4

Mark, one of Julio's friends, tells you the following.

> It was actually a very long car ride (well over 500 miles, crossing several states), and at least as uncomfortable for his two buddies as it was for Julio. Mark called Julio's mother when they arrived on campus, and he had the presence of mind to ask her about Julio's mental health history. (Currently on her way here, she is temporarily unavailable for questioning—she has no cell phone and no plans to stop along the way.) Mark plans to study engineering; he presents what he knows in verbal bullet points:

• For several weeks, Julio had been feeling down. His mom thought he was nervous about college and leaving home for the first time; he'd rarely even been out of the state before. Mark says, "She told me that he'd lost his appetite, couldn't sleep, and didn't even seem interested in organizing his stuff to take with him. For a couple of weeks, he just sat there in his room." She said that a few months earlier he'd had a similar episode, which started about the time a girlfriend broke up with him. Then she'd worried that he'd been drinking—several bottles had disappeared from the family's liquor cabinet.

• But 10 days ago or so, he'd snapped out of it. Now, brim full of optimism and good spirits, *still* he hadn't slept much. "Only now, he seemed not to need it. That's what she told me," Mark said. "And though he talked more than usual, he hadn't said anything that was, you know, nutty? Except that maybe he didn't *need* to go to college, that he'd learned enough in high school? She said she took that as a joke, but after our car ride, I wonder. Y'know?"

• When he first started kindergarten, his mother had to stay in the classroom the whole 4 hours, until it was time to go home. Otherwise, little Julio would weep inconsolably. "That would probably count as separation anxiety disorder now," offers the infirmary nurse, who is thumbing the pages of a nifty text that explains DSM-5.

• Years ago, the mother's younger brother—Julio's uncle—suddenly became hugely excited and disappeared from home. Weeks later, when he finally telephoned from a neighboring state, he said that he been called to the ministry of the family's church, to bring about "a new order of social justice and lower taxes." He eventually hanged himself in jail, where he'd been taken "for his own protection."

You know what I'm going to ask next: I want to know what you would include in your differential diagnosis for Julio, and why

____

____

____

____

____

____

Note D

Here's how I view Julio's differential diagnosis, and it isn't astrophysics. It's pretty much what you'd expect—and pretty much what you've written down, I'll bet.

◊ Substance/medication-induced mood disorder
◊ Mood disorder due to another medical condition
◊ A bipolar disorder

◊ Major depressive disorder
◊ Separation anxiety disorder
◊ Other anxiety disorders, such as panic disorder

The first two diagnoses are there because they are *always* on top of my differential list, as I've emphasized throughout the book. Major depressive disorder is in the mix because of the incident in Julio's history that sounds as though he had experienced an episode; a bipolar disorder is there because it sounds very much as though his mood is currently on the upswing. And separation anxiety disorder belongs on the list because the nurse could be right: Julio may well have deserved that diagnosis when he was 5.

By the way, perhaps without realizing it, we've employed a diagnostic principle here: Collateral history sometimes beats the patient's own.

Step 5

And now what's your best diagnosis for Julio? Please justify your choice. And, no matter how much I usually like it, I won't accept *undiagnosed* for Julio. In his case, there is only one really good choice we can justify.

Rant

Although I've used the term several times, I don't think I've yet explained just why I am so inordinately fond of *undiagnosed.* I value it because it allows us to state without equivocation that we believe there is something wrong, but that we don't yet have enough information to say just what that might be. Using it doesn't commit us to any course of action except gathering more information, and it doesn't condemn the patient to carry a diagnosis that might be incorrect—and hard to expunge from health records, should that become necessary.

Furthermore, *undiagnosed* serves as a beacon to warn other health care providers that more interviews, more facts, more thought, and maybe more time are needed before deciding which diagnosis (if any) is warranted.

Undiagnosed but ill is invoked far too seldom by mental health clinicians. OK, it doesn't work in the case of Julio. But it often works for me, and it will for you too, if you remember to use it.

Note E

Of course, before settling on any other diagnosis, I'd want to be sure that both substance/medication-induced and medically related mood disorders have been ruled out. Assuming that this is done, I'd make my best diagnosis (like yours, I suspect) a bipolar disorder, currently on an upswing. From what his mother told Mark on the telephone, his mood had shot skyward at least a week earlier, and he'd slept less (he felt he didn't need sleep), talked more, and seemed grandiose in that he thought he'd learned all he needed in high school.

As for major depressive and separation anxiety disorders, Julio clearly would have carried those diagnoses in times gone by. But now they have been superseded. There's another diagnostic principle here: Recent history beats ancient history.

Step 6

We've skipped a bit lightly over the type of bipolar disorder we'd diagnose for Julio. So let's think about that: Just how do we differentiate between bipolar I and bipolar II? It would be great if you could provide some operational guidelines. Something to do with symptoms, consequences, and duration? (If you'd like some hints, you can refer to the two relevant tables in Chapter 3, page 39.)

Bipolar I

Symptoms: ______________________________

Consequences: ______________________________

Duration: ______________________________

Bipolar II

Symptoms: ______________________________

Consequences: ______________________________

Duration: ______________________________

Note F

Of course, the descriptions of Julio's symptoms could apply to bipolar I *and* bipolar II disorders, either of which would find the patient's mood on the upside of normal. The difference is not one of direction but of degree, as indicated by time (duration) and severity of the symptoms. What we are talking about here is really the type of episode Julio is having right now: Is it manic or hypomanic?

A hypomanic episode can be as brief as 4 days, whereas a manic episode must be present for at least a week before it can be diagnosed. And of course, symptoms are more intense for a manic episode than for a hypomanic one. By definition, a hypomanic person is not psychotic and does not require hospitalization. (However, symptoms during the hypomanic episode must be intense enough that an observer will notice that the patient has changed.)

Julio's mom, reporting through Mark, noted that his upswing in mood had begun more than a week ago; on the road trip, he was so high that he needed restraining. Indeed, it seems clear to me that he is headed for hospitalization. Although I don't see any symptom that is unequivocally psychotic, the fact that he required restraints is enough to persuade me that we should call his episode manic, not hypomanic. As such, we would have to say that his diagnosis is bipolar I disorder, current episode manic. Of course, a patient with bipolar I can have a hypomanic episode, but if the reverse ever happens, we have to change the bipolar II diagnosis to bipolar I.

Again, I encourage you to check those Chapter 3 tables for a close comparison of mania with hypomania, and of bipolar I with bipolar II.

Rant

By the way, what do you make of Julio's uncle, the one who was psychotic and eventually died? Of course, we cannot say with certainty, but it sounds to me as though he had a manic episode, probably followed by a depressive episode that resulted in his suicide. Although family history doesn't serve as a criterion for *any* DSM-5 disorder, it can be a strong indicator that we should consider whenever it comes to hand.

Besides family history, several other features can suggest ultimate bipolarity in a patient who has (so far) shown only depression:

- Youthful onset (first depressive episode by the patient's mid-20s)
- A history of psychosis, worsening with the use of antidepressants
- Severe guilt and suicidal feelings

All of this should remind us that although DSM-5 serves as a guidepost for making diagnoses, it isn't a stop sign. It should never deter us from harvesting information from other sources in our attempts to peer into a patient's future.

The Takeaway

Our experience with Julio reaffirms the importance of obtaining information from collateral resources. We have also explored some of the methods of interview control for coping with a patient who cannot relate a coherent history without rambling. We've noted that recent history beats history long gone by—again underscoring the importance of obtaining accurate, current information from those who know the patient well. (Yes, that's another diagnostic principle: Collateral information sometimes beats the patient's own.) In regard to Julio's diagnosis, we've explored the differences—matters of degree, not direction—between bipolar I and bipolar II disorders. And in a Rant, I've noted that the later development of bipolarity in a patient with a current major depressive episode can be heralded by features not mentioned in DSM-5 criteria.

We've also considered the conditions under which we should *not* talk with informants, and the importance of maintaining confidentiality when we *do* speak with them.

Break Time

In the Chapter 2 Break Time (page 30), I've mentioned the film *A Beautiful Mind,* based on a true story. In this movie, the viewer experiences mathematician John Nash's visual hallucinations as real; the point in the story where they are revealed as products of his own mind comes as a shock to the viewer.

A film that deals with similar themes is *The Truman Show,* in which Jim Carrey portrays young Truman Burbank, whose life plays out as the subject of the most popular television program of all time. His home is on what turns out to be a huge movie set—cameras hidden everywhere—created by his father, a television executive who never wanted Truman in the first place. The crisis of the story comes when Truman learns the truth of his existence and attempts to escape.

The story is an engaging twist on the experience of paranoid patients, who turn ordinary perceptions and beliefs into a harsh unreality. Truman, on the other hand, has for all of his 30 years been the focus of an actual deception and only gradually comes to appreciate what everyone else in the world already knows.

11

Small Bites—Kylie

Step 1

"This thing has gotten beyond me. Even when my weight is OK, I'm still all lumpy."

For the past 4 years, Kylie has had problems with eating. Her story began with her sophomore high school gym class, when she thought she seemed fatter than most of the other girls. Even today, she believes there was some truth to this—she remembers being teased about "love handles," and thinks that she might have "jiggled a bit" when she ran. "Whatever the truth of the situation," she says, "I swore I'd never again put myself at risk for verbal abuse based on my weight."

And with this, Kylie breaks down in tears.

So how do you proceed? The first thing you might say is the traditional "Could you tell me more about that?" That's probably what I'd start with, too. But suppose it only leads Kylie to ramble, more or less repeating what she's already said? And to weep still more? Then you'll need a different approach entirely.

What I'd like you to think about is the sort of data you should go after when you are probing for specific details of someone's complaints. I'm thinking in terms of little morsels of information—small bites, really—that you harvest not with open-ended questions, but with ____________. (Using my broad hint, please complete this sentence.)

Note A

In Chapter 9, in the case of Inez, we've observed the value of closed-ended questions in helping us to manage time when interviewing a new patient. And now here's the other situation where they can be so useful: in ferreting out the data you need to confirm diagnostic criteria. Then they can also confirm specific negatives and so eliminate from consideration all manner of issues, including physical abuse and neglect. In a word, use closed-ended questioning to serve as probes for obtaining further information. And that's probably what's called for now, with Kylie. Indeed, after my none-too-subtle hint, that's what you probably scribbled into the blank just above.

Closed-ended questions—they can be answered "yes" or "no," or in a multiple-choice format—don't encourage creativity in a patient, but neither do they leave much room for evasion. "Just the facts, Ma'am," as Sgt. Joe Friday would have said on *Dragnet,* a police procedural series that was popular a couple of centuries ago. And to get the facts, you have to know something about the possible disorders you are trying to uncover.

Ordinarily, I try to use closed-ended questions later in an interview, once I'm pretty sure that free speech has encouraged the patient to offer up the main themes of the consultation. And even after I've started using these short-answer questions, I try to remain alert for any later chance to interject something else that's open-ended. "Mix it up" might be the motto of the middle and later portions of the initial clinical interview.

Two precautions: First, I always try to ask short-answer questions carefully—that is, in a way that doesn't sound like rapid-fire interrogation. A respectful manner, a reassuring smile, and an occasional restorative pause will help maintain the feeling that you and the patient are a team seeking information, not two parties to an inquisition. Second, be careful not to ask leading questions. "You don't ever overeat, do you?" is the sort of query that can pretty much swallow up honest answers.

Step 2

So we've agreed to try questions that should yield short answers to specific questions. The trouble is, there's a world of possible topics out there, so what exactly do we address? Clearly, we need a focus.

That will depend a lot on our first impressions of the case—an initial, quick-and-dirty assessment that every experienced professional makes within the first few moments of an interview. You can think of it as a sort of tentative list of initial impressions that you employ to guide your quest for information. It will be crude, based on limited information and perhaps a clinical hunch, and it won't be anything that's complete enough to dignify with the term *diagnosis* (differential or otherwise).

So let's make some preliminary choices, based just on our Step 1 information for Kylie: For what sorts of disorders would you seek more information? In the list below, put an asterisk on the two or three types of issues (I sometimes call them *areas of clinical interest*) you think you'd like to pursue, and then compare your choices with mine in Note B.

- Difficulty thinking (especially delirium and dementia; DSM-5 calls them *neurocognitive disorders*)
- Substance use
- Psychosis
- Mood disturbance, especially depressive, manic, and hypomanic episodes
- Excessive anxiety, avoidance behavior, and arousal
- Physical complaints (including problems with sleeping and eating, and the somatic symptom disorders)
- Social and personality problems

Note B

Kylie has already disclosed the issues of her weight and problematic eating. For sure, that points us toward physical complaints, specifically the eating disorders. Her focus on physical symptoms would encourage me to consider a somatic symptom disorder as well. She has also been tearful, so I'd also want to consider mood disorders (as I do almost always!); some patients don't even realize they are depressed until they are questioned about moods and behavior.

That's three areas to think about—a pretty good start, though other possibilities could turn up later. But remember, this isn't a differential diagnosis, only a preliminary list of categories to consider. We haven't listed any specific disorders, and we haven't included substance use and other medical disorders.

With experience, you'll start making mental lists of issues to pursue from the very first moments of your interaction with any new patient. But you won't confuse them with an actual differential diagnosis. Will you?

Step 3

Now, using our list of principal suspects, what questions do we need to ask? That is, what specific information will we want to obtain next? I'm thinking, and I hope you are too, of a series of a dozen or more probes specifically related to eating and weight. Each of them will take a small bite of the information we'll need to establish a diagnosis.

Of course, this process requires that you know something—quite a bit, really—about the disorders you seek to rule in or out. When I was a student, the amount of information I lacked about various disorders was enormous, so I had to interview for a while, then read up to see what I'd missed, then go back to the patient with more questions. That's perfectly feasible if you have a captive population such as hospitalized patients, but it is a lot slower if you only work with outpatients. Then you might have to wait a week or more to pick up data you passed by the first time around.

But for Kylie, we'll take the same sort of shortcut we've used for Douglas in Chapter 4. Of course, you can obtain the specific information you need for any condition from the relevant chapters of a textbook. As with previous patients, we'll use the numbered and underlined passages later.

> In her efforts to slim down, Kylie had succeeded spectacularly by her junior year.[1] From her highest-ever weight of 135 pounds (she stands only 5 feet 3 inches tall), she had whittled herself down to 97 pounds, with strict dieting every day and prodigious exercising.[2] But even at that weight, she thought that the "love handles" still showed,[3] so she began using laxatives and diuretics[4] supplied by a classmate. Although she managed to lose another 5 pounds, her mirror confirmed her worst fears: She still looked fat.[5] By this time she was eating only once a day, an amount that she now estimates at about 400 calories.[6] Even some of that she would throw up; she had learned how to vomit at will.[7]
>
> She joined the Health Club,[8] an organization of girls at her school who exchanged diet tips and supported one another for weight loss. A few years earlier, after several

members were found to be passing around diet pills, school administrators had ordered the club to disband. In effect, they drove it underground; its meetings were secret and unsupervised. Now teachers and parents had no input at all into students' use of medication and other aids to weight loss.

Kylie's weight dipped to 85 pounds,[9] alarming her parents so much that they admitted her to a local hospital's special treatment unit for eating disorders.[10] Six months of education and fear (during Kylie's stay on the ward, another patient about her age died of malnutrition) had had their effect: Since discharge, she's maintained her weight at a healthy 117 pounds.[11] Her menstrual periods, absent for nearly a year, began once again.

To protect her from adverse consequences of further association with other girls in the Health Club, Kylie's parents went the last mile—in fact, 50 of them: They moved to another community[12] at the opposite end of the county. Kylie graduated from school there, but she never lost the feeling that something was wrong with the shape of her body.[13]

Below are some of the questions eliciting the part of her history that Kylie has just related. Mark the number(s) of the underlined passage(s) corresponding to each question; some questions may refer to more than one underlined passage. Each question helps us nibble away at Kylie's history.

- Over what period of time has this part of the problem existed? ______
- How often does it occur? ______
- How much do you eat during any meal? Total per day? ______
- Do you consciously limit how much you eat? ______
- Are you afraid of gaining weight? ______
- How do you feel about how you look? Do you think you are too heavy? ______
- How do you think this matches with your actual body shape and size? ______
- What are your current weight and height [to compute body mass index (BMI)]? ____
- What was your lowest weight? ______
- What did you do to keep yourself thin? Dieting alone? Exercise? Any purging (using laxatives or causing yourself to vomit)? ______
- What treatment or other remedies have you sought? ______

Note C

And here are my answers to the Step 3 questions.

- Over what period of time has this part of the problem existed? 1
- How often does it occur? 2
- How much do you eat during any meal? Total per day? 6
- Do you consciously limit how much you eat? 6
- Are you afraid of gaining weight? Covered in Step 1
- How do you feel about how you look? Do you think you are too heavy? 3, 5, 13
- How do you think this matches with your actual body shape and size? 13
- What are your current weight and height [to compute BMI]? 2, 11
- What was your lowest weight? 9

- What did you do to keep yourself thin? Dieting alone? Exercise? Any purging (using laxatives or causing yourself to vomit)? 2, 4, 7, 8
- What treatment or other remedies have you sought? 10, 12

Of course, as we look at the larger picture, the important things here aren't the answers Kylie has given, but the sorts of questions we've used to probe for the information. With time, you'll amass a similar set of probes for each of the many disorders you encounter in the course of a clinical practice.

Step 4

Now let's continue with Kylie's history. Brace yourself: At the end, I'll ask you to endure the same sort of exercise.

> After high school, Kylie took a business course, then found work in the secretarial pool of a large insurance company. As soon as she could afford to, she moved away from home into a tiny studio apartment. Once she was free from the watchful eyes of her parents ("They were always prying"), her eating habits quickly deteriorated.
>
> About a year prior to her current evaluation,[14] she began consuming large quantities of food within a brief period of time[15] ("I'd practically inhale it"). At the movies, she might consume a "family-size" tub of popcorn and a giant cola drink;[16] at home, she would gobble her way through a quart of frozen yogurt ("full-fat") during a rerun episode of *Friends*. "Hungry or no, I'd scarf it down till I was stuffed,"[17] she says. "Once, during a rerun of *Prime Suspect*, I ate an entire box of Froot Loops; I think it gives new meaning to the term *cereal killer*." Because she still morbidly fears becoming overweight, she almost always causes herself to throw up most of what she has eaten.[18]
>
> Recently, these eating episodes have occurred as often as two or three times a week,[19] and they extend beyond snack time to her regular meals. "When I eat alone, I've put away as much as a 1-pound package of spaghetti and two cans of sauce. I don't binge every day, but once I start, I can't seem to stop.[20] My doctor says I'm healthy[21]—and isn't *that* a laugh!"
>
> After she's cried for a bit ("I'm just so frustrated"), Kylie recomposes herself. During the balance of the interview, she even manages a smile. She says she's both embarrassed and ashamed, but she denies feeling depressed.[22] She's never been suicidal. And though she admits freely to her problematic eating habits, she denies ever using alcohol or street drugs.[23]

Below are the questions eliciting the second part of Kylie's history. As in Step 3, mark the number(s) of the underlined passage(s) corresponding to each question (some questions may refer to more than one selection). This time, there could also be questions that are not asked (mark these N/A). And yes, a lot of them are the same as those in Step 3, but they apply to a different time period. In our business, there's a lot of repetition.

- Over what period of time has this part of the problem existed? ______
- How often does it occur? ______

- How much do you eat during any meal? Total per day? ______
- How quickly do you eat? Do you ever gobble your food? ______
- Do you eat until you are uncomfortably full? ______
- Do you eat when you aren't hungry? ______
- Do you eat alone (perhaps because you're embarrassed about what you eat, or about your eating behavior)? ______
- Do you ever eat in binges? ______
- How much do you consume at a time? ______
- Do you have a sense of lack of control over your eating? ______
- Are you afraid of gaining weight? ______
- How do you feel about how you look? Do you think you are too heavy? ______
- What do you do to keep yourself thin? Dieting alone? Exercise? Any purging (using laxatives or causing yourself to vomit)? ______
- Please tell me about your mood, substance use, and general health. ______

Note D

And here are my answers to the Step 4 questions.

- Over what period of time has this part of the problem existed? 14
- How often does it occur? 17
- How much do you eat during any meal? Total per day? 15
- How quickly do you eat? Do you ever gobble your food? 17
- Do you eat until you are uncomfortably full? 17
- Do you eat when you aren't hungry? 17
- Do you eat alone (perhaps because you're embarrassed about what you eat, or about your eating behavior)? N/A
- Do you ever eat in binges? 15
- How much do you consume at a time? 16
- Do you have a sense of lack of control over your eating? 20
- Are you afraid of gaining weight? 18
- How do you feel about how you look? Do you think you are too heavy? Covered in Step 1
- What do you do to keep yourself thin? Dieting alone? Exercise? Any purging (using laxatives or causing yourself to vomit)? 18
- Please tell me about your mood, substance use, and general health. 22, 23

Step 5

Now please formalize the differential diagnosis, and write it down in a safety order (as we've done for Brad on page 27). And, just to keep things interesting, rather than falling back on the generic "substance this-or-that," make a stab at deciding which substances would be likely (during either intoxication or withdrawal) to produce changes in appetite and eating habits.

Note E

Do you find any surprises in what I've listed below as Kylie's differential diagnosis? How does it compare with your own?

- ◊ Cannabis intoxication
- ◊ Stimulant withdrawal
- ◊ Tobacco withdrawal
- ◊ Substance/medication-induced depressive disorder
- ◊ Depressive disorder due to another medical condition
- ◊ Major depressive disorder (and other primary mood disorders)
- ◊ Anorexia nervosa (AN)
- ◊ Bulimia nervosa (BN)
- ◊ Binge-eating disorder
- ◊ Somatization disorder (from DSM-IV)
- ◊ Personality disorder

Note that DSM-5 includes no such diagnosis as substance/medication-induced eating disorder or eating disorder due to another medical condition. That's partly why, even with barely any depressive component in Kylie's history, I've included depressive disorders in these categories on the list. (OK, it's also because I usually include mood disorders. They're ubiquitous.)

Step 6

And now, no surprise: I'd like you to write down your final, best diagnosis. And could we see your reasoning (maybe a note or two next to each choice in Note E) for ruling these various disorders in or out?

Note F

Although each of the three instances of intoxication or withdrawal I've listed includes appetite changes in its criteria set, right away we can discard them all—along with substance-related depressive disorder. That's because we have good information that Kylie hasn't abused substances of any sort. (Well, other than when she was using diet pills, but those days are in Kylie's distant past.)

We'll similarly throw out the possibility that another medical condition has led to depressed mood; it was never very likely anyway, and the (reported) testimony of Kylie's physician pretty much rules it out. We can summarize these decisions with this diagnostic principle: When you hear hoofbeats in the street, think horses, not zebras. That is, common things occur commonly, but rare diagnoses are just that: rare. Besides, we'd have tough work to sustain any mood disorder diagnosis, mainly because the duration of her depressive symptoms has been too brief.

So let's skip down to somatization disorder—for which Kylie has had far too few somatic symptoms to qualify. (I'll explain my preference for DSM-IV somatization disorder over DSM-5 somatic symptom disorder in Chapter 15.) Personality disorder? Although it is always something to keep in mind, that would be a real problem to diagnose right now; we should heed the diagnostic principle of avoiding a personality disorder diagnosis when the patient is acutely ill. And *that* brings us to the main course of the meal, so to speak: three possible eating disorders.

To do them justice, we should consider the two time frames indicated in Step 3 and Step 4. When, as a high school student, she first began to worry about her weight, Kylie had all of the symptoms necessary for the diagnosis of AN. She restricted her food intake so severely (to as little as 400 calories a day) that her weight dropped to 85 pounds. Even when starving herself, she feared gaining weight, and she *still* thought that she looked fat. (Even her periods had stopped; that was a DSM-IV criterion for AN, but because it made it hard for males to earn the diagnosis, this criterion was dropped in DSM-5.) Because vomiting was one method she used for weight control, she earns the subtype of binge-eating/purging type. At her height of 5 feet 3 inches, her low weight yielded a BMI of just 15.1 (people of normal weight will score in the range of 18.5–24.9). During high school, then, Kylie was on the border between a rating of severe and extreme AN.

Afterward, living on her own (Step 4), Kylie has begun to eat in binges, during which she consumes prodigious quantities of food. After these short bursts of consumption, she usually throws it all up. She admits to the lack of control over her eating behavior ("once I start, I can't seem to stop") These behaviors occur several times a week and have gone on for a year. Her self-evaluation is still focused on her body shape and weight ("I'm still all lumpy" is her Step 1 chief complaint). She therefore qualifies now for a diagnosis of BN, and *not* binge-eating disorder, in which a person's massive overeating is *not* accompanied by compensatory behavior such as purging, fasting, or excessive exercise. With episodes occurring two to three times a week, DSM-5 criteria suggest a severity score for her BN of mild. However, that is a minimum level; because of her degree of emotional discomfort, we'll exercise clinicians' prerogative and raise that to moderate.

So we've managed to come up with two diagnoses for Kylie: AN followed (chronologically) by BN. List them both, with an eye to treating one and preventing any recurrence of the other. I've chosen to list the current diagnosis first.

◊ BN, moderate
◊ AN, severe (by history)

Rant

Suppose your only source of information about a patient's possible personality disorder is—the patient. What sorts of question could you ask to obtain information that is both relevant and accurate? Here are a few you could use:

"Describe yourself for me. That is, what sort of a person do you think you are?" [Be on the alert for answers that show excessively high or low evaluations, or that contradict what you know already.]
"What were you like when you were younger?" [Especially watch for lifelong characteristics, such as "I've always made friends easily."]
"What do you like best about yourself? What do you like least?"
"How do you view the world? For example, would you say it is friendly and welcoming, or threatening and cruel?"
"How well do you get along with other people?"
"How would you describe your mood, most of the time?"
"How well would you say you normally control your temper?"

The Takeaway

Kylie's story demonstrates how we can use closed-ended questions as probes to obtain specific answers and fill in missing parts of a history. The process is aided by an initial, quick-and-dirty impression (it's *not* a differential diagnosis!) that experienced clinicians use to guide them in their quest for relevant information. It's derived from a list of possibilities I sometimes refer to as *areas of clinical interest.* We've noted that because familiarity with the symptoms of each possible disorder greatly facilitates gathering the information needed to make a diagnosis, clinicians may need to consult the relevant textbook chapter for information on what symptoms to expect in people with eating disorders.

Along the way, we've warned against the use of leading questions ("You don't binge-eat, do you?") and against a focus on rare conditions when more common ones may explain circumstances and symptoms (when you hear hoofbeats, think horses, not zebras). Another diagnostic principle we've mentioned is that of avoiding a personality disorder diagnosis when the patient is acutely ill. Still another is this: Always consider the [very common] mood disorders.

Finally, we've noted that we don't have to accept the recommended severity level for any disorder: We are the clinicians of record, and it's our clinical judgment that matters.

Rant

Until you stop to think about it, you might not appreciate just how often bodily functions appear in the criteria sets we use to make mental health diagnoses. Do stop just for a moment and try to think of a few examples. Then you can take a look at those I jotted down one afternoon while awaiting a visit from the Muse (see the table on page 127). Remember, these are only the characteristics that are contained in the criteria sets, not in the associated features included in every DSM-5 text description.

And here are a few additional entries that the table doesn't cover: nystagmus with alcohol intoxication; flushing of the face with caffeine intoxication; and speaking (is speaking even a body function?) in speech sound disorder, childhood-onset fluency disorder (stuttering), selective mutism, and frontotemporal neurocognitive disorder.

The table and related items underscore how deeply integrated are body and mind in the maintenance of health. In fact, I once wrote a whole book that explored how physical illnesses could masquerade as mental symptoms. The reference is listed, well, in the References and Suggested Readings.

Break Time

Some years back, using odd moments of free time (and evidently in an odd frame of mind), I surveyed every issue of *The New Yorker* magazine to identify every cartoon with a subject that involved mental health issues. In all, there were more than 1,800 cartoons from the magazine's inception in 1925 to 2010. Of that number, almost half (OK, 48%) were in some way related to alcohol.

In the early years of publication, showing people who were acutely intoxicated was apparently considered pretty side-splitting. Back then, two out of every three cartoons concerned with the use of substances (alcohol or drugs) featured people whose evident staggering and crooked smiles seemed to shout, "I'm under the influence."

But by 1985, all that had changed. In the most recent 25 years of my survey, only about a third of the cartoons exhibited actual intoxication. In the majority, people might be shown sitting at a bar rationally discussing almost anything (but especially politics); alternatively, a tavern or bar might serve as an excuse for a twist on a meme, such as "Home of the bottomless martini." Clearly, our national psyche has changed, and for the better; the sophisticated readers of *The New Yorker,* at any rate, have come to appreciate that alcoholism is due not to moral failure but to illness.

In a related development taking place around the same time, the magazine's overall focus on mental health cartoons shifted from making fun of the patient to skewering clinicians. It's been that way ever since. Evidently, in the 21st century, psychologists and psychiatrists offer richer targets than do their patients.

Physical Symptoms as Criteria for Mental Health Diagnoses

	Eating/appetite	Elimination	Breathing	Heartbeat	Sleeping	Erection and orgasm	Sweating and fever	Pain	Involuntary movements	Changes in weight
BN, binge-eating disorder	×									
AN	×									×
Avoidant/restrictive food intake disorder	×									×
Major depressive episode and disorder	×				×					×
Persistent depressive disorder	×				×					
Premenstrual dysphoric disorder	×				×			×		×
Manic and hypomanic episodes and bipolar disorders					×					
Panic attack and disorder			×	×			×	×		
GAD					×					
Anxiety disorder due to AMC			×	×						
Substance/medication-induced anxiety disorder			×	×						
PTSD and ASD					×					
Encopresis and enuresis		×								
All sleep–wake disorders					×					
Frontotemporal NCD	×								×	
Lewy body NCD					×				×	
NCD due to traumatic brain injury									×	
Various sexual disorders						×				
Substance (various) intoxication									×	×
Substance (various) withdrawal				×	×		×	×	×	×
Sleep apnea/hypoventilation (various)			×		×					
Sleep terrors			×	×	×		×			
Somatic symptom disorder, conversion disorder								×	×	
Genito-pelvic pain/penetration disorder								×		
Autism spectrum disorder								×	×	
Developmental coordination disorder									×	
Stereotypic movement disorder									×	
Tic disorders, including Tourette's									×	
Catatonic disorder and specifier									×	
NCD due to Parkinson's									×	

Note. BN, bulimia nervosa; AN, anorexia nervosa; GAD, generalized anxiety disorder; AMC, another medical condition; PTSD, posttraumatic stress disorder; ASD, acute stress disorder; NCD, neurocognitive disorder.

12

Swan Song—Liam

Step 1

"I don't really think I should even be here," says Liam. He appears to be quite elderly, but perhaps the fact that he is lying on his back in the emergency room makes him seem older than his years. A note from the emergency medical technician who brought him in says, "We found Liam slumped against the bathroom door. Next to his head, over the knob, was a long loop of towel. He told us, 'I may have slipped on the wet tiles and fallen.'"

Liam's face is pale; his once-ginger hair is now nearly all white. You glance at the darkening marks (ligatures?) under his chin. "Could there be anything else? Please tell me exactly what you've been thinking," you ask him.

He looks past you as tears well in his eyes. But he says nothing.

How can you persuade an obviously ill but remarkably reticent patient to open up about suicidal thoughts? Here are several possibilities. Among them, one in particular seems unworkable for Liam. Can you spot it, and say why?

- ☐ Try to normalize the situation by pointing out that many people in desperation have ideas like this.
- ☐ Gradually work up to it, starting with "Have you ever wished you were dead?"
- ☐ Point out that continued silence could have unwanted consequences—such as a hospital commitment.
- ☐ Try to reduce his guilt by emphasizing the misery Liam must have felt.
- ☐ Just jump in and ask if he's ever had suicidal ideas.
- ☐ Ask about any history of "dark times" when he might have had desperate thoughts.
- ☐ Skip this particular line of inquiry for now, ask about something else, and return to this subject later.

Note A

First, let's note how our suspicions are raised by two observations: the marks on Liam's neck, and his emotional reaction when you ask for more information. (Besides tearfulness, patients who want to hide something may refuse to meet a clinician's gaze or hesitate before answering.) Any of these behaviors suggests that we use this diagnostic principle: Signs beat symptoms. You'll find it helpful every once in a while.

So how could you draw Liam out? Threats (of unwanted consequences) might do the job, but they might also do a number on your professional relationship, and perhaps on your self-image as a mental health professional. Besides, why would you threaten someone with whom you are trying to form a relationship? This is the one choice I'd steer clear of. But to drop the other shoe quickly, anything else on the list could be a reasonable choice.

You can ease a patient into a discussion of suicidality by offering some protective cover. One method is to point out that many people who are burdened with their problems think about death, which can then prompt a consideration of thoughts about hurrying things along. This approach pushes the experience of having suicidal thoughts—which can cause patients to feel like freakish outliers—into the mainstream of human existence. You could say, "Many people who have [the given mental health problem] at some point wish they were dead, or even think of suicide. Have you ever felt so bad you've had thoughts like these?"

Another way of working up to a discussion of suicide would be to "start low and go slow." In effect, you avoid the shock of jumping into cold water. So you might ask, "Have you had desperate thoughts? Wished you were dead? Considered ending your life? Planned your own death?" This incremental approach probably benefits the (novice) interviewer more than the patient, but it's still a reasonable way to proceed, and it may aid the process of drawing out the patient.

Trying to reduce guilt offers yet another strategy by putting current feelings into the context of all the misery the patient has experienced: "You've had so much trouble with [the problem in question], have you ever had thoughts about ending your life?"

Actually, forthrightly asking, "Have you ever had thoughts of killing yourself?" is a well-recommended way of phrasing the question; it is clear, concise, and offers little room for misinterpretation. And of course, it is a truism that asking about suicide will *not* recommend it to someone who has previously had no such idea. In fact, getting suicidal thoughts out into the open may actually help lighten the patient's emotional burden.

But suppose the answer to your straightforward question about recent suicide ideas is "No." You're stuck, right? Well, not really. Follow it up by asking whether there have been any past thoughts, plans, or attempts. (Some experts recommend that we always try to lessen anxiety and break down resistance by *first* inquiring about past history of suicide behavior—even for a patient who seems likely to endorse a current wish to die.)

Once you've extracted an admission of death wishes or suicidal thoughts, ask for amplification: "Please tell me exactly what you've been thinking." (Of course, you should then use probes that will reveal plans, mode, means, specific intent, and any factors that might *lessen* the likelihood of an attempt.)

With a given patient, you can never be sure which tactic will ultimately yield this vital information. But eventually something will work; keep at it.

Step 2

"I think it's important that we try to be frank here," you say. "You seem reluctant to discuss this, and I can understand that it's hard for you. We'll start with something different, but if at any point you feel you can't answer honestly, just say, 'I'd rather not talk about that right now.'" Liam glumly nods his head and with evident effort, engages in the discussion.

He is 73 years old. He was formerly an operatic bass–baritone, but for some years now, he has been unable to sing. "I've got 'old man's voice,'" he complains. "I'm not even fit to sing 'Old Man River,'" he adds with a mirthless chuckle. His speech *is* rather croaky, and he frequently pauses to clear his throat.

Besides problems with vocalization, he admits that arthritis makes it hard even to move around in his flat. His internist, whom Liam rarely sees, has expressed concern about his serum cholesterol and a cardiac arrhythmia that seems to be worsening. In response to a question, he admits, "Some days I drink too much. I can get to the point that I don't even remember what happened the night before, but that's only happened once or twice." His wife used to praise him for always being so careful about drinking; indeed, until the last few months, he'd rarely drunk even wine or a beer and had never experienced a hangover. But she died just before Christmas, and since then, he's had "no one to remind me to keep a lid on. Since I started feeling so depressed, I've pretty well lost the drive to 'just say no.'"

After a few minutes, a little of the tension has seeped out of Liam's demeanor; now he speaks with less hesitation. He volunteers that he's never made friends easily; he was always afraid that they would find him boring and wouldn't want to associate with him. He offers this: "Most of our friends were really *her* friends, so it was easier just not to have them at all. In fact, it's a miracle I ever got married in the first place. Trudi was very good for me. I always said that." Liam doesn't go to church, never has—"I'm a lifelong atheist."

"Do you still really want to die?" you ask. And when he nods his head, you add, "And why now?"

Liam responds, "I just don't see much hope that things will change in the future. I mean, what's the point? I have no kids to live for, no grandkids to enjoy. So when I got a notice from the landlord that my rent was being raised again, I thought, 'That does it!'"

"Do you feel that way, quite strongly?" you ask.

Liam nods, and drops his gaze. "It's like one of those recurring tunes that plays in your head—a theme with variations, but it's never completely out of mind."

Liam denies that he is especially impulsive; his intent was to plan it all out. "I've made sure my affairs are in order. Redrew my will last month—should make the folks at my public radio station happy, anyway," he says with a wry chuckle.

A few weeks ago, "for no new reason other than I had passed my sell-by date," he made his one previous suicide attempt, for which he used not a noose but an overdose of the pain pills left over from Trudi's final illness. He guesses that he was unconscious for several hours; the paramedics who responded told him he'd been lucky. ("Hah!" he editorializes.) After he regained full consciousness, he'd been "pretty unhappy" at being still alive: "I swore I'd make a go of it next time."

No, he hasn't considered using a gun—he neither owns one "nor do I want to give the NRA the satisfaction of a sale." He also hasn't considered drowning himself ("Where, in City Park? My bathtub?"). Cutting would hurt too much, but he's thought he might leap from a tall building—"Plenty of those around."

Then he adds, "To be frank, I'm not at all afraid of dying. Finally, today, I just decided it was time."

To another question, Liam answers, "I might want to go on living if I didn't feel so bloody awful. Most days, I feel like I have bags of rocks tied to my legs—for hours at a time, it's too much even to drag myself around the house. So I just sit there, rooted in my chair. I'm too weary to do anything but sleep. It's the only thing I have going for me," he adds. "I can sleep 10, 12 hours a day. Most days I do."

When awake, he spends a lot of time eating. "There's an empty something inside me that I can't seem to fill up, no matter how much I eat. Awful for my diabetes. I've turned my lovely doctor into a world-class nag."

When Liam was still in grade school, a (much) older sister, suffering the heartache of a failed romance, swallowed a massive overdose of Tylenol. She lingered for days before eventually succumbing to liver failure. "For years they called it accidental, but I knew she did it on purpose, because she told me." And his mother might have had a postpartum depression after the birth of his youngest brother.

Although Liam's speech is halting, at first nearly to the point of muteness, he gradually becomes more vocal as the interview progresses. Eventually his affect brightens, and he volunteers details before they are requested. He even smiles a time or two and attempts the odd joke.

Now he lives alone on Social Security and a tiny savings account, plus occasional residuals from a few old opera recordings. "For a time I tried teaching, but I just didn't have it in me to go head to head with students," he says. "It felt I was casting artificial pearls before genuine swine."

Liam chuckles again, this time with some conviction. Then he uncrosses his legs and tilts his body forward, literally leaning into the discussion.

Now here's a tough assignment, but it has important implications. I'd like you to make a list of the questions that we should ask in attempting to evaluate any patient's suicidal behavior. Actually, you can do pretty well for Liam if you just go through the long run of narrative above (in Steps 1 and 2) and underline the relevant sections. You'll find a few questions as asked, but some further information is evident in Liam's responses to questions—or perhaps even anticipated questions. All are vital in the complete workup of a suicidal patient.

Note B

We get a head start (in Note A) with "Please tell me exactly what you've been thinking." It is open-ended, inviting the patient to say whatever comes to mind. Considering how a suicidal patient has likely been feeling and behaving, the engine of that train of thought will likely have quite a bit to do with plans for a foreshortened future. Also note how you've tried to forestall any temptation Liam might have felt to tell less than the truth: You've asked him to say nothing about a given topic, rather than making something up.

Here are some of the questions we need to ask that specifically target suicidal thoughts and attempts. Most of them have been covered either directly or by inference in the Step 2 material, as I've indicated in brackets after each item.

"How often do you think about killing yourself? How long do these thoughts last?" [Liam notes that suicide is "never completely out of mind."]

"How intense are these suicidal thoughts?" This would be an expression of what is sometimes called *subjective intent.* You could ask for a rating on a scale of 0–10, where 10 equates to "Absolutely sure I'll take my first chance to go through with it." [You should pursue this with Liam.]

"Why do you want to die?" [Liam: "I just don't see that much hope that things will change . . . "]

"What hope do you see for the future? What would make you want to continue living?" [Liam: " . . . if I didn't feel so bloody awful."]

"Have you made any preparations?" These could include making a will, giving away possessions, and arranging for the care of pets. Each of these might be viewed as an expression of *objective intent.* Rehearsal of carrying through with the attempt would be another aspect of preparation. [Liam's "intent was to plan it all out," and he adds that he has revised his will.]

"Do you have access to a firearm?" But don't assume that family or friends will follow through with firearm safety. [Liam has definitely not considered using a gun.]

"Besides [the most recent attempt], what other methods have you considered?" Run through the possible methods to cover them all: hanging, shooting, jumping, pills or poisons, cutting, suffocation. [Liam rejects shooting, cutting, and drowning; leaping remains a possibility.]

"Are you an impulsive sort of person, or do you generally like to plan things out?" [Liam denies being impulsive.]

"Why did you make an attempt at this time [precipitant]?" [Liam's "rent was being raised again."]

As regards a prior attempt:

"What were the reasons [motive]?" [Liam notes "no new reason" for his one previous attempt.]

"How serious was it [outcome]?" Consider medical seriousness (physical sequelae) and psychological seriousness (for example, was it timed so that it was likely to be discovered)? [Physical: Liam was unconscious for hours, and the paramedics said he'd been lucky. Psychological: Liam vowed to "make a go of it next time."]

"How do/did you feel about having survived [reaction]?" or "What were your feelings when you found you wouldn't die? Relief? Distress at not succeeding?" [Liam was "pretty unhappy" at being still alive.]

Step 3

Now how should we judge Liam's potential for another suicide attempt, or worse?

Let's frankly admit that clinical judgment is useless at predicting the future. One study reported that of those patients who ultimately died of suicide, 84% had been assessed as having either low risk or no risk at all. Other studies have found that the ability of clinicians to predict outcomes doesn't improve much throughout their professional lives, regardless of how much training and clinical experience they have had. We need a different approach.

The task becomes more manageable if we focus not on trying to determine the probability of suicide, but on protecting our patients from their own actions. That approach helps diminish the burden of any clinician whose crystal ball is on the fritz. The process known as *actuarial modeling* is the currently favored approach to evaluation. It utilizes numerous factors that have been demonstrated to correlate with eventual suicide. Below, I've provided a bulleted list of many of these factors. First, though, here's what I'd like you to do:

1. After each element in this list, circle either M (modifiable, at least potentially) or N (nonmodifiable).
2. Then place a checkmark beside those items that apply to Liam.
3. Finally, how serious an overall risk would you say Liam represents (on a scale of low–moderate–high)?

Now here's my list of risk factors for eventual suicide:

- Access to firearms: M/N
- Age: M/N
- Command hallucinations: M/N
- Depression: M/N
- Family history: M/N
- Gender: M/N
- Hopelessness: M/N
- Impulsivity: M/N
- Living alone: M/N
- Panic or severe anxiety: M/N
- Personality disorder: M/N
- Physical illness: M/N
- Prior suicide attempt: M/N
- Race: M/N
- Recent personal loss: M/N
- Recent suicide of friend or relative: M/N
- Substance use: M/N
- Being unemployed: M/N

How many checkmarks did you attach to this list for Liam? ____________________
How serious would you assess Liam's risk as being, overall? ____________________

Note C

Let's review the characteristics that warn of a future successful suicide. We'll start with those that patients are stuck with—the ones that are nonmodifiable, regardless of effort. Note the checkmarks on the factors we've identified for Liam.

- Age. Older people have a much greater risk of killing themselves than do those who are years younger. Liam is 73 years old, looks and acts his age or even older, and draws Social Security. ✓
- Gender. Perhaps the most solid fact in suicidology is that men are three to four times more likely to die by suicide than are women. On the other hand, by about the same margin, women are more likely to make a nonfatal suicide attempt. ✓
- Race. Based on his pallor, his once-red hair, and his name, we can guess fairly confidently that Liam is of European American descent, and possibly Irish. Especially in the United States, white/European American people are more likely to die of suicide than are those of other racial backgrounds. ✓
- Family history of mental disorder and suicide. It is a well-established fact that, all else being equal, a positive family history of suicide confers additional risk—it's at least double—for an individual patient. This factor may be especially useful to alert clinicians when they must advise a person who has made an attempt or who has suicidal ideation, but has no current evidence of mental illness. The risk from family history is even stronger for teens and young adults. Liam's sister did commit suicide; it was hushed up, and it occurred during his formative years. ✓
- Recent suicide of a friend or relative. Adolescents are especially likely to imitate the suicidal behavior of others.
- Personality disorder. More than half of those who die of suicide reportedly have a personality disorder. Especially at risk are those with borderline personality disorder (which some studies have identified in up to one-third of completed suicides) and those with antisocial personality disorder. Determining whether this factor applies to Liam would require further interviewing, both with him and with any possible informants.
- Prior attempts. Data show that those who have made at least one previous attempt have a far greater chance of a future successful attempt. Liam has already made one that we know of. ✓

And now risk factors that potentially can be modified:

- Living alone. Liam is widowed and childless. The absence of supportive family or other close relationships is an important signpost. ✓
- Recent loss. Important examples include recent job loss and the breakup of an intimate relationship. The effects of loss, such as Liam's bereavement, can potentially be ameliorated by therapy. ✓
- Being unemployed. Nothing beats gainful employment for making your life feel useful. ✓
- Physical illness, incorporating the concept of functional impairment. Physical illness and impairment are especially prevalent in older people, though they can affect anyone who has, for example, multiple sclerosis, Huntington's disease, stroke, systemic lupus erythematosus, HIV/AIDS, cancer, or a seizure disorder. Of course, physical illness is a risk factor that can only partly be modified: Although Liam probably can-

not change the fact that he has arthritis and diabetes, treatment might be able to alter the degree to which these affect his life. ✓

- Use of alcohol or other drugs. Liam has admitted to drinking heavily. Even apart from the diagnosis of, say, alcohol use disorder, someone who is acutely under the influence is more likely to make a suicide attempt. This may be a factor in a third or more of completed suicides. ✓
- Hopelessness. This correlates more strongly with eventual suicide than with suicide in the near term. Closely related is the perception of being a burden to other people, mostly family. Liam has openly expressed feelings of hopelessness. ✓
- Impulsivity. Some people act on the spur of the moment. Note that, once thwarted, most would-be bridge jumpers are still alive years later. Liam denies that he is impulsive.
- Depression. Whether it occurs in the context of major depressive disorder or of bipolar disorder, a current severe depressive episode is one of the most powerful elements in the decision to commit suicide. ✓
- Panic or severe anxiety. Studies have found that these two emotional states increase the likelihood of a suicide attempt, especially in someone with a mood disorder.
- Command hallucinations. Not surprisingly, this factor is most often encountered in individuals who have schizophrenia. Patients are more likely to obey hallucinations that they associate with an identifiable source.
- Access to guns. We don't have to explore here the politics of this highly contentious (in the United States) issue; we'll just go with the data. And the data demonstrate that the majority of suicides, especially in men, are by gunshot. The availability of firearms in the home is a significant risk factor, especially if coupled with an individual patient's impulsivity, substance use, or depression. Fortunately, Liam doesn't have ready access to a firearm, or even want to obtain one.

Because each of the foregoing elements contributes to the risk of suicide, each should be carefully assessed in patients who have expressed thoughts about death, and especially about committing suicide. However, even in the aggregate, they cannot predict who is in imminent risk of completed suicide. Evaluate them in the spirit of preventing suicide, not predicting it.

Applying Liam's data to the risk list without an excess of precision, I'd say that in the absence of treatment, the likelihood that Liam will try again, and succeed, is far too high to ignore.

Rant

For decades, mental health professionals have used suicide prevention contracts, whereby patients agree orally or in writing to avoid self-harm for a stipulated period of time. Several writers have suggested that the principal benefit of such a contract is to make a *clinician* feel more secure. These same writers note that contracts generate a false confidence: There is scant objective evidence that they protect patients from their own actions, or providers from legal proceedings.

However, suicide contracts do present several ways in which a clinician can come to grief. For one thing, they place the burden of decision making on someone who very likely cannot think clearly, and who has come for evaluation in part because of an inability to cope with feelings. Is it reasonable to expect a person who is ambivalent about the value of life itself to sign a promissory note and then adhere to it? For those in the throes of desperation, behavior that appears feasible one moment may seem unendurable the next. Furthermore, a suicidal patient may come to regard the clinician not as a caregiver, but as an adversary who will attempt to thwart the desired final act—in other words, someone to be gotten around, perhaps by signing an agreement the patient has no intention of honoring. For me, the next-to-bottom line is this: These are people who should not be required to enter into a contract for their very lives.

And here is the very bottom line: Sometimes you may have no other device at your disposal. Then, I suppose, you use what comes to hand, but only until you can implement something better in the way of averting disaster. Whatever you do use, document your reasoning, all the while realizing that a no-suicide contract may be something your patient cannot fulfill and you cannot afford.

Step 4

But before moving on, we should try for yet a bit more information, of a different sort. That is, can we think of any factors that might help *protect* a patient like Liam from future suicide attempts? Of course, we could write down the opposite of some of the Step 3 factors that *favor* suicide. But studies have reported some issues you couldn't deduce from the previous list. They are not nearly as numerous as the risk factors, but perhaps that only reflects a need for more research in an area that isn't sexy.

I'll make this multiple-choice. Just put a checkmark in the box for each factor below that you believe should protect against an ultimately successful suicide attempt in someone who has been treated for a recent unsuccessful attempt. You might place another checkmark after those items that apply to Liam.

- ☐ Family support
- ☐ Children at home
- ☐ Pregnancy
- ☐ Religion
- ☐ Cultural proscription against suicide
- ☐ Denial of suicide intent at discharge from hospital
- ☐ No-harm contract
- ☐ Prospect of an upcoming happy event

Note D

To cut to the chase, each of the first five conditions has been shown to protect against an ultimate suicide; the remaining three have not.

Let's start out by admitting (again!) that, even with the best information, we clinicians aren't very good at predicting who will die of suicide, and especially when. For example, if before discharge you survey 100 patients who have been admitted for a suicide attempt and ask, "Are you suicidal now?", the vast majority will answer "No." But studies have found little comfort in this answer: Even a few days before the final act, those who die by suicide are quite likely to deny having suicidal ideas (one study found a 73% rate within 7 days). So neither the presence nor the absence of suicidal ideas is an efficient predictor of who will eventually commit suicide. The same can be said for having a plan: Suicidal ideas either with or without a plan fail to foretell the future. As we've noted, something similar can be said for predicting *when* a suicide will occur: Having suicidal ideas is more closely associated with suicide down the road than with its acute risk for the near future.

Asking about suicidal ideas is likely to reveal only what a patient wants you to hear. Denial may serve to gain the patient release from the hospital, or to turn down the heat of close observation sufficiently that a plan can be enacted later. Similarly, someone who claims to look forward to some future event (such as a wedding or a family reunion) is not less prone to eventual self-harm. And, please, place no faith in any no-harm contract a patient might agree to. Again, there is no evidence that these pacts prevent suicide; they serve mainly to soothe clinicians' anxiety, sometimes with the unhappy consequence of relaxed vigilance.

That said, let's consider Liam in the light of those factors that correlate with protection against suicide.

- Family support? Of course, Liam has no close family. Or friends, for that matter.
- Children at home? Nope.
- Pregnancy? (!)
- Religion? No joy there; he's an atheist.
- A cultural proscription against suicide? Culture most likely serves as a proxy for religion or relationship to family, both of which we've already mentioned—and found wanting—for Liam.

In the end, apart from sheer luck, I can find nothing that would help protect Liam from making a future attempt.

Step 5

Now I'd like you to write down your differential diagnosis for Liam. Again, I've provided blanks—and, it's almost needless to say, please follow the safety principle. Put an star after the diagnosis you consider most likely.

____

____

____

____

____

____

Note E

No surprise: I've organized my differential diagnosis for Liam around the most important symptom—depression.

- ◊ Depressive disorder due to another medical condition. Of course, other than the fact that Liam *has* other medical conditions, the evidence is sparse. Diabetes mellitus and depression have often been found to co-occur, though the etiological relationship is not clear.
- ◊ Substance/medication-induced depressive disorder. Liam also drinks alcohol. But as best we can tell from his own account (and he seems to be a pretty accurate observer of his own mental state and behavior), his heavy drinking began only after the onset of his depression. Before initiating treatment, I'd like to see whether his mood improves any in the absence of alcohol. But for now, I'd reject this diagnosis in favor of something else.
- ◊ Uncomplicated bereavement. Of course, Liam has been bereaved a few months ago. But the fact of an important personal loss shouldn't deter us from making a diagnosis of major depressive disorder, if the requisite symptoms are present. Otherwise, we would risk deferring or rejecting completely effective treatment for a remediable condition. As DSM-5 itself notes, the predominant emotional content of bereavement is that of feeling empty or of having lost something valuable, not the persistent depressive feeling state that is typical of depressive disease. Other features can help discriminate the two conditions; I've put some of this into the table on page 139.
- ◊ Bipolar I or II disorder, current episode depressed. One fact pretty much eliminates this possibility: Liam has had no history of mania or hypomania.
- ◊ Persistent depressive disorder. We won't consider this further, inasmuch as Liam simply hasn't been ill long enough.
- ◊ Major depressive disorder. For weeks or longer, Liam has had depressed mood, changes in sleep and weight (a proxy for appetite), low interest, fatigue, feeling worthless, death wishes, and suicidal ideas. Without a doubt, his symptoms have caused distress. His chronology has allowed us to downplay drinking as an etiology. That completes the requirements for major depressive disorder as our final best diagnosis. ★
- ◊ A neurocognitive disorder with depression. Liam admits to having memory problems when he's been drinking; are there other times? This diagnosis is one that would require more testing—and perhaps more time—to clarify.

Rant

Let's talk about cause and effect. When something big happens (for example, an earthquake) and something else follows (a building collapses), we can be pretty confident when we claim a cause-and-effect relationship. Doing so helps us view the environment as an orderly place—something we can understand and depend on, perhaps even predict, and ultimately control. So it should come as no

Comparison of Uncomplicated Bereavement with a Major Depressive Episode

	Uncomplicated bereavement	Major depression
Principal mood (affect)	Emptiness or loss	Depression; cannot anticipate joy or happiness
Thought content	Preoccupied with thoughts of departed person	May feel worthless, unable to cope
Occurrence vis-à-vis mental content	In waves, increasing with thoughts of the departed person	Not associated with specific thoughts
Triggers for low mood	Thoughts of the dead	May occur unprovoked
Time course	Usually decreases over days or weeks	May persist for months
Relief	May be interspersed with positive emotions, even humor	Not so much
Thoughts of death	If any, focused on the person who has died	Focused on ending the patient's own life
Vegetative symptoms[a]	Usually not	Often occur
Impairment of daily activities	Usually not	Usually occurs

[a]*Vegetative* is a very old word that refers to the maintenance of life. Classic vegetative symptoms are anorexia, insomnia, weight loss, constipation, loss of sexual interest, and fatigue.

surprise that we might also try to figure out a causal relationship between other events that occur in close proximity to one another. For example, if we're exposed to someone with a cold, and 3 days later we start sneezing, we think we know where to cast blame.

With mental health patients, we use these temporal relationships (or we should!) to help determine when and whether to offer treatment for a given set of symptoms. That's what we've been up to with Liam: trying to learn whether we need to address his depressive symptoms with psychological or somatic treatments—perhaps modifying his social situation would help? Suppose we could be sure that he became depressed first, *then* started drinking. We'd be inclined to begin whatever form of treatment seemed appropriate for a major depressive disorder. But if we find that his mood symptoms started only *after* he had been drinking heavily for a long time—let's say, weeks or months—then we'd probably decide that he's suffering from an alcohol-induced depressive disorder and hold off on an offer of antidepressant medications. After all, there's no point in further intoxicating (with medications) someone whose main problem may stem from intoxication in the first place.

Step 6

In the patients we've encountered so far, we've paid little attention to specifiers that can apply to the various mood disorders. You've probably already noticed something a little peculiar in Liam's symptoms—his sleepiness, his perhaps excessive appetite, the fact that he seemed to brighten as the interview progressed. These symptoms (well, some of them are signs) are not exactly typical behavior for a depressed person. What can they mean? And should we express them in his final diagnosis? The answer has to do with a specifier. The one-word blank I hope you can fill in is *with* ______ *features.* (I've buried a hint in this paragraph.)

Note F

Liam's sleep has been prolonged, and his weight has increased; he's said that he eats a lot to fill up the inner void. Each of these changes is in a direction opposite to that of a patient with a classic depressive episode; each suggests that we might need to specify his depressive episode as—here's the one word I was searching for—*atypical.* This could have implications for the type of treatment he should be offered (certain antidepressants work better than others).

Here are the two main requirements for the specifier that carries the official name *with atypical features*:

1. The person's mood must be reactive to stimuli, improving with the presence of friends or the prospect of something pleasant happening. Liam's affect has brightened even in the course of a conversation with *you.*
2. Then the mood episode itself must be characterized by at least two of these four symptoms:
   - Increased appetite or weight gain
   - Increased sleep
   - A sensation of leaden paralysis of limbs
   - Excessive sensitivity to rejection of others that has persisted for most of the person's adult life (not just during periods of depression, though it may worsen during depressive episodes)

The interview with Liam suggests that he has probably experienced each of these four, and so his final diagnosis would be major depressive disorder, recurrent, severe, with atypical features.

The Takeaway

With Liam, we have considered how to broach the subject of suicidal ideas and past attempts—and, once the ice has been broken, how to pursue them: What questions do we need to ask? We've compiled a long list of risk factors, many of which are potentially modifiable, for eventual suicide. Some of Liam's symptoms are considered atypical for depressive syndromes, and in the final step, we've discussed how to express them in diagnostic terms. His demeanor in the face of denial of symptoms has encouraged us to use this diagnostic principle: Signs beat symptoms. However, we've acknowledged that we clinicians aren't very good at predicting which patients will die of suicide, or when; rather, we need to focus on steps that might help prevent it.

Break Time

Even through his pain, Liam shows tiny flashes of humor. That brings to mind (mine, anyway) the question of humor and what makes something funny. Through the ages, there have been several theories.

The philosopher Thomas Hobbes opined that in humans' constant competition with one another, they look for the shortcomings of others. Laughter expresses an individual's abrupt realization (Hobbes called it *sudden glory*) of being superior to others.

The *relief* theory of humor was popularized by Sigmund Freud. It posited a physiological basis in which laughter releases tension and *psychic energy*, the mysterious force that helps us suppress taboo feelings.

The third influential theory, *incongruity*, was originally formulated by the philosopher Immanuel Kant—who suggested, in essence, that a well-crafted joke completely fuses two disparate elements.

My own view of what makes something funny I call *connect the dots:* We laugh when we ourselves identify the nexus between two or more elements. If we must work a little to understand just how the elements are joined, we feel clever and reward ourselves with laughter. Let's consider an example:

A *New Yorker* cartoon shows a rabbit parent admonishing an abashed-looking juvenile rabbit. The parent says, "I'm not hopping mad, I'm just hopping disappointed." Here's how I deconstruct the humor: We recognize the rabbit parent and child, and we associate them with our own child-rearing experiences. Of course, we know that rabbits hop; we recall the phrase "hopping mad" (it originated in a poem written in 1675, though no one except readers of the *Oxford English Dictionary* remembers that today). Viewing the cartoon, we note the wonderfully abashed expression on the young rabbit's face, and we connect two senses of the word *hopping* with the disappointment felt by the parent—and by extension, perhaps by us with our own offspring. And then, pleased with our own cleverness, we laugh.

13

Age-Old Questions—Melissa

Step 1

Without knocking, the accompanying attendant throws open the door to Melissa Hudson's room and swoops in.

"Here we are! Hello, Melissa, dear. How are we today?" In a clearly audible aside, the attendant remarks, "Isn't she sweet? Even her name, Melissa. It means 'sweet.'"

Hmm, right away we have an issue. Is this how we should address any patient, especially someone who is an inpatient on a hospital ward, and especially one of advanced age? Should we always use first names, or last name and title? Or should we mix it up? Perhaps we should just respect the patient's own wishes. Just what form do *you* use to address a patient?

Note A

As a very young student, I learned that, unless working with a child or an adolescent, clinicians should address every patient by last name and title—"Mr. Khan" or "Ms. Greenblatt." Throughout my career, I've scrupulously followed that injunction. Even when a patient has asked to be called by first name only, I've resisted, usually electing to use first and last names, with an honorific. So I'd summon such a person from the waiting room with a smile and "Mrs. Jeannette Hancock." How could Mrs. Hancock—Jeannette—respond, but to smile back?

One reason for this obsession with formality, as explained to me decades ago, is that all patients, and especially those in mental health—and *really* especially those who are hospital inpatients—by their very status occupy a one-down position. Using a first name only, particularly when the clinician expects to be called by last name and title, only further emphasizes the power differential, in which the patient is the perpetual loser. The disparity seems especially noticeable with a patient who is older than the clinician, or when a patient belongs to some ethnic or religious minority group and the clinician does not. Another reason: Hospitalization is itself an infantilizing experience; yet, paradoxically, one of its goals is often to help patients become more self-reliant and regain full societal participation. We could encourage maturity, the thinking went, by referring to patients in a manner befitting adult status.

But that was then. Over the past half century, society has moved on, and we've become less formal in many of our interactions with one another. These changes have encouraged me to rethink some of my prejudices (but not all). I now acknowledge that it is possible to develop warm and respectful relationships with patients by using a variety of approaches, and that clinicians can be flexible in their mode of address.*

So my current recommendation is this: Knock first (that'll never change!), and then use last name and title, unless the patient requests otherwise. I'll try not to give the evil eye to younger staff members who habitually use first names, even with older patients. And I'll ask your understanding if, for the sake of uniformity with the rest of this book, I sometimes refer to our patient, Melissa, by her first name, however sweet (or not) the practice seems to me.

Rant

There isn't a lot of research on how we should address our patients, but a couple of articles a few years ago noted that, too often, clinicians failed to introduce themselves when meeting patients or relatives. *And,* whereas the patients interviewed were divided on whether to use first or last names, they were united in preferring clinicians to use both of their own names when introducing themselves at the beginning of the first session ("Hi, I'm Leslie Frey, and I'd like to interview you today"). Finally, don't forget to shake hands. These are the niceties of a relationship that, in the rush to complete a task, it seems we too often let slide.

Step 2

Let's begin again. You knock on the door to Melissa Hudson's room; you wait a few moments. Hearing no response, you call out your name (first and last!), announce that you are about to come in, and cautiously open the door.

An elderly woman sits on the bed. Her silk pajama top is misbuttoned, so that one shirttail hangs inches below the other. Melissa makes good eye contact and answers every question—though not every response is strictly relevant. She talks mainly about her childhood, her siblings, and the house her family occupied when she was 12. At one point, she answers your question about her mood by reminiscing about her young adult relationship with her husband ("It was idyllic"). When pressed, she claims her mood has been "just fine." Later, when you ask how well she's been sleeping, she recounts an anecdote concerning the fifth birthday of their son, her only child. Now on the cusp of old age himself, he occupies the lone chair in the room.

*United States federal privacy regulations (HIPAA) require that we not reveal personal information about patients. Though the use of first and last names is not prohibited, how we call out names in a waiting room is an issue for individual institutions to wrestle with, and is beyond the scope of this book.

I can think of two principal ways to understand Melissa's ramblings. One is rooted in pathology; how might you characterize the other one? Fill in the blank: It could be ____.

Note B

Every interviewer values the crisp, clear, cogent responses that some patients provide instinctively. They convey information in a manner that is at once effective and efficient. But for one reason or another, the response we get instead is sometimes rambling and long-winded, perhaps bordering on the incoherent. This may be especially the case with people of advanced years.

Of course, as with any other patient, you should approach every senior citizen with the presumption that this person is fully competent. If you need to spend extra time with older patients, it's partly that they have lived longer, so they have accumulated more life experiences they need to unpack. These can include the many losses that inevitably attend advancing age. Too, by the time your patient's eighth or ninth decade rolls around, the act of reminiscing may have assumed the role of comfort food for the psyche. In short, an older person's discursive speaking style may have no pathological significance at all.

The other underlying cause of a patient's rambling, of course, could be that the responses are symptomatic of a mental disorder, whatever that turns out to be. And that possibility is where we should focus our attention now.

Step 3

So how should you respond to Melissa's circumstantial rambling? Check all that apply.

- ☐ Ask more closed-ended questions.
- ☐ Move immediately to a formal mental status evaluation (MSE), as described in earlier chapters.
- ☐ Ask an informant to help you out.
- ☐ Resign yourself to spending (a lot) more time obtaining the history.
- ☐ Ask Melissa to describe how she spends a typical day.

Or did you have something else in mind?

Note C

Here's my short answer: Any of the responses you might have checked above could help; which one(s) you choose would depend in part on your own interviewing circumstances (time constraints, perhaps) and the severity of a given individual's psychopathology.

Some people simply require more time (and lots more patience) to interview than others do. If you are working with someone who can lay out a history with the clarity and efficiency of a textbook vignette, count yourself lucky. If not, then you must resign yourself to spending the extra time required to obtain a full history. That will likely entail using some of the techniques for guiding and shaping an interview—such as making a clear statement of your needs ("Our time is getting a bit short, so we'll have to move along") and asking closed-ended questions.

However, in Melissa's case, the rambling is probably a sign of her illness, so dealing with her behavior may be complicated. Assuming that she does not take well to your attempts to control the conversation, you might decide to proceed with one of the other techniques.

You could move right on to aspects of the formal MSE. Eventually you'd want to do that anyway, and if you aren't obtaining much information, now might be a good time. So switching to an evaluation of orientation, attention span, recent memory, and insight and judgment could be in order. If you take this tack, introduce it with something to suggest that you don't suspect her of some sort of mental deficiency: "Clinicians need to ask all their patients to do certain tasks; I'd like to ask you some routine 'quiz questions' now." You can use air quotes if you wish, but don't call them "silly questions," as I've heard from many beginning interviewers. (If they're silly, why ask them?)

Or you could ask Melissa to explain how she spends a typical day. Not only might you get an idea of her activities, but you should also be able to use her responses to estimate attention span and recent memory.

Then again, you could ask an informant. And for the sake of obtaining the history, it may come down to this in the end. Even patients who are generating what appear to be coherent, reliable responses can occasionally make mistakes in what they report—we all need to be checked up on, once in a while. Fortunately, Melissa's son is available; perhaps he can help.

In any event, you will undoubtedly end up spending far more time in evaluating Melissa than most patients will require.

Step 4

Based largely on information from her son, the following picture emerges. (I've added paragraph numbers to facilitate our analysis in Note E.)

> 1. Even well into old age, Melissa pursued a lifestyle that was vigorous and self-reliant. She occupied a variety of niches: cleaner for a janitorial service (beginning while she was still in high school); then young wife and mother; still later, an aide at her children's elementary school. The principal there encouraged her to attend college. Eventually she obtained her credentials and taught elementary school for more than 30 years. When she retired, she began to write, and by her mid-90s she had penned a series of adventure books for young readers.
>
> 2. "Mom was the hardest-working woman in three counties," Jason, her son, tells you with evident pride. "Nothing was ever handed to her on a silver platter; she worked for every dime she ever got, and for every certificate of merit and letter of appreciation. When she retired from teaching, they poured in—hundreds of them from parents, other teachers, fellow writers, even the neighbors."
>
> 3. But one day 6 years ago, not long after her 90th birthday, she'd told Jason, "I think I'm done. That's the last thing I'm going to write." She had waved a hand at the

small stack of books on her desk, presentation copies of her latest. "I just don't have the oomph any longer." Jason had said he understood that after all these years she had earned her retirement.

4. In truth, for a couple of years now, Jason has thought Melissa was slowing down. He'd first noticed it during a phone call they'd had while he was on an extended business trip. Lizzie, Melissa's "baby sister," had been visiting, and "Mom seemed confused about who had come, and at just whose house we'd all gathered." When Jason returned home, he realized that confusion had become a way of life for his mother. "She had trouble remembering things. Like, she was interested in genealogy, and showed me a book that mentioned an ancestor of ours who'd come to America on the *Mayflower.* 'What a wonderful find!' she exclaimed. I didn't have the heart to point out that last year she'd shown me the same passage in the same book. She'd even underlined it at the time; now she didn't even recognize her own scrawl."

5. But Melissa kept herself clean and tidy, and she'd chat animatedly with family members whenever they came to call, though she sometimes didn't recognize their behavioral cues when they needed to leave. "She'd stay seated and keep right on talking while they were putting on their coats," Jason observed. "Before, she'd always been so socially alert and appropriate."

6. Last year, Jason and Lizzie had accompanied Melissa to an appointment with her internist, who conducted a careful examination that included a formal MSE. The Mini-Mental State Examination (MMSE) yielded a score of 24 out of 30. Finding no evidence of a stroke or other obvious cause for memory loss, the doctor said she was probably developing Alzheimer's disease. Lizzie exclaimed that no one else in the family had ever been diagnosed with dementia.

7. But Melissa had been able to stay in her house, struggling on with some help in the form of Post-it lists that she'd stuck up in every room—shopping (what to buy and where to buy it), times when different cleaning chores were due, a compendium of family birthdays. Jason said, "She told me that the lists kept her from neglecting the basics."

8. By the time another half year had passed, she'd slipped to the point that even those reminders failed her. Now she'd frequently repeat what she'd just said, and she sometimes even swore at neighborhood children who were playing hopscotch on the sidewalk in front of her house. "It was as though she'd had a personality transplant," Jason explained, "and the one that everybody loved had been replaced by someone entirely different."

9. Lately, even with the help of her lists and a caregiver who arrives every morning to cook her meals and help with the cleaning, Melissa cannot manage to keep up her household. Just bathing, dressing, and feeding herself require all her focus. Now she's back in the hospital for a neurological workup and a social work referral for placement.

10. During the interview, Melissa makes eye contact for just a moment, but then her gaze drifts away. She unbuttons and rebuttons the pajama top she's wearing. To any question, she gives one- or two-word answers that are sometimes on point, though just as often not. Her speech is clear but often monosyllabic; she frequently seems unable to find the word she wants, and substitutes "That thing, you know" for the item or idea she wants to express.

11. Melissa admits to feeling depressed; she says that she sees no future for herself and hopes she can die soon. "But I'd never do anything about it. I wouldn't want to,

um, to do . . . well, that thing, you know. To everyone." She denies ever experiencing hallucinations or delusions. On the MMSE, she now scores only 16.

So I'd like you to write down your differential diagnosis for Melissa. Put an asterisk on your best diagnosis.

____

____

____

____

____

Note D

Melissa's symptoms could be related to a neurocognitive disorder (NCD), or possibly to some sort of mood disorder—she does have some symptoms of depression, after all. Therefore, I'd include several diagnostic possibilities:

- ◊ Depressive disorder due to another medical condition
- ◊ Substance/medication-induced depressive disorder
- ◊ Substance/medication-induced NCD
- ◊ Major depressive disorder
- ◊ NCD due to another medical condition (perhaps traumatic brain injury?)
- ◊ NCD due to Alzheimer's disease*

I'll admit that, as usual, the first two bulleted items only underscore the point that first I *always* consider substance use and other medical conditions. They often don't pan out, but I would hate to overlook such a possibility, even once. For me, the last two on the list are the most promising choices.

Step 5

It's time now to bite the bullet and figure out the diagnostic requirements for an NCD—for *any* NCD, not just one due to Alzheimer's. After we've answered four essential questions, we'll apply them to the information accumulated from our previous encounters with Melissa. Here is what we need to know for NCD:

1. What noteworthy *change* has occurred in the patient's condition? There must be a decline from the patient's previous level of cognitive ability. It can involve any of several areas, including complex attention, executive functioning, memory and learning, use of language, perceptual–motor skills, and social cognition. Of course,

as the NCD worsens, more and more areas will be involved, and the degree of involvement will increase.

2. What *evidence* for the change is required? To verify this loss in cognitive ability requires two sorts of evidence: (a) The patient (or the informant, or even the clinician) is worried about it; *and* (b) the patient's performance is impaired, as documented by psychological testing (preferred) or by clinical assessment.
3. Can we rule out all *other possible causes* for the symptoms? Other mental disorders (mood disorders, psychosis, delirium) must not account for the findings.
4. How do the symptoms *affect the patient's life*? If the decline is modest and the person can still live independently (can manage finances and medications, for example), we call it *mild* NCD. If the decline is so pronounced that the person can no longer manage independently, we label it *major* NCD.

So now I'd like you to evaluate Melissa against these four criteria. The easiest way would be to underline passages in her history (mainly, these will be in Step 4) that support your decision that she does (or does not) fulfill each of these conditions.

Rant

Melissa's substitution of "that thing" for more precise terms is one of the early symptoms that recent research has found in the speech of people who are on the way to becoming demented. Two other early symptoms are repetitive speech and a reduced number of unique words used. (These findings are based on two studies: of the speech of Ronald Reagan when he was U.S. president, and the later writings of two British novelists, Agatha Christie and Iris Murdoch. Both studies included the speech of control subjects: George H. W. Bush for Reagan, and P. D. James for the two writers.) Recently, researchers have found that football players who may be at risk for chronic traumatic encephalopathy have similar evidence of reduced linguistic complexity.

For clinicians and their patients, of course, the importance of this sort of analysis lies in the possibility for recognizing NCD early, before the emotional and behavioral toll can set in. We can observe substitutions ("the thingamajig") in our patients' speech, and we can ask informants whether they have noted other alterations in the speech pattern of their loved ones—even those who are not presidents or famous writers.

Note E

One by one, this is how I see Melissa's history in the light of the requirements for a diagnosis of NCD. The numbers given for the pieces of evidence below are the paragraph numbers in Step 4.

1. The change. Her memory was impaired enough that at first she had to augment it with Post-it notes (7); her social cognition (for example, her failure to recognize cues from her visitors) had also slipped (5).
2. The evidence. Melissa, her internist, and her son were all concerned about her cog-

nition (4); on the MMSE (11), she earned about half the score of a person whose mental functioning is normal.

3. The alternatives. Her internist (6) could find no evidence of other disorders likely to be affecting her mental state. She has had some symptoms of depression, but not nearly enough to justify a diagnosis of major depressive disorder. Her ability to maintain attention seems pretty good, actually—too much so to sustain a diagnosis of a delirium. And we have no evidence at all for suspecting psychosis.
4. The effects. Her everyday activities have become increasingly affected, but at first, by using lists, she was still able to live independently (7, 9).

You'll note that the symptoms for NCD fit reasonably well into the mantra we've recited in previous chapters: "inclusion, exclusion, duration, distress." In this case, *duration* must be understood to mean not just the length of the time that's gone by, but rather the change that has taken place over time.

Also note that we haven't yet pinpointed the cause of her condition. For that, we'll have to go to Step 6.

Step 6

Let us stipulate that Melissa has no other disorder of the sort that can cause symptoms of NCD. (The list is long; you can check out the various possibilities in DSM-5 or in any relevant textbook.) Of course, we worry about traumatic brain injury (at Melissa's age, largely from falls), but we have no evidence of any such occurrence. That leaves Alzheimer's disease the major candidate for her diagnosis. What must we do now to confirm it?

The DSM-5 requirements for this diagnosis are somewhat hard to decipher, enough so that I'm going to create a table to help us sort through them. Without it, it's *really* hard to get a feeling for just how to discriminate the two dichotomies—severity and likelihood—for NCD due to Alzheimer's.

So, using the roman numerals (which I've employed to avoid confusion with my own Step numbers), please march through the table on page 150 to determine Melissa's diagnosis at two points. Wording of these diagnoses will take the form of "[major][mild] NCD due to [probable][possible] Alzheimer's disease." What is your determination for Melissa . . .

1. At a time approximated by the end of paragraph 7 in Step 4?
2. At the very end of Step 4?

Note F

To confirm Alzheimer's disease as a cause of NCD, we must not only consider major and mild forms of the disease, but decide whether our level of certainty is high enough to term the diagnosis *probable* or only *possible*. Our table should help us unwind this tangled skein.

THE EARLIER EVALUATION

From Melissa's history (Step 4, paragraph 6), we can say that she's definitely had a gradual onset with progression of her cognitive difficulties. Her relatives' concern plus her MMSE

The (Somewhat Complicated) Requirements for Diagnosing Neurocognitive Disorder (NCD) Due to Alzheimer's Disease

Requirement	Major NCD due to Alzheimer's		Mild NCD due to Alzheimer's	
	Probable	Possible	Probable	Possible
I. Concerns and test results	Concern about a decline in cognitive functioning *plus* confirmatory testing			
II. Onset	Insidious, with gradual progression of disability			
III. Number of cognitive domains affected[a]	Two or more		One or more	
IV. Degree of decline and impairment in cognitive function	Significant decline in cognitive functioning		Modest decline in cognitive functioning	
V. Interference with independent living	Unable to perform daily activities without assistance		Can carry out daily activities, perhaps with greater effort or help from reminders	
VI. Positive genetic evidence (testing or family history) for Alzheimer's disease	Major NCD due to probable Alzheimer's disease	—	Mild NCD due to probable Alzheimer's disease	—
VII. Steady, gradual decline with no extended plateaus; no evidence of mixed causation;[b] evidence of decline in memory and learning	All three factors present: Major NCD due to probable Alzheimer's disease	If any of these three is missing: Major NCD due to possible Alzheimer's disease		All three factors present: Mild NCD due to possible Alzheimer's disease

From *DSM-5 Made Easy* by James Morrison. Copyright © 2014 The Guilford Press. Adapted by permission.

[a]Cognitive domains include complex attention, executive functioning, learning and memory, language, perceptual–motor, and social cognition.

[b]Any evidence for mixed causes forces a diagnosis of NCD due to multiple etiologies.

of 24 get us past rows I and II of the table. Even relatively early, Melissa had problems in more than one cognitive domain (for sure, memory and social cognition), so according to row III, we could still be dealing with either mild or major NCD. However, her level of cognitive decline at this point was modest (IV), and she could still carry out her daily activities, using the Post-its and other assists (V). These two findings confine us to the "Mild NCD . . . " columns of the table.

Based on Ruthie's comment in the narrative, we have no known genetic evidence, so row VI would not apply. However, suppose that Melissa *did* have a strong family history or genetic testing that proved positive for Alzheimer's disease. Then we could say that she had mild NCD due to probable Alzheimer's disease. But this was not the case, and indeed it will usually *not* be the case.

On to row VII, where we must consider the presence or absence of three factors. And sure enough, the course of Melissa's illness was one of steady, gradual decline without plateaus or sudden drops; there was no evidence of mixed causation (such as strokes or falls that could have contributed to her symptoms); and she did at this point show evidence of decline in memory and learning (she couldn't keep in mind that she'd already read, and marked up, a favorite book). The presence of all three row VII factors persuades us that hers was an instance (at this evaluation) of mild NCD due to possible Alzheimer's disease. If she'd lacked any of these three elements, we'd be forced to state that she had mild NCD due to an unspecified cause.

THE SECOND EVALUATION

By the end of our Step 4 history, Melissa has at least two affected cognitive domains, and her cognitive functioning has declined significantly (IV), directing us to the "Major NCD . . . " columns of the table. She cannot function independently, even with Post-its and other types of assistance (V). There are still no data from genetic testing, but the three row VII factors are all present, so her present diagnosis is major NCD due to probable Alzheimer's disease. (If even one of those three factors were to be missing, we could only say that she has major NCD due to *possible* Alzheimer's disease.)

Step 7

Sure, this has been a slog for us, but it's worse for Melissa and her family. And our diagnostic journey isn't quite over yet. We still have to determine what specifiers to append.

There are a couple of choices—for degree of severity, and for the presence or absence of behavioral disturbance. The behavioral specifier should be considered for all patients with NCD, regardless of whether the diagnosis is major or moderate NCD and regardless of etiology. But severity (mild, moderate, severe) is a specifier that we can only apply to patients who have major NCD. That's logical, since by its very name, mild NCD already proclaims its own level of seriousness.

- Major NCD severity is judged on the basis of the person's activities of daily living:
- If the person can still handle basic activities such as feeding and dressing but has trouble with what DSM-5 calls "instrumental activities" such as doing housework or managing finances, the severity level is *mild.*
- Trouble even with the basics? Score *moderate.*
- Full dependence on the care of others yields, of course, a rating of *severe.*

So did Melissa, at her first evaluation, have a behavioral disturbance? And at her second evaluation, please state whether she has behavioral disturbance and whether her severity is *mild, moderate,* or *severe.* Here are your choices:

	Behavioral disturbance?	Severity
First evaluation	Yes–no	—
Second evaluation	Yes–no	Mild, moderate, severe

Uh-oh, there's one other thing: We've noted that at the very end of her (Step 4) second evaluation, Melissa is quite depressed. Should she have an additional diagnosis of a mood disorder? Watch out! There's a trick lurking in this terminology.

Note G

We'll start with the second evaluation, which is the more complicated. By the time she is seen in the hospital (Step 4, paragraph 11), she requires help with meal preparation, but she can still handle her basic care functions of feeding, bathing, and dressing herself. So I'd rate her impairment from major NCD due to Alzheimer's disease as mild. Note carefully again the difference between her diagnosis when first evaluated (mild NCD) and her second diagnosis (major NCD with a severity rating of mild). This is, let's be frank about it, more than mildly confusing.)

As for the behavioral disturbance, I think you're going to be surprised. Of course, at the first evaluation she had none. But by the second evaluation she is clearly depressed, and for DSM-5, that counts as a behavioral disturbance—as do any symptoms of psychosis, agitation, or apathy. Go figure.

By the way, what about an independent diagnosis of mood disorder? I think we should pass on that one, because the mood symptoms are already covered in the specifier for behavioral disturbance. Here's an example of the value of Occam's razor, which advises us to select the simple explanation from among competing hypotheses. It's one of my diagnostic principles.

So here (at last) is a final diagnostic statement for Melissa:

- ◊ At evaluation 1:
  - ♦ Mild NCD due to possible Alzheimer's disease, without behavioral disturbance
- ◊ At evaluation 2:
  - ♦ Alzheimer's disease
  - ♦ Major NCD due to probable Alzheimer's disease, mild, with behavioral disturbance (depression)

Note that at the first evaluation, because we've said that she has NCD due to *possible* Alzheimer's disease, we do not give her an additional diagnosis of Alzheimer's. In the second evaluation, she does rate a line of diagnosis stating unequivocally that we believe she has Alzheimer's.

The Takeaway

Our experience with Melissa has prompted a discussion of how to address a patient during a conversation—especially one who is an inpatient on a mental health unit. I've said that I usually prefer not to use first names, but that over the years I've come to be less dogmatic about this. We've also talked about the (sometimes) challenging nature of work with older patients, about the possible need for asking closed-ended questions, and about how to structure an interview when time is short. We've navigated the diagnostic requirements for NCD, and the often convoluted criteria for a further refinement of NCD due to Alzheimer's disease—with and without specifiers. Finally, we've used the diagnostic principle of Occam's razor to simplify our explanation for her behavior.

Break Time

Great literature is loaded with stories of people who have mental health problems. As clinicians, one of our pleasures is to read how various authors have viewed patients like those we encounter every day. So we can experience psychosis, anxiety states, mood disorders, and even somatic symptom disorders in the works of the greats: Dickens, Melville, Hawthorne, Trollope, and many others. But have you thought about this: In classic literature you rarely—if ever?—encounter someone with dementia. There the very old may be eccentric and perhaps crotchety, but are apparently sentient to the very end.

An alleged exception: Scrooge's vivid hallucinations were once ascribed by a columnist (a psychiatrist writing in *The New York Times Magazine,* of all places) to Lewy body dementia, now called NCD with Lewy bodies in DSM-5. Such patients can also have symptomatic tremor (which is described for Scrooge, though also at one point for Bob Cratchit!) and stiffening of gait (Scrooge has that one, too). However, by definition, the tremor of Lewy body dementia comes *after* the cognitive decline has begun—and, most tellingly, Scrooge spends many years after his nocturnal adventures living well and doing good, with no further reported hallucinations. Therefore, I'm going to summarily reject NCD with Lewy bodies for Dickens's most famous creation.

More recent fiction does feature some characters with dementia/NCD. One of the principal figures in Jonathan Franzen's novel *The Corrections* develops parkinsonism with subsequent symptoms of cognitive decline. And you can find more examples of dementia in other contemporary novels: *The Madonnas of Leningrad* by Debra Dean, *Still Alice* by Lisa Genova, *Animal Dreams* by Barbara Kingsolver, and *The Wilderness* by Samantha Harvey. However, each of these works has been published fairly recently. The greats of the previous several centuries seem to have avoided cognitive disorders, perhaps because it is so hard to evoke a compelling character in someone who is gradually losing touch with what makes us interesting as people.

Of course, it is possible that I have simply not encountered examples of dementia that do exist in older fiction. If you find one, please write.

14

Family Secrets—Norman

Step 1

"He won't come in. I've asked, but he says he won't see a shrink."

Norman's wife, Sheila, is on the line, calling from the privacy of her bathroom. "Norman mustn't learn that I'm calling you; he'd be terribly distraught. Maybe you could come here? Tell him you're a friend of mine?"

Well, how do you approach a prospective patient who resists seeking treatment? Is it OK to do any of the following things?

- ☐ Have a secret telephone conversation with the person's spouse (which is what's happening now)?
- ☐ Trick the patient into an evaluation, such as by making a home visit under pretext of seeing someone else?
- ☐ Call the police?
- ☐ Obtain more information from the informant?

Check those you think would be OK.

Note A

The ethical center of the question is the principle of *beneficence*—that is, your professional duty to provide what will help the patient. The problem is that there may be several "goods" competing for your attention, among them the patient's health and the well-being of people other than the patient. Remember that you also have a duty to avoid harming the patient in any way; this is another ethical principle, called *nonmaleficence*. When a patient is competent (more accurately, when a patient has not been judged incompetent), it is important to preserve the patient's right to make health care decisions. This ethical principle is called *autonomy.**

A clandestine phone call from a relative poses no problem with a patient who refuses to be seen. At this point, you are only obtaining information from someone who desires to give it. When, or if, you do evaluate the patient, there is no requirement that you disclose the content of your conversation with the spouse. You can say, "I'm not telling her what I've discussed with you, and vice versa—unless you request that I share what you've told me."

The problem with trying to keep secret the very fact that you have met with a relative is, of course, that secrets have a way of escaping. Should that happen, there could be consequences harmful to the patient (and the patient's relationships with friends and relatives), to your therapeutic relationship, and perhaps even to your professional credibility.

Tricking the patient into an evaluation, however, is almost certain to create problems. For one thing, because you'd encounter a natural limit to the sorts of clinical information you could learn, you might accomplish little more than you would from speaking solely with the informant. But the big problem is that you'd risk poisoning any future relationship, if the patient does decide to accept care. Trust is fragile and, once broken, hard to mend.

Of course, if you have reason to believe that the patient (or someone else) is in danger, you may have a duty to notify the police or whatever other government agency might be appropriate—adult protective services, for example. But in the absence of any threat of imminent harm, blowing the whistle wouldn't be an appropriate choice, either.

Under these circumstances, your best course might be to learn as much as possible from the spouse or other informants. Even if you didn't interview the patient, collateral information could enable you to advise the informant how best to proceed. However, I'd emphasize the tentative aspect of any conclusions by saying something like this: "Here's how things look to me at this point. This is what I'd say about someone—though not this individual, whom I don't actually know—who has similar symptoms. But remember, I haven't even examined Norman, so I cannot make an actual diagnosis that we can hang our hats on."

And of course, trying to treat someone you have never met would be way beyond dicey. In this chapter's section in the References and Suggested Reading, I've included an interesting article that goes further into these questions.

Step 2

Sheila settles into a chair in your office. She is carefully dressed, calm, and poised, and she expresses herself clearly.

"Every 2 months, I spend a long weekend in Dallas, visiting my mother," she begins. "Two weeks ago Monday, when I got back late, here's what I found."

She then describes the behaviors that had, virtually overnight, transformed Norman. "Always before, he's been someone who's, well, rather stoic—not terribly com-

*The fourth ethical principle usually cited is that of *justice*, by which we mean that we must try to assure that the benefits of society are distributed equitably. These benefits are usually grouped into three categories: scarce resources (*distributive justice*), respect for individual rights (*rights-based justice*), and respect for morally acceptable laws (*legal justice*).

municative, you know? But when the taxi dropped me off Monday evening, he cried so hard he had to gasp for breath. He clung to me and said, over and over, how frightened he was. His eyes were rolling from one side to the other, and he looked disheveled and positively terrified. When I was growing up, I'd never seen anything like it in my younger brothers—and I have four of them. I could hardly believe that this was Norman."

Although she queried him repeatedly, he insisted that nothing untoward had happened. "He said he'd awakened in a total panic Saturday morning. At first he thought he might die—then he felt that he *had* died. For the next 2 days, he hardly slept at all. And he said he hadn't eaten, either. Now that I was back, he'd only sit on the edge of the bed and moan, and hold his head in his hands, and say that he was afraid he'd died."

Tuesday and Wednesday, Norman didn't go in to work. Repeatedly, Sheila urged him to see his doctor, but he refused every time. "He wouldn't say why, but I could tell he was afraid—of what he might be told, I can only suppose. When he did get up, he mostly sat around in his grubby gardening pants and Googled his symptoms. He found someone local who claimed to be a therapist, who said that acute anxiety was something that she could help with."

Sheila paused. "He went to see her once. Afterward, for the first time, he mentioned the voices." The voices, Norman told Sheila, had informed him he should hurt those who were trying to hurt him. "'Shooting is too good for them,' he claimed they'd said. After that, the *therapist*"—Sheila encloses the word in air quotes—"refused to see him again. Said he was too sick, that he might have schizophrenia."

Whoa! Right now, what's the next question you should ask? Hint: It is safety-oriented.

Note B

What I'd do next is to put down my pencil and ask, "Does Norman have any access to firearms?"

The chances that he'd actually follow through on his ideas about harming anyone (including Sheila, himself, or any caregiver) are probably low, but they are not zero. Any health care provider who ignores this issue does so at significant peril. Of course, every household has knives; that risk cannot be eliminated. But firearms can be locked up or, better still, placed in the safekeeping of a friend or relative.

Rant

Note the line above about putting down my pencil.

Although I've always taken notes, I'll admit freely that if I'm not careful, the practice can get in the way of forming a relationship. But it's possible to take notes and still maintain eye contact most of the time—which I strongly recommend.

However, nothing says, "You are talking to a stenographer," like a clinician who taps away on a keyboard throughout the crucial initial evaluation. This is an element of electronic recordkeeping we have yet to resolve satisfactorily.

There are two sorts of notes you might make. One is to jot down a few details (names, dates, places) that might otherwise escape you. The other is to remind you to cover certain issues. Generally, you'll use one-word cues to issues the patient has brought up. That's the sort of note that I'm recommending you focus on when you talk with anyone, whether a patient or an informant.

Step 3

Sheila says she's afraid of guns and would never have one in the house; no friends or relatives own one, either. She now thinks that the whole experience has "freaked him out" so badly that Norman just might come in for an evaluation after all.

But what, she wants to know, *is* wrong with her husband? Could he have schizophrenia, as the therapist suggested? And if not . . . ?

So—yes, you know what's coming—what would be on your list of possibilities for Norman? OK, your list of *tentative* diagnoses, inasmuch as you've never even met the man. I'm not going to ask you to justify each one, just to list them. That should be pretty easy, and I've left lots of blank lines for creativity.

Note C

Here's my *tentative* (or working) list of possible diagnoses—those that would guide my investigation, should I ever meet Norman:

- ◊ Substance/medication-induced psychotic disorder
- ◊ Psychosis due to another medical disorder
- ◊ Substance/medication-induced anxiety disorder
- ◊ Anxiety disorder due to another medical disorder
- ◊ Panic disorder

◊ Depressive disorder with psychosis
◊ Brief psychotic disorder
◊ Schizophreniform disorder
. . .
◊ Schizophrenia

Notice that schizophrenia appears dead last on this list. In fact, by using an ellipsis to separate it from the other possibilities, I've tried to indicate just how improbable I'd consider it—for Norman, or for anyone at this point in time. Of course, it isn't impossible. In the field of mental health, nearly anything *could* happen. But with the diagnostic interview, we attempt to learn what's likely so we can prepare for the future.

Step 4

So now let's respond to Sheila's Step 3 question. What would be your reason for rejecting a diagnosis of schizophrenia *at this time*? (I can think of three important reasons, and they all have to do with the diagnostic requirements for that diagnosis.) I've started you off with some broad hints:

1. (Number of symptoms) ______________________________
2. (Mode of onset) ______________________________
3. (Duration) ______________________________

Note D

Here are the reasons we can all but rule out the diagnosis of schizophrenia *right now*.

1. The diagnosis of schizophrenia requires, first and foremost, at least two basic symptoms of psychosis. They are the A criteria of DSM-5—delusions, hallucinations, disorganized speech, disorganized behavior, and negative symptoms (such as flat affect or lack of motivation); refer back to Brad's history in Chapter 2 (Note F, page 26) for a refresher. At this time, we don't know that this is the case with Norman. Sheila reports that when she came home, he thought he might have died, or he was afraid he had died. No one seems to have asked him, "Are you really dead, or does it just *feel* that way?" That's a big difference. To count as a symptom of schizophrenia, a delusion must carry conviction. (If it doesn't, it's not an actual delusion.) Also, Norman has reportedly heard voices, but we don't know anything about their quality. Does he recognize them, talk back to them? Do they issue commands? Does he admit that they only exist in his head? At this point, we simply do not know.

2. People with schizophrenia typically become ill gradually—*insidiously* is the word often used—over a period of months or even years. However, Norman's symptoms have developed abruptly, perhaps literally overnight. That can happen in schizophreniform disorder, but it's a big red flag warning us off the diagnosis of schizophrenia.

3. Finally, schizophrenia is a disorder that we *cannot* diagnose short of a *minimum* 6-month duration. In and of itself, that requirement is enough to keep us from making the diagnosis. For now.

Once again, schizophrenia is one of those diagnoses (along with Alzheimer's dementia and a few others) so serious that I keep it forever at the bottom of my differential diagnoses—until, after ruling out everything else, I simply have no other reasonable choice.

Step 5

Two days later, Sheila and Norman arrive together for an appointment. Sheila waits while you interview Norman privately. Almost immediately, he breaks down sobbing. You pass him a box of tissues and lean forward slightly (demonstrating your interest and sympathy) as he struggles to gain control.

"Those voices," he says, "they were my conscience testing me." He says he knows now that they "weren't real; they existed entirely in my head." But it worries him that "part of my own mind could urge me to harm another person. I mean, where does *that* come from? I've always been a total pacifist."

You do the safety check again, ascertaining that he has no intention of actually hurting himself or another person. And you confirm that he has no access to firearms. Then you ask the big question: "How do you think all this got started?"

Norman drops his gaze for a moment, then straightens in his chair and looks you full in the eye. "I guess I'd better level with you." You smile just a little and nod a silent encouragement to continue.

Sheila had departed for her long weekend, leaving Norman feeling bereft and rather sorry for himself. Marijuana has recently "gone legal" where he lives, and he felt so lonely, he thought he might just renew his youthful acquaintance with the drug. In college, he'd tried it exactly twice. Not only was he "underwhelmed" by its effect, but when Sheila found out (at that time, they were just beginning to date), she'd threatened to break up with him if he ever did drugs again. But after she departed for her mother's, trying a little pot seemed like a tiny rebellion that might help fill the expanse of time yawning ahead.

However, he didn't want to smoke—pot, or anything else. "Terrible for your lungs," he points out, with just a whiff of righteousness. So he obtained some tetrahydrocannabinol oil, which he stirred into the box-mix brownies he'd bought at Safeway.

"Of course, I had no idea what I was doing—especially how much I should be using," he explains ruefully. "But they tasted OK, so I just ate a couple. And then one more. And then I sat down to see what would happen." He pauses a couple of beats. "I sure found out!"

So the issue of a substance-related disorder has suddenly come to the fore. It makes me want to know: Just what sorts of mental disorder symptoms can we usually expect from the various substances people misuse? I've put several possibilities into a form, on page 160; I'd like you to put a checkmark in each box that you think represents a likely result of using each class of substance, during either intoxication (I) or withdrawal (W). Go ahead and use any book or online resource you like: This stuff is hard to keep in mind, and it isn't always

Type of symptoms	Alcohol and sedatives		Cannabis		Hallucinogens and inhalants		Stimulants and cocaine		Opioids	
	I	W	I	W	I	N/A	I	W	I	W
Anxiety/panic										
Depression										
Psychosis										
Sleep										

something that yields to logic. But checking off the boxes in this form may help drive it into your memory.

Note E

Below is how I'd fill out the form. Of course, some choices will occur more frequently than others. Note that psychosis can be induced in at least five different scenarios. This suggests just how vigilant we must remain in searching for substance use etiologies of psychotic symptoms. It's just one more reason why I *always* place substance use (along with other medical disorders) at the very top of my differential diagnoses.

Step 6

And now we should at last be able to reduce Norman's diagnostic possibilities to just a couple of choices. They are . . . what? Please write them down.

____

____

Type of symptoms	Alcohol and sedatives		Cannabis		Hallucinogens and inhalants		Stimulants and cocaine		Opioids	
	I	W	I	W	I	N/A	I	W	I	W
Anxiety/panic		✓	✓		✓		✓	✓		✓
Depression	✓	✓			✓		✓	✓	✓	✓
Psychosis	✓	✓	✓		✓		✓			
Sleep	✓	✓	✓	✓			✓	✓	✓	✓

Note F

Because we've been broad-ranging in writing our initial differential diagnosis in Note C, we have already included two substance/medication-induced disorders (mood and psychosis). Of course, at first we've had no idea that Norman might have taken *anything* potentially intoxicating, let alone what it might have been. But because of our ingrained diagnostic habits, we've written down that suspicion in our working list of possibilities. Hurrah for us! Our working diagnoses will now be these:

◊ Cannabis-induced psychotic disorder
◊ Cannabis-induced anxiety disorder

The Takeaway

We have begun our evaluation of Norman by discussing a couple of issues that should guide all clinicians: the ethics of tricking a patient who doesn't want care into being seen, and the requirement that we not make a diagnosis for people we have never met. We've stated the four ethical principles that underlie every health care encounter: beneficence, nonmaleficence, autonomy, and justice. And, once again, we've emphasized a prime responsibility of any health care provider: to ensure the safety of everyone, patient or not, with whom we become involved. Often, we've noted, that means asking about the availability of firearms. We've responded to another clinician's too-hasty diagnosis by reviewing the A criteria for schizophrenia, and we've touched upon the onset and duration requirements.

Then we've tackled the distribution of anxiety/panic, depressive, psychotic, and sleep symptoms during intoxication with, or withdrawal from, several substances of abuse. The form is a bit complicated, so we probably won't remember all of it in detail; rather, it's useful just to recall that these substance classes are pretty broadly capable of creating havoc with the mental health of anyone who misuses them—even if only once. It's another affirmation of the importance of always putting substance use and medical disorders into the differential diagnosis for just about any set of symptoms.

Oh, yes—and I've also subjected us all to a Rant about taking notes and yet maintaining good eye contact.

Break Time

Making diagnoses is all well and good—when it comes to our patients. But there are situations where, though it's tempting to spout off with what we know, or think we know, we should be extremely chary about exhibiting our expertise. Here's a short list of good opportunities to keep silent:

- When the person in question is a friend or relative (in that situation, the risks of diagnosis are enormous)
- When it is a political or other public figure (most of what we "know" we glean from the op-ed writers, and they may be writing from a position of some bias)
- Anyone for whom we have only a scrap of information
- Anyone, for that matter, with whom we haven't done an actual interview

This issue has deep roots. It goes back at least to the U.S. presidential election of 1964, long before many clinicians working today were even born. To be sure, only 20% of psychiatrists answered a magazine survey about presidential politics. But of those who did, nearly half stated the opinion that Barry Goldwater, the Republican nominee for president that year, was not fit to be president. The article cited conclusions based on supposed clinical insights into Goldwater's mental state.

The poll had been commissioned and published by Ralph Ginzburg, who could fairly be characterized as an *avant-garde* writer (a magazine he later founded and edited even bore that term as its name). Clinicians who were drawn to his sort of publication might have been atypical of the broad spectrum of mental health care workers. (Subsequently, Goldwater sued Ginzburg and was awarded damages to the tune of $75,000—peanuts now, perhaps, but a fair chunk of change over 50 years ago.)

The ultimate outcome was the perhaps long-overdue rule (popularly called the "Goldwater rule") from the American Psychiatric Association that forbids psychiatrists to comment on a person's mental state without first conducting an examination of that person—and, of course, receiving the individual's authorization to make the conclusions public. It's an argument that arose again, even in the popular press, early in 2017.

In any event, when you are asked what you make of Senator *X* or Mayor *Y*—and, believe me, it happens all the time—what *can* you say?

First, I'd point out that this is a person I've never met, for whom I have little information, and with whom I haven't done an interview. And if I had, I'd hasten to add, it would probably be privileged information, so I wouldn't be able to talk about it.

Next, I might say, "Here is the information I'd need before I could even hazard a guess." Then I'd talk about the various points of personal history and the mental status evaluation that would be necessary to make any mental health diagnosis.

If the question is about a specific diagnosis, then I might say, "And here are the features you should look for. If you don't have access to that information, then the diagnosis is not tenable." And I'd be pretty darned circumspect about making any diagnosis myself.

For other comments and ideas about the Goldwater rule and mental disorders in public figures, see the articles cited in References and Suggested Reading for this chapter.

15

Rejections—Olivia

Step 1

The note from Olivia's referring doctor sets the scene:

> *For 5 years, I've treated Olivia for intractable, atypical migraine. She's tried every conceivable drug, every preventive measure, all to no avail. At her request, and with my facilitation, for the last 2 years she has been supported by a monthly disbursement from her private disability policy. Several times I've tried to suggest other approaches to her distress, but she responds with argument and refusal to cooperate with anything I've put forth. Some months ago, I referred her to a psychologist for testing; after the first few minutes, she became enraged and walked out. I've begun to wonder how great a role her personality may be playing in her symptoms. Finally, I told her that I would continue to see her (and approve her disability payments) only if she agreed to keep this appointment for consultation.*

Now, when you meet Olivia, you ask, "What seems to be the problem?" She responds, "You're supposed to tell me what's wrong—so do your job, already!" She folds her arms across her chest and leans as far back as her chair will permit.

After this rather ill-mannered challenge, how would you proceed?

- ☐ Ask the same question, with the assumption that she didn't hear right.
- ☐ Ask it in a different way, with an explanation.
- ☐ Focus instead on the feelings expressed.
- ☐ Sit quietly and wait for her to say something.
- ☐ Stand up and say, "I hope you have a nice life. Goodbye."

Note A

As tempted as you may be to invoke the last suggestion (thereby terminating the interview), let's step back for a moment and ask ourselves: Is "What seems to be the problem?" absolutely the best introductory question?

In fact, there isn't a lot wrong with the way the question is phrased. It may only elicit complaints from someone who is supersensitive and, perhaps, spoiling for a fight. But that's just the situation you face with Olivia. If instead you were to ask, "Please tell me why you came here," there'd be less room for complaint—about you, at any rate. But it's an easy slip of the tongue, and I can imagine saying something similar myself, in an unguarded moment.

That said, resistance this early in the interview indicates a serious potential roadblock. You will have to navigate around it with extreme care. *Pussyfooting* might not be too extreme an expression.

I would respond with a second request for information, but one that adds an explanation: "Of course, I have a note from your doctor. But to figure out what's wrong, we'll need to explore your point of view." Notice that this little speech manages to combine several features:

- It acknowledges that you do have collateral information . . .
- . . . while refuting the idea that the written note is sufficient. You've thereby moved to shut down one avenue of distraction.
- It identifies with the patient by using her own phrase (" . . . what's wrong").
- By using the first-person plural ("we'll need to explore . . . "), you are aligning your goal with hers.
- It offers Olivia another opportunity to speak.

That's a lot of benefit squeezed into two dozen words! And of course, you can use body language (perhaps leaning forward and frowning in a worried sort of way) that conveys concern and concentration.

However, even these efforts could still meet further resistance, perhaps in the form of another direct refusal to participate. (By the way, patients can resist interviewers in lots of other ways. We'll discuss some of them later.)

In such a situation, I'd try this often-successful method: Ignore the substance of the comment (for now) and focus on the emotion that seems to be driving it. I might say something on the order of "Wow! That's a lot of emotion. Perhaps you could tell me how you are feeling right now." Of course, you might get an explosion that's hard to contain, but the blast should throw up some useful chunks of fact and feeling. From the debris, you can select something to pursue further.

If this doesn't work—if you harvest only stony silence—then offer a multiple-choice series of emotions that the patient might be experiencing. For example, you might try, "I think I hear some frustration. Is that it?" Note that by starting with an emotion that doesn't carry any hint of blame, you offer the patient a chance to express her feelings as an understandable response to a difficult, perhaps even intolerable situation. If you still aren't successful, try another step in your series of emotions: "Maybe it's anger." And, yes, I'd be content at that point to just sit for a few more moments, hoping that Olivia will offer a further comment—*something* that can form the basis for a conversation.

Only after all of these attempts have failed would I throw in the towel and suggest that she come back later, if she decides she would like to talk about her issues.

Step 2

For the next 15 minutes, a torrent of information pours forth. There's far too much to reproduce all of it word for word, but below are extracts from what Olivia says concerning several of the themes.

> "It hurts sort of, you know, all over my head. Like, I feel I'm going to explode. Look!—That *is* my best description! No, I don't have any shooting pains, it's just general. Sort of dull and sharp. Can't you understand? Even my own doctor doesn't believe me! Do you think I *like* being sick all the time?
>
> "Of *course* I've felt depressed! Under the circumstances, who wouldn't? It's so bad that my food intake has dwindled to a trickle. What?—No, my weight has been about the same. But I sleep horribly, hardly a wink all night. Just last week, I was up all night three nights running. Of course I'm tired—I could really use a nice long coma!
>
> "The migraines are more insistent now; they sometimes come on with almost no provocation, though often it's when I'm under a ton of stress. I've had a lot of trouble with them, for years now. And my general physical health? Well, I don't feel like discussing it right now. Too depressing to contemplate.
>
> "It's enough to drive me to drink, except that I swore I never would again. Don't ask.
>
> "No, I can't discuss this stuff with anyone in my family. They're all pretty upset with me, but it's not my fault. The migraines have me under such stress. The other day my sister said, 'Don't blame the headaches; you've always been difficult.' She's such a bitch!"

As I've mentioned in Step 2 of Chapter 11 in regard to Kylie (page 118), *areas of clinical interest* is my term for the various types of problems mental health patients experience. Feel free to categorize them any way you want, but these seven different areas seem to cover most of the ground pretty well:

- ☐ Difficulty thinking (cognitive problems, especially dementia; DSM-5 calls them *neurocognitive disorders*, as we've seen in Chapter 13 with Melissa)
- ☐ Substance use
- ☐ Psychosis
- ☐ Mood disturbance, especially depressive, manic, and hypomanic episodes
- ☐ Excessive anxiety, avoidance behavior, and arousal
- ☐ Physical complaints (including problems with sleeping and eating, as well as the somatic symptom disorders)
- ☐ Social and personality problems

Of course, you can probably name some disorders that don't fit all that comfortably into one of the categories above. In case you're having trouble, here's a little boost:

- Sleep and appetite disorders (insomnia and hypersomnia, for example, and anorexia and bulimia nervosa) are physical conditions that are rather different from chest pain and diarrhea.
- Kleptomania and pyromania are compulsions, in a sense, but also social problems.
- To a degree, conditions such as dissociative amnesia and dissociative identity disorder defy ready categorization.

Now, from the clues that have erupted from Mt. Olivia, what can you find that might help guide the rest of the interview? You could underline each chunk you collect, and then check off the relevant area of clinical interest in the list of these areas above. Then compare your findings with what I've identified in Note B.

Note B

OK, so my areas of clinical interest aren't perfect—and if you feel more comfortable adding a separate "all other" category, that's your call. Based on the extracts from Olivia's Step 2 speeches, however, here's *my* call on the clinical areas that we need to investigate further in a subsequent interview:

- Mood disturbance. Olivia has some depressive symptoms; although she denies weight change, she's experienced loss of appetite, trouble sleeping, feeling tired, and, of course, depressed mood (not to mention her affect, which is just about the most irritable I've ever encountered).
- Substance use. There's actually only a hint here, but it's underscored by her reluctance to elaborate; we'd need to flesh out the details. Of course, substance use is everywhere in the population and often figures in the etiology of other emotional and behavioral disorders, so we should consider it for every patient. But what we've heard from Olivia so far suggests that we should take an extra measure of care in this department.
- Physical complaints. Even if she hadn't had migraine, I'd want to learn something more about Olivia's physical health. Especially prevalent in younger women are the somatic symptom disorders; failing to diagnose one is a cardinal error that's made over and again in clinics worldwide.
- Personality problems. From Olivia herself and her doctor's note, we can gather enough hints of difficulty getting along with other people that I'd want to pursue this area, too.
- Social problems. Even apart from personality issues, relationship issues can bedevil any patient. For Olivia, these would seem a real possibility, based on how she describes her relationship with her sister.

This isn't really all that hard to figure out, is it? Although it's simple, it is truly important: Picking up on any hints of what's important to the patient is key to gathering all the relevant information while at the same time gaining the patient's trust and developing rapport.

Step 3

Here is the information elicited from Olivia. Note that I've reduced it to the (boring) format that's usual for mental health writeups. What isn't usual is that I've labeled each major section, to make clear what sort of information is being addressed. (Some categories of information—you'll find a more detailed breakdown back in Step 2 of Chapter 1, on page 8—I've included without special labeling.)

- *Chief complaint and introductory information.* Olivia Rosenthal is a 35-year-old married woman who comes to the office with this complaint: "You're supposed to tell me what's wrong—so do your job, already!" Other than a detailed note of referral from her physician, she is her own chief informant. Within the limits of her manifest irritability and hostility, she appears reliable.
- *History of the present illness.* For several years, Olivia has been treated for what her physician terms "atypical migraine headaches." Currently, about three times a week she experiences headaches so severe that she must draw the shades and take to her bed. These headaches last several hours, during which she cannot tolerate sounds, smells, or bright lights; even a pillow touching her head induces exquisite pain. She has been treated with a variety of drugs to prevent migraine, and with at least three tryptan-type medications for acute episodes. Usually she responds well at first, but within weeks the treatment will lose effectiveness; several times, she's developed devastating, debilitating side effects. Her physician has tried to suggest a possible emotional component to her problem, but she vehemently rejects this interpretation. She has reluctantly agreed to this evaluation as a requirement for continuing her migraine medication and the documentation necessary for her Social Security disability payments.

Olivia says she's been sickly "throughout my adult life, and much of my childhood." Here are some of the symptoms she's had, none of which her physician could explain after evaluation: amnesia for a 3-week period 11 years ago; inability to walk without staggering for several days at age 29; paralysis of her entire left side for one day "due to a kidney infection"; recurrent abdominal pain; several spells of vomiting; episodes of abdominal bloating; menstrual periods that have been "incredibly painful and never regular"; vomiting throughout all 9 months of her first pregnancy; total inability to experience orgasm, "except once when I was 17 and drunk"; back pain that intermittently requires chiropractic treatment; joint pain (knees and left elbow); muscle spasms of her legs and feet; painful urination 18 months ago that was successfully treated with naturopathic herbs; and shortness of breath (chest X-ray and electrocardiogram normal). On two occasions, she felt briefly "pinned to the bed and covered in a cold fear" with a paralysis the source of which a neurological consultation failed to discover. Bursitis recently limited range of motion in her left shoulder. Despite these complaints, her current general physician finds no evidence of serious medical disease, other than the migraines. She says that she is allergic to Demerol and nickel.

Olivia once drank alcohol heavily. A decade ago, her drinking led to blackouts and repeated fights with her husband. Although she had no legal or employment problems, she admits to driving while intoxicated on at least two occasions. ("I wasn't caught, but it frightened me so badly that after the second time, I resolved never to drink again.") Although she often thinks about drinking, her fear of what would happen should she "cave to the craving" has prompted complete abstinence for the past 10 years. She has never used street drugs, beyond a couple of hits of marijuana when she was a teenager, and she's never smoked tobacco or used e-cigarettes.

For several months, Olivia has been depressed, possibly in reaction to her impending divorce from her husband of 16 years. "Nearly all the time" for the past 3–4 weeks, she has been distressed by crying spells, loss of concentration, and decreased interest in her usual activities. She has had low energy, marked trouble getting to sleep, poor appetite (though no weight loss), ruminations about dying, death wishes, and suicidal ideas. She denies ever having had manic symptoms. When she was 27, she had a "nervous breakdown" during which she hyperventilated, felt depressed, and was treated with antidepressants for several weeks. At first she responded well to the antidepressants, but later they seemed to make no difference. "My mood then was pretty much the way it is now."

- *Personal and social history.* Olivia was born in Peoria, Illinois, where her father worked in construction; her mother was at home. She is the third of five siblings, "so I always had someone to play with." When she was 10, her parents separated and subsequently divorced; 3 years later, her mother remarried. Olivia never got along well with her stepfather, though she admits that he was generally kind to her; she denies ever being abused, either physically or sexually. On three occasions, she was picked up by the police for running away. She was several times truant from grade school and had some physical fights in high school, but has had no legal problems since then. She did poorly throughout school and dropped out midway through the 11th grade to take a grocery store clerking job, which she quit when she married at age 19. Since then, she has been at home. She was reared as a Roman Catholic, but now claims no religious affiliation ("and little interest"). She's never served in the military.

Mini-Rant

In context, military service, which is usually included along with other parts of personal and social history, seems superfluous. Unfortunately, clinicians too often leave it out, even when it may be relevant.

- *Family history.* Her mother and father both abused alcohol, as did a brother, two paternal uncles, and "all" of her maternal uncles and aunts. A sister has never been well and suffered a "nervous breakdown" during which she attempted suicide.
- *Mental status evaluation.* Appearing to be about her stated age, Olivia is a slightly overweight woman dressed in a nearly transparent blouse with a deep neckline. She seems somewhat anxious at times during the interview, but remains very verbal throughout. Speech is dramatic but clear, coherent, and relevant to the content of her thought, with no loosening of associations. Her affect is full range—or greater: She becomes tearful at times, but within a few moments she will smile or even laugh. Once she asked whether "a tranquilizer might help."
- She describes "hallucinations" that have occurred intermittently since age 27. Once she heard her mother calling her name; another time, it was the voice of her husband calling to her. There were no other abnormal contents of thought such as delusions, phobias, obsessions, or compulsions. She denies having panic attacks, but seemed interested in learning about the symptoms.

- She can recite seven numbers forward and five backward. She names five recent presidents in reverse order and without hesitation. She performs the months-backward test flawlessly. She is fully oriented for person, place, and time. She realizes that something is wrong with her, but insists that it is all physical; she says she would reject psychotherapy, suggesting judgment that may be defective.

OK, what's Olivia's differential diagnosis? (That's the last part usually included in the writeup.) Yes, I'd like you to write it down first, and I hope you're long on persistence. I've arranged my diagnoses according to the areas of clinical interest we've discussed in Step 2, but feel free to create yours as you wish.

Physical symptoms

Mood disorder

Substance use

Personality issues

____

____

____

Note C

Whew! With four areas to consider, and a list for each, this could drag on for a bit! I'm going to pour a cup of cocoa and grab a plateful of cookies, because I know *I'll* be here for some time while we discuss this complicated differential diagnosis.

Let's start with the migraines and other physical symptoms, which is where Olivia's complaints began.

- ◊ First, I'd include actual migraines and other physical causes of disease, because that's where I always start.
- ◊ There are several conditions in a class that DSM-5 calls *somatic symptom disorders.* The first is a specific diagnosis that DSM-5 confusingly calls *somatic symptom disorder.* (I'm not perseverating; it's just that the latest edition of the official psychiatric manual uses the same term for the general and the specific—like "New York, New York, so good they named it twice.") DSM-IV called the specific condition *somatization disorder;* clinicians from another era used the term *Briquet's syndrome.*
- ◊ Another is *somatic symptom disorder, with predominant pain,* where pain is the main symptom.
- ◊ Yet another would be hypochondriasis—oops! Sorry, DSM-5 has renamed that one too. Now called *illness anxiety disorder,* it still identifies people who have minimal symptoms but are overwhelmingly worried about being sick.
- ◊ And still another would be *conversion disorder,* where the patient has symptoms of sensory or motor dysfunction that, due to the limits of anatomy and physiology, simply can't be caused by an actual medical disorder. Typical conversion symptoms include tunnel vision and seizures that occur in the absence of abnormal activity on an electroencephalogram.
- ◊ You could also make a case (not a good one, but the goal of a differential diagnosis is to be inclusive) for *factitious disorder.*
- ◊ Could Olivia be *malingering*—that is, consciously making up symptoms for some concrete benefit?

Now to the question of mood disorder. I'll admit that throughout all my cases, there's a certain sameness in the differential diagnosis of mood symptoms. That's OK, because it means that we don't have to make it all up anew every time we talk about the differential diagnosis for depression.

- ◊ Depressive disorder due to another medical condition.
- ◊ Substance/medication-induced depressive disorder.
- ◊ Major depressive disorder. This comes quickly to mind—it is common and, well, popular.
- ◊ A bipolar disorder, current episode depressed.
- ◊ Persistent depressive disorder (dysthymia).
- ◊ Adjustment disorder with depressed mood.
- ◊ "Normal" depression, whatever that is—let's just say a mood that is low but not pathological. But it's the sort of sadness that could be connected to the ongoing misery of a personality disorder, or to a once-in-a-lifetime unhappy experience that doesn't rise to the level of an adjustment disorder. In effect, this is a nondiagnosis that is very close to *no mental illness.*

We move on now to the substance use possibilities.

- ◊ Alcohol use disorder, which could be either current or by history only.
- ◊ Alcohol intoxication.
- ◊ Alcohol withdrawal.
- ◊ The misuse of other substances, either prescription medications or street drugs.

And, finally, the personality issues.

- ◊ I've already mentioned borderline personality disorder, which I would consider a real possibility for Olivia.
- ◊ She is rather dramatic, so we should also include histrionic personality disorder.
- ◊ Personality traits that don't meet criteria for any stated disorder. DSM-5 would call them *other* or *mixed.* These labels are highly unsatisfactory, but the concept belongs on the list.

These are the high spots, though you could probably garnish this Dagwood sandwich of a differential list with a few other disorders. If you want to add some ingredients, please go right ahead while I finish my cocoa.

Step 4

Now, with our differential diagnosis in mind, what's the best diagnosis, and why? Keep in mind that your best step (as always) would be to write down your thinking, so you can compare it with mine. I've left several lines, because sometimes there are multiple "best" diagnoses.

___

___

___

Note D

For Olivia, there simply isn't *one* best diagnosis—there are several. That is, no matter how much we want to wield Occam's razor, we cannot explain all of her symptoms on the basis of a single disorder. (Quick review: *Occam's razor,* or the *parsimony principle,* advises us to choose the simplest explanation possible for all the data.) For example, her mood disorder can't be a physiological consequence of drinking that stopped far in the past. It also probably isn't the result of a personality issue that began years earlier. When you cannot explain everything on the basis of one disorder, you have to make multiple diagnoses. (Yes, this is another diagnostic principle.)

Again, let's commence with Olivia's index complaint, the headaches. Of course, she could have a peculiar type of migraine that her other clinicians haven't been able to get a handle on, but after all the testing, all the time and effort spent by various health care providers, and her lackluster response to multiple treatments that usually succeed with migraine, in the end we have to reject actual migraine as a likely possibility. As to malingering—consciously making up symptoms for some primary gain (such as qualifying for disability?)—there's no hard evidence to back up this hypothesis. Also, and very importantly, malingering is a diagnosis that should come at the rock bottom of any differential list, after all else has been examined and discarded. We aren't there yet, not nearly.

So let's consider the somatic symptom disorders. Illness anxiety disorder (formerly known as hypochondriasis) is easily ruled out: Although Olivia has had many clinician appointments, she appears to have the serious symptom of overwhelming headache, and patients with illness anxiety disorder don't have serious somatic symptoms—only serious concern about being ill. Although she has had some conversion symptoms (paralysis and staggering gait, for example), conversion disorder is another diagnosis we should make only after ruling out all other possibilities. As we'll see, for Olivia, we can't. Factitious disorder? Nope, I don't think she's faked her symptoms. Also, once more, this is a perennial next-to-last-on-the-list diagnosis that I seldom invoke, and then only with strong evidence in hand.

Furthermore, Olivia does qualify for another preemptive condition: somatic symptom disorder. By DSM-5 criteria, she'd need only one serious physical symptom (in her case, headaches), as long as she also has serious concerns about health or the investment of a great deal of time in health care. That description appears to fit Olivia's situation perfectly.

Rant

Olivia has had numerous other physical complaints. Enough, in fact, that she could qualify for the old DSM-IV diagnosis of somatization disorder, which requires a lot more symptoms and has been much better validated than has somatic symptom disorder. In brief, here are the requirements for this useful, if rather complicated, disorder.

Starting before age 30, Olivia has had many physical complaints, for each of which (1) she has sought treatment or (2) she has been materially impaired in work, social, or personal functioning. Overall, there must be at least eight such symptoms, portioned out as follows:

• *Pain symptoms (four or more required).* Olivia has had headaches, abdominal pain, excessively painful menses, back pain, knee and left elbow pain, muscles spasms, shoulder pain (bursitis), and painful urination. Other possible pain symptoms include pain in the chest or rectum, and pain related to other body functions such as intercourse.

• *Gastrointestinal symptoms (two or more needed, excluding pain).* Olivia has had abdominal bloating and spells of vomiting. Other possible symptoms include recurrent nausea, diarrhea, and intolerance to several foods.

• *Sexual symptoms (at least one required, excluding pain).* Olivia has had vomiting throughout pregnancy and inability to experience orgasm. Others could include irregular menses and excessive menstrual bleeding.

• *Pseudoneurological symptoms (at least one required).* Olivia complains of having experienced paralysis and staggering gait. Other possible conversion symptoms include double vision, blindness, numbness, hallucinations, loss of voice, urinary retention, deafness, seizures, amnesia (or other dissociative symptoms), and loss of consciousness.

And once malingering and factitious disorder are ruled out, Olivia would, I believe, meet the requirements for this complicated but highly useful disorder of somatization.

Now let's move on to Olivia's depression. I'd love to be able to say that it is part and parcel of her somatic symptom disorder. That would allow us to invoke the diagnostic principle of Occam's razor. Alas, although mood and other mental symptoms were included in the original descriptions of Briquet's syndrome, a well-defined and carefully researched forerunner of somatization disorder, they are nowhere to be found in the descriptions of contemporary somatic symptom disorders. Olivia has done some drinking in her time, but none for the past 10 years or more. So we'll have to hang her depression on something else from our list of differential diagnoses.

This actually turns out to be pretty smooth sailing. She easily meets the inclusion criteria for a major depressive episode and for major depressive disorder. She's had at least five symptoms of the nine that are listed for the episode (see the table in Chapter 1, page 11, for a review). Now let's talk about exclusions. She's not had an episode of mania or hypomania, so she doesn't qualify for a bipolar disorder, and the depressive symptoms haven't persisted for the 2 years required for persistent depressive disorder (dysthymia). Adjustment disorder with depressed mood? What would be the antecedent stressor? Surely not her concern about diagnosis, which would be a really good example of circular reasoning. And "normal" depression? Again, the fact that her life has been deeply affected suggests otherwise. That eliminates other possible causes of depression.

As for substance use, there's actually not too much going on there—or rather, it doesn't seem to be current, if we accept at face value what she tells us. (We'd be on safer ground if we could get some corroboration from people who know her well, to affirm that she could not currently qualify for alcohol intoxication or withdrawal. Somehow, though, once you've gained her cooperation with the interview, what she has said seems believable.) We do know that, years ago, Olivia consumed alcohol even though she knew that it caused her to drive when under the influence. She also repeatedly fought with her husband. That's two symptoms, the bare minimum needed to make a diagnosis of alcohol use disorder, though now in sustained remission (DSM-5 points out that her ongoing craving for alcohol doesn't preclude remission status). We should include the diagnosis for Olivia as a warning to subsequent clinicians about what medications to avoid, and as an indicator that she could still have the potential for subsequent substance misuse. Her two experiences with marijuana mark her as having once been a teenager—nothing more.

And, finally, what about her personality issues? Of course, rejecting blame and stating that her relatives are all upset with her could characterize several personality disorders, but there is something more specific. Histrionic personality disorder is often found in people who have a somatic symptom disorder, and Olivia has several of its characteristics: emotional lability, physical appearance contrived to call attention to oneself, and exaggerated emotional expression. Her first speech sample (in Step 2) sounds a little vague; ordinarily, I'd want longer excerpts from a patient's speech to see whether it often wanders and lacks focus, but for the sake of the exercise, let's assume that we do have a representative sample. Is she easily influenced and seductive? Again, we'd need more information. In good conscience, I'd say that we don't have enough to make a firm diagnosis, but we do have enough to stimulate further investigation. In particular, I'd want to interview her at greater length once I'd gotten to know her better, and to get information, if possible, from those who already know her well. And all of this would I want to pursue in full recognition of this diagnostic principle: Be chary of making any personality disorder diagnosis in a patient who has unresolved major mental health issues.

Here is my complete lineup:

- ◊ Alcohol use disorder, mild, in sustained remission
- ◊ Major depressive disorder
- ◊ Somatic symptom disorder

Step 5

Now how would you list these three diagnoses? That is, in what order should you write them down in the patient's chart or in a letter to the clinician who has referred her? Are there any principles that can guide us? Does it matter? Why? Here are some choices:

- ☐ Alphabetical order
- ☐ Chronological order
- ☐ Ordered by importance for treatment

Using one of these principles (or something else), write down the order in which you would list the three final diagnoses from Note D:

1. ______________________________

2. ______________________________

3. ______________________________

Note E

There is a very simple reason why order in a list of diagnoses is important: Lots of people, even some clinicians, are more or less list-averse. Show them several possible diagnoses, and they pay attention to just one—the first one. If that's ever the case, then I want them to focus their attention on what I consider to be the most important for my patient. Let's see how this might play out for Olivia.

For her, I'd list somatic symptom disorder first, partly because she's had it for such a long time. We know that people who somaticize tend to start doing so as teenagers or young adults, and that they often continue doing it for many years. They use their physical symptoms to cope with life stressors; being ill is how they see themselves, and often how they are seen by the world. So emphasizing this disorder by listing it at the top makes good sense.

However, the principle of importance for treatment is also an important consideration. Consider Olivia's own therapeutic history. (Although this is not a book about treatment, remedy is implied in every diagnosis we make.) Over the years, numerous clinicians' direct attempts to attack her depression have largely failed, sometimes after an initial apparent success. Failure of the same treatment that has apparently resolved a prior episode is not the usual experience of patients who have, say, major depressive disorder without any antecedent condition. Listing Olivia's mood disorder second hints at the wisdom of trying something different from the usual combinations of drugs and psychotherapy.

You can make other arguments to support the importance-for-treatment approach. Sometimes we can effectively manage one disorder only after we have successfully addressed the first—as when a patient whose severe substance use prevents a therapeutic focus on, say, anxiety symptoms. Or, once disorder *A* has been dispatched, condition *B* may simply fade away. That's sometimes the experience with a personality disorder whose symptoms later disappear, once major depression or alcohol use has been dealt with.

Whichever principle you follow, Olivia's alcohol use disorder, which is no longer active, should come a distant third. We've kept it in the mix because, following Olivia's own wisdom, we must always, always keep in mind the fact that drinking was a problem for her once, and it could become a problem again.

As far as a personality disorder is concerned, I don't think we have enough evidence yet to make it a firm diagnosis. If we did, I'd put it dead last, which is where I usually (but not always) place personality disorders.

Finally, let's just note that the alphabetical method succeeds only as a framework for information retrieval. Otherwise, we might as well file it under *Useless*.

By the numbers, then (the DSM-5/ICD-10 code numbers, that is), here's how I'd list Olivia's diagnoses:

- ◊ F45.1 Somatic symptom disorder
- ◊ F32.1 Major depressive disorder, moderate, single episode
- ◊ F10.10 Alcohol use disorder, mild, in sustained remission

And somewhere in the concluding parts of the write-up, I'd indicate that she has personality traits that could suggest histrionic personality disorder, with further evaluation recommended.

In the medical profession, at least,
the opposite of Occam's razor is *Hickam's dictum:*
"Patients can have as many diseases as they damn well please."

The Takeaway

At the beginning, Olivia is unhappy—*really* unhappy!—about being referred for evaluation. With consummate skill, we have coped with her resistance and persuaded her to accept ongoing mental health care. We've also demonstrated how important it is to explore a patient's medical history thoroughly, while also paying careful attention to the areas of clinical interest throughout the interview. We've invoked the principle that multiple diagnoses should be considered when a single one cannot explain all of the facts. We've discussed the differential diagnosis for patients with a lot of somatic symptoms, and we've concluded that the DSM-IV diagnosis of somatization disorder may be preferable to a DSM-5 diagnosis. We've also demonstrated the elements of a mental health evaluation writeup. And although we've discussed Occam's razor, we've had to leave it on the shelf, unused.

Break Time

Take a few minutes to turn (or click through) the pages of your newspaper and notice all the stories that concern mental health issues.

It's well worth keeping up with how these issues are portrayed in the popular press, in film, on TV, and on the Internet; these resources are where our patients get much of their information about illness (and about us). Over the years, I've sometimes been surprised at just how much a patient does know about a particular disorder—sometimes more than I do.

You'll find oceans of ink (electrons) used to relate findings that pertain to mood disorders; psychosis; autism, attention-deficit/hyperactivity disorder (ADHD), and other disorders that typically first appear in kids; and eating disorders. Multiple personality disorder (as it used to be called) is sexy and gets a lot of play; Alzheimer's isn't sexy at all, yet it gets even more. And of course, substance misuse is in the news 24/7.

But somatic symptom disorders? Not so much. And that's a great shame, because a lot of patients have some form or other of these disorders, and often not even their clinicians realize it.

16

To Tell the Truth—Pierce

Step 1

Pierce hesitates at the door. His eyes flick from one object to another, finally lighting on you. As he enters, he seems unsure whether he should pull the door shut; finally, he leaves it slightly ajar and slowly crosses to the chair you indicate. His pullover hoodie bears the logo of a local sports team, which is on its way to the playoffs. As you both settle into your chairs, you note his evident discomfort and mention the team.

"Yeah," says Pierce. He breaks into a crooked, strangely attractive grin, and leans forward. "This weekend's game should decide who goes to the playoffs. A friend gave me an extra ticket, if you're interested." He fishes a crisp ticket from his shirt pocket, lays it on the desk, and pushes it toward you.

Wow! Not even a full minute into the appointment, and already we need to discuss two topics: (1) small talk as lubrication for the interview process, and (2) the proffer of a ticket for the big game. What are your thoughts about these two issues—thumbs up or down on each, and why?

Small talk:

☐ It lubricates the machinery of conversation.
☒ It's a distraction; use it if it seems necessary, but don't consider it necessary.
☐ Avoid it! It's a time waster.

Free ticket or other gift:

☒ Always a bad idea—run from it!
☐ Let's not be overly doctrinaire; under some circumstances, you could accept it.

Note A

The first issue—small talk—is barely any problem at all; perhaps it's an issue more of style than of substance. But for what it's worth, here's what *I* think.

When patients seek help, they generally have one thing in mind: a pressing health care issue. With rare exceptions, at this moment they are not concerned with road conditions, the state of the economy, the weather—or the prospects for the local sports team. Of course, if a clinician begins an interview with a topic that's peripheral to the real reason for the appointment, it is with the intention of creating a relaxed atmosphere that will ease anxiety and promote the patient's sense of acceptance and safety. However, in my opinion, that emotional nirvana is better achieved by disclosing the problems that have necessitated the appointment in the first place. It's the difference between draining a festering wound and applying a bandage to hide it. That's why I always begin the first session with a new patient by saying, with no other preamble, something to the effect of "Please tell me why you are here."

Of course, if you could have deflected the first issue, the proffered gift might not have come up at all. And that, using our unerring retrospectoscope, would have been an entirely good thing. For you are now on the cusp of needing to accept (or reject, which can also be a problem) a favor from someone with whom your relationship should be all business.

As it stands, you are teetering on a boundary that defines the distance clinicians must maintain between themselves and their patients. This separation exists to prevent any chance that we will act in any way other than to support the health and well-being of those seeking care. That is, we clinicians must always put aside our own interests in the service of those who come to us for help. Although accepting a ticket to a sports event might seem a minor deviation from this standard, it is a step onto a slippery slope we must always work to avoid.

Rant

Let's talk some more about boundary violations. At first, I thought it would be a good idea to arrange the various types according to degree of potential harm. That turns out to be pretty difficult, if not impossible, since the degree of potential harm depends so much on the actual act, the circumstances, the patient, and the specific consequences. In the end, I've decided just to list, with a bit of explanatory material for each, the boundary types described by Gabbard and Nadelson in their seminal 1995 article (listed in the section for this chapter in References and Suggested Reading).

- *Sexual situations.* This one needs very little elaboration. An absolute proscription, it must be followed, without exception, by all clinical providers, male and female, at all times with every patient. It embraces (*sic!*) three sorts of situations. The first type is *sexual impropriety,* in which a clinician makes sexual comments or refers to a patient's appearance, regardless of intent. Comments a clinical provider believes to be humorous or trivial may be viewed as demeaning or embarrassing by patients, who often don't feel powerful enough to push back. The second type is *sexual transgression,* in which the clinician touches (perhaps even kisses) the patient in a manner that does *not* include actual, genital contact. The third type is *sexual violation,* defined as any overtly sexual act, regardless of who initiates it.

• *Dual relationships.* These include both friendships and financial arrangements that can imperil clinicians' ability to act solely in the interest of their patients. As Gabbard and Nadelson point out, the implied lack of objectivity is one reason why clinicians do not treat their own relatives.

• *Gifts and services.* Services might include babysitting or working in the clinician's office, possibly in lieu of payment for treatment. For one thing, office work could disclose the contents of other patients' clinical records. Of course, gifts can go both ways between patient and clinician; either direction carries a potential obligation that can distort the fulfillment of duty implicit in that relationship.

• *Timing and duration of appointments.* An instance would be to keep one patient waiting while spending added time with others. On an occasional, urgent basis, it is expected; we've discussed an example in the case of Fritz in Chapter 6. As a regular occurrence, however, it should be avoided. And seeing patients only during regular office hours, when other staff members are available, avoids any potential discomfort on the part of a patient who may feel vulnerable at being alone with a clinician in an otherwise deserted building.

• *Language.* Using erotic or seductive terms, or making personal observations about a patient's physical appearance, must be avoided. Even pet names or cute forms of address, such as "Honey" or "Dear," can cause discomfort. (Other than with children, I try always to refer to patients by last name and title, as I've discussed in regard to Melissa in Chapter 13.)

• *Self-disclosure.* Here's an issue where the boundaries are not so clear. We sometimes try to forge relationships through the exploration of common backgrounds and interests, such as growing up in the same town or attending the same school. These associations can be helpful to a relationship and are usually innocuous. However, revealing intensely personal material—especially the clinician's own emotional, social, or other problems—warps the strictly professional nature of a clinical relationship and can lead to enmeshment. And issues such as politics and religion should be reserved for private social gatherings outside work—if even then.

• *Physical exams and other physical contact.* Mental health clinicians don't often personally perform physical exams. If they do, it should be only with appropriate draping and a chaperone present in the room. More common is the issue of touching. A handshake at the beginning of a first session is both expected and accepted; physical contact in other circumstances is a bit more dicey. Touching an arm or hand when a patient is upset is something many clinicians will allow, but where do you draw the line? A hand on the back? An arm around the shoulder? Frontal hugs? Uh-oh, we're sliding into a serious problem area; once we're there, we may have no clue where to draw the line.

Overall, you can appreciate how important boundary issues are. They present decisions that you should give time to considering—before the need ever arises.

Step 2

You refuse the ticket (with thanks, and perhaps an explanation that your office policy wouldn't permit you to accept) and ask, "Why did you come in today?"

"You may be the only one who can help me," Pierce responds. "The last shrink I saw was a jerk; clearly, you're not like that." There's that crooked smile again.

"So tell me your story," you respond.

He breathes out a short sigh and his gaze drifts a bit. "It's a little complicated," he says, "but here goes."

Pierce needs help with his disability application. Several months ago, he was visiting in a part of town he doesn't normally frequent (" . . . but I was just minding my own business. Really!") when his car blew a tire, and he swerved into a power pole.

"I must've struck my head, because I lost consciousness for a few moments. When I came to, some people had gathered around my car. They didn't seem to like me very much, I guess, because a couple of them opened my car door, dragged me out, and began to pummel me. Then I *really* lost consciousness—I was out for 10 or 20 minutes."

When the police eventually arrived, they stuffed *Pierce* into the back of a patrol car! "One of the cops even kicked me! I mean, aren't they supposed to be *protecting* me?" Tears fill Pierce's eyes.

Wait a minute! He's driving along, minding his own business, when he has a relatively minor accident. Yet passers-by attack *him*? And the police first abuse him, then they arrest him? Nothing here adds up! How would you respond to a patient who tells such a confusing, apparently illogical story? I've provided a few alternatives:

- ☐ "That doesn't even seem possible! Don't you want to rephrase that?"
- ☐ "I must not have heard you right—you didn't say they arrested you?"
- ☐ "I'm confused: You were injured, and yet they arrested you. Can you help me understand this sequence of events?"
- ☐ Ask, "Is there someone else I could call for clarification?"
- ☐ Or you could simply ignore the issue for now, with the idea that it will all sort itself out in the end.

Note B

Let me state at the outset that, whenever possible, I try to avoid confrontations with a patient, especially those that occur during an initial interview. Early in a relationship, if hard feelings develop while you are trying to sort things out with the patient, you don't have a reservoir of good will to fall back on. However, in a case like this one, where the facts as you understand them just don't compute, your job is to try to root out the truth. (There's a diagnostic principle in play here: Watch for contradictory information.)

However, *confrontation* doesn't have to mean that you go to war. And the way I'd confront a situation like this one is to state it in terms of my own perplexity (as though I were the one who could be wrong), leaving wiggle room for the patient to avoid the appearance of deception. The form is this: "I'm a little confused here. On the one hand, *X;* on the other hand, *Y;* and those two seem mutually exclusive."

OK, I might state it in simpler language, but you take my point: I'm asking the patient to help clarify *my* misunderstanding. In so doing, I take care not to point my finger or otherwise imply wrongdoing or misstatement on the patient's part. And I most certainly want to avoid any implication that Pierce is lying.

What if, despite your careful choice of words, the patient remains adamant and your perplexity persists? Then you should move on to cover other parts of the interview, but with an ear tuned to a critical evaluation of all else you hear. At the end, if the conflicting bits haven't been resolved, do what you can to obtain information from collateral sources.

Now let's backtrack just a bit and consider Pierce's opening comment in Step 2: "You may be the only one who can help me." Of course, its intent could be completely innocuous, but this sort of flattering statement seems like an almost seductive attempt to bend you to the patient's perspective. For the wary clinician, however, it will have the opposite effect: to heighten the sense that there is something to note, to watch, to probe, but never to embrace unexamined. Opening gambits of this sort may be used by people who have long since learned their effectiveness in recruiting others to their point of view. Our job as alert, discerning professionals is to resist such siren calls to vanity—while leaving space to discover that, after all, it was perhaps offered without any such intent.

Rant

Are there times when it is OK *not* to trust your patient? Well, to put it another way, sometimes it's right to be pretty darned suspicious. This holds for patients who are currently incarcerated; those who have a past history of extensive lying (everyone lies to some extent, but we're talking about major-league prevarication); and those who have something obvious to gain, such as financial reward or relief from some obligation or punishment. The diagnosis of certain mental disorders should also sound the warning gong: Antisocial personality disorder is one; recurrent, active substance use (especially of illicit substances) is another. Otherwise, though, I try to follow this maxim: Trust the patient. And to that, I'd add the corollary, purloined without apology from nuclear arms inspectors: Trust but verify.

Step 3

So you say, "I'm a little confused here. You were injured in an accident, and total strangers responded with an unprovoked attack on you? And then you were arrested? I wonder if there's more to this story that I need to hear."

At this, Pierce's eyes again well up, and he comes clean. He had been lying—by omission—to conceal the shameful parts of this history. He drinks, and he was drunk when he drove up and over the curb, striking a 5-year-old girl who was pushing her dolly in a pram. Fortunately, only Disney Princess ended up trapped by the front tire of Pierce's car.

That was over 2 months ago. As a result of the combination—a traffic accident and two enthusiastic beatings—Pierce has sustained several ongoing problems. His license was summarily suspended, so he must take the bus to work. That means a 2-hour ride each way. And he faces possible jail time. And a lawsuit filed by the child's parents.

"No wonder I have nightmares." Pierce dabs his eyes with a tissue. He has bad dreams at night; and often during the day, he'll have recurring visions of the little girl lying on the sidewalk, not moving. "A glancing blow, thank God!" says Pierce, with real fervor. Since the accident, he cannot drive at all, of course, but now he won't even ride in another person's vehicle. "It's too terrifying even to get into a car," he explains. "Too humiliating. I richly deserved those beatings I got. I'll tell you, sometimes I wish they'd killed me."

He goes on to say that now, he doesn't do much of anything but work and go home. "I've stopped dating. Figured I might as well—I can't seem to get along with anyone any more. I can't keep my mind on anything, and I don't think I'll ever get my sex interest back. I just fly off the handle at the slightest thing. And if someone drops a book behind me? I'll jump a foot. I'm not depressed, like, you know, feeling horrible day in and day out, but I sure just wish it would all go away."

"And have you stopped drinking?" you want to know.

"Well, then, there's that." Pierce again sighs and glances away.

So what *do* you want to ask as you probe for the details of Pierce's drinking—as it was before the accident, and as it is now? In Note C, I've included a potful of issues to bring up. Depending on how you phrase your questions, you may come up with fewer (or even more) than I did. However you divide things up, try to write down as many important areas for inquiry about substance use as you can. (In the case of Douglas in Chapter 4, we've spoken of the newspaper reporter's traditional use of "who, what, when, where, why, and how" to elicit facts about any story. You might keep these points in mind as you clarify your understanding of Pierce and his many problems.)

Time out for a weaseling note from Morrison

I recognize that it can be really hard to play the game of "Guess what I'm thinking," which, in essence, is what I've asked you to do here. Up to this point in the book, I've mostly tried to avoid requests for guesswork and mind reading. In most of the questions I ask, I prefer to give some sort of a hint—such as multiple-choice options. So spend a few minutes trying to think of as many questions as possible. Then move on to Step 4, where I've thrown you a lifeline.

I'll start you off with two general questions:

"What substance(s) do you use?"
"How often do you use each of these substances?"

____

____

____

____

Now add some questions to determine the consequences of use:

____

____

____

____

____

____

____

And, finally, come up with some questions to elicit what steps the patient has taken in an effort to stop:

____

____

____

____

____

Note C

After some thought, have you run dry, so to speak? It wouldn't surprise me, especially if you are a relatively new mental health caregiver. Move on to Step 4.

Step 4

Now read the additional history just below; see if it provides hints that help you augment the questions you've come up with on your own. Many of the sentences there I have underlined and marked with superscript numbers, as I've done in a few earlier chapters. These indicate statements that should suggest the questions you'd use as probes to determine the extent of Pierce's substance use problems. Once you've finished reading, you can go back to what I assume are the several blank lines at the end of Step 3, and fill in some more of the probing questions you would need to ask of Pierce (or anyone else you were interviewing about the effects of substance use).

> Pierce says that for the past several years, he's been drinking "heavily, way too heavily, <u>like nearly every day," and that it has even increased since the accident.</u>[1] <u>"And that wasn't the first time I drank and drove, though it's the first time I've ever had any sort of legal issue.</u>[2] <u>It's only beer, but it's been an awful lot.</u>[3] Even for me," he says, his voice breaking.
>
> <u>For several years, he has consumed about a six-pack a day, every day.</u>[4] <u>"Sometimes less, more often—it's more, I'm afraid," he admits.</u>[5] For example, last month on his 28th birthday, a friend gave him <u>a case of his favorite local microbrew.</u>[6] The two of them shared a couple of cans; then, despite his resolve to nurse the rest, <u>Pierce polished off most of the case that evening while watching a women's basketball game.</u>[7] "<u>I seem to</u>

need it for survival.[8] I know I drink too much, but whenever I try to cut down, something happens, and I just lose my resolve."[9]

That isn't all he's lost. His girlfriend (for 5 years, ever since grad school) recently told him that she was "cutting me loose. She couldn't deal with the fact that I was more interested in drinking than in her.[10] And I've been absent from work often enough[11]—hung over, mainly, but also the fire's sort of gone out of my belly, I guess you'd say.[12] The promotion I thought was mine went instead to some woman they'd hired right out of college."[13] He doesn't feel embittered; he is smart, educated, and has retained his perspective on his own behavior.[14] "I have no one to blame but myself.[15] I know that I've got to make a change in my life—maybe even take something like Antabuse."[16]

For a time—a very brief time—he set rules for himself about when he would and would not drink ("I blew right through all of those—even had vodka for breakfast on a few occasions").[17] Thoughts about joining are about the only steps he's ever taken toward Alcoholics Anonymous (AA).[18] "I'd like to control it enough that I only drink for special occasions.[19] Trouble is, when you're an alcoholic, every occasion is special!"[20]

On the bright side, he's never even experimented with other substances—except pot, which "of course" he'd tried back in high school[21]—"It never did anything for me." He's never suffered from withdrawal symptoms ("no little green people, no shakes or vomiting"),[22] and he doesn't think his internist is even aware of his problem.[23] Of course, he's been "down because of the accident, but otherwise, mood's been pretty good.[24] Other than the thing with my girlfriend." He does admit that his mother has been after him[25] to take care of himself. "She worried I'm going to go the way of her father, who died drunk, frozen in a snowdrift."[26]

Now compare your list of questions from Step 3 with the questions I'd like to raise with Pierce in Note D.

Note D

Finally, here are the questions I'd use to dig out information regarding a patient's substance use. The material in brackets indicates possible responses. The numbers in parentheses indicate which underlined passages would suggest that bit of information. The first two questions are the ones I've already mentioned:

"What substance(s) do you use?" (3, 6, 21)
"How often do you use each of these substances?" [Times per day/week/month?] (1, 4, 5)
"For each substance, when did your use start?" (4)
"How much of the substance do you consume each time?" (4)
"What is your usual route of administration?" [Oral, smoking, injection, snorting?]
"Have there been medical issues as a result?" [Blackouts, vomiting spells, cirrhosis, ulcers?] (22, 23)
"Have friends or relatives suggested that you use too much?" (10)
"Have any of your relatives had substance use issues?" (26)
"What have been the effects on your mood?" (14, 24)
"Have you ever felt you've lost control over when and how much you will drink/use?" (7, 8, 9)

"Have you noted any changes in your motivation to get things done?" (12)
"Have any psychotic symptoms ever resulted from using?" [Illusions, hallucinations, delusions] (22)
"What have been the effects on your work?" [Missed work, reduced performance, being fired or laid off?] (11, 13)
"What effects have you noted regarding your family life?" [Discord with spouse/partner or other relatives, separation, divorce?] (25)
"What effects have there been on your other social contacts?" [Loss of friends, verbal or physical fights?] (10)
"Have you had any previous legal difficulties?" (2)
"How badly do you want to quit using?" (16)
"Has a doctor—or anyone else—ever warned you to quit?" (23, 25)
"Do you think of yourself as an alcoholic/drug addict?" (20)
"What attempts have you made to control your use?" [Setting rules for when you will/won't drink or use; joining AA or NA; use of drugs such as Antabuse, methadone, Suboxone?] (16, 17, 18)
"What success have you had at trying to quit?" (10)

Step 5

After that rather convoluted quest for data, let's move on to something simple: Pierce's differential diagnosis. As usual, please include all those conditions you consider possible. I'd also appreciate a note or two about each, in which you state how likely (or unlikely) for Pierce you consider each disorder you've included to be.

MDD caused by subs. use
Subs use R/t MDD
PTSD

Note E

My differential diagnosis for Pierce would include the following:

- ◊ Alcohol-induced depressive disorder
- ◊ Depressive disorder due to another medical condition
- ◊ Posttraumatic stress disorder (PTSD)

- ◊ Major depressive disorder
- ◊ Persistent depressive disorder (dysthymia)
- ◊ Alcohol use disorder
- ◊ Personality disorder

Of course, there's precious little support for some of these possible diagnoses. You can probably figure out why I've gone ahead and included them, but for the sake of completeness, I'll justify each selection. Evidence for PTSD and alcohol use disorder is pretty strong, so I'll discuss their formal requirements later.

Depression is often found in people who have PTSD or who misuse substances, so I've included several mood disorders on my list. For all his tribulations, Pierce claims he isn't seriously depressed, but we must be careful not to dismiss the possibility out of hand; lots of people with mood disorders fail to recognize just how bad they feel. I'll cite this diagnostic principle yet again: Always consider mood disorders. It is a category we should keep up our diagnostic sleeves, ready to hand.

What about a personality disorder? At first, I wasn't going to include it at all, both because I didn't see a lot of evidence in favor of one and because we hardly need one to explain Pierce's symptoms. However, as I began to write this paragraph, I realized that I really should follow what I preach: Because I even thought of it, I have to put it in. However, every so often, even when a patient qualifies for the diagnosis of a personality disorder at first interview, the patient no longer qualifies once the main mental disorder has been effectively treated. So, whether or not you've included a personality disorder in your differential diagnosis, I won't argue with you. But a really complete differential diagnosis would at least include the possibility.

Step 6

Pierce has been severely traumatized; symptoms have ensued. He may meet criteria for PTSD. But what does that mean, exactly? I could ask you to try to conjure up the different categories of requirements, which in DSM-5 are highly complicated, both for PTSD and for its sibling, acute stress disorder (ASD). But I don't want to risk traumatizing my readers. Instead, from one of my own books, I've boldly ripped off a table (see the facing page) that makes the comparisons a little easier. What you can do is to make a checkmark beside each requirement for adult PTSD and for ASD that Pierce fulfills. For now, we'll ignore the list for childhood PTSD.

Note F

When you consider that there are separate versions of PTSD for adults/adolescents and for young kids, and when you add in ASD, the PTSD and ASD criteria sets are perhaps the most complicated in all of DSM-5. But if we take these diagnoses in small bites and pop everything into a convenient table, we can make sense of it—and even perhaps remember what's required for a diagnosis. OK, let's get to it.

Comparison of Child and Adult Posttraumatic Stress Disorder (PTSD) with Acute Stress Disorder (ASD)

	Child (<7 years) PTSD	Adult PTSD	ASD
The trauma	☐ The trauma can be incurred by directly experiencing, witnessing, or just learning of an event; it can have occurred to the patient or to a friend or relative; if death or the threat of death, it must involve violence or accident.		
		(Trauma can be repeated exposure to repugnant aspects; see text.)	
Symptoms	*Intrusion symptoms (1/5)*[a]	*Intrusion symptoms (1/5)*	*All symptoms (9/14)*
	☐ Memories	☐ Memories	☐ Memories
	☐ Dreams	☐ Dreams	☐ Dreams
	☐ Dissociative reactions	☐ Dissociative reactions	☐ Dissociative reactions
	☐ Psychological distress	☐ Psychological distress	☐ Psychological distress *or* physiological reactions
	☐ Physiological reactions	☐ Physiological reactions	
	Avoidance/negative emotions (1/6)	*Avoidance (1/2)*	
	☐ Avoidance of memories	☐ Avoidance of memories	☐ Avoidance of memories
	☐ Avoidance of external reminders	☐ Avoidance of external reminders	☐ Avoidance of external reminders
		Negative ideas (2/7)	
		☐ Amnesia	☐ Amnesia
		☐ Negative beliefs	
		☐ Distortion → self-blame	
	☐ Negative emotional state	☐ Negative emotional state	
	☐ Decreased interest	☐ Decreased interest	
	☐ Detachment from others	☐ Detachment from others	
	☐ No positive emotions	☐ No positive emotions	☐ No positive emotions
	Physiological (2/5)	*Physiological (2/6)*	
	☐ Irritability, anger	☐ Irritability, anger	☐ Irritability, anger
		☐ Recklessness, self-destructiveness	
	☐ Hypervigilance	☐ Hypervigilance	☐ Hypervigilance
	☐ Startling easily	☐ Startling easily	☐ Startling easily
	☐ Poor concentration	☐ Poor concentration	☐ Poor concentration
	☐ Sleep disturbance	☐ Sleep disturbance	☐ Sleep disturbance
			☐ Altered sense of reality of self or surroundings

(continued)

[a]Fractions indicate the number of symptoms required of the number possible in the list that follows.

	Child (<7 years) PTSD	Adult PTSD	ASD
Duration	☐ Duration: >1 month		☐ Duration: 3 days–1 month
Distress/ disability	☐ Distress or functional impairment		
Exclusions	☐ Not due to substances or to another medical condition		
			☐ Rule out brief psychotic disorder
Specifiers	For onset after 6 months: Specify *with delayed expression*		
	If there are dissociative symptoms: Specify *depersonalization versus derealization*		

Note. Adapted from *DSM-5 Made Easy* by James Morrison. Copyright © 2014 The Guilford Press. Adapted by permission.

As you have probably noted, besides the boilerplate, five main points are needed for inclusion.

- ✓ *Stressor.* Of course, there must be a traumatic event. It has to be one that the patient has experienced personally or that has affected a close associate; if it involves actual death or the threat thereof, it must be caused by an accident or some other form of violence. For ASD and for adult PTSD, trauma can be repeated contact with horrible details of the event (such as collecting body parts)—but it cannot be based only on repeatedly viewing, say, the cable news account of a tragedy. Without a doubt, Pierce has been traumatized—first by the accident he caused that could have taken a child's life, then by at least one beating.
- ✓ *Intrusion symptoms.* The event must, in effect, come back to haunt the patient. That is, there will be intrusive recollections, dreams, flashbacks and the like. Only one of these experiences is needed. Pierce has had both nightmares and repeated images (memories) of the little girl he struck with his car.
- ✓ *Avoidance.* The patient tries to tamp down these memories or feelings, or avoids places and events that might bring the trauma to mind. Only one avoidance symptom is required. Pierce isn't allowed to drive, but he won't even get into a car to ride with someone else.
- ✓ *Negative ideas.* Included here are worsening of mood or thinking that is associated with the trauma. These symptoms can include trouble remembering parts (or all) of the event; loss of interest in usual activities; detachment from other people; inability to feel love or other positive emotions; the opposite—ongoing negative emotional states (anger, fear, guilt, horror, shame); pessimistic beliefs (such as "My life will be short" or "I'm a terrible person"); and distorted thoughts about the patient's responsibility for, or the consequences of, the event. Two of these negative thoughts or emotions are required. At a minimum, Pierce has cut himself off from other people (his girlfriend), and he has lost interest in sex and other activities—all he does now is to work and go home. However, I wouldn't call his self-blame inappropriate.
- ✓ *Physiological/arousal symptoms.* Also in association with the traumatic event, the

patient must experience symptoms that reflect changed arousal or reactivity—irritability, increased startle response, excessive vigilance, disturbed sleep, or trouble concentrating. Oh, yes, and recklessness or behavior that is potentially self-destructive. At least two symptoms in this category are required. Pierce has at least three such symptoms: He's irritable, startles easily, and has poor concentration. And, aside from nightmares, we don't yet know enough about his sleep.

After all that, there's still the usual boilerplate stuff (yes, the rest of the diagnostic mantra) to get through. The symptoms must:

1. Last at least 1 month for PTSD (less than 1 month for ASD).
2. Cause distress or significantly interfere with typical functioning.
3. Not be due to the physiological effects of using substances or of another medical condition.

I think we can add those necessary checkmarks for Pierce to the table on pages 187–188. Whew!

It's interesting to compare the requirements for PTSD in adults with those for young kids and with those for the diagnosis of ASD in everyone. Although the symptoms we rely upon for diagnosis are essentially the same in all three lists, *fewer* are required for children, and *more* are required overall for ASD. Also note from the table the distribution of symptoms required for inclusion in each of these diagnoses. You'll never remember all of this stuff, but you can at least keep in mind the five *types* of required information with the mnemonic SPAIN:

- Stressor
- Physiological symptoms
- Avoidance symptoms
- Intrusion symptoms
- Negativity

Or it may be easier to remember it as PAINS.

Step 7

If we are to decide whether Pierce also has an alcohol use disorder, what standard should we use? Let's proceed this way: I'm going to write down the 11 classic symptoms that characterize any type of substance use disorder. From the Step 4 narrative, just write down the superscript numbers of each passage that seems to suggest any of these 11 characteristics. Then, in Note F, compare what you've found with what I think does or does not qualify Pierce for alcohol use disorder. (In case you're having a sense of *déjà vu*, this *is* the same list you've encountered in our discussion of Fritz in Chapter 6.)

- Using more. Many patients use more of their substance of choice than they intend.
- Control issues. The person wants to control use or repeatedly fails in attempts at control.

- Time investment. Many people, especially those who use drugs other than alcohol, spend much of their time ensuring continuity of their supply.
- Craving. A lasting desire for the substance has been linked to dopamine release in chemical dependence and other addictive behaviors such as gambling.
- Shirking obligations. Patients may abandon their roles at home, in the community, or at work in favor of substance use.
- Worsening social or interpersonal relations. Use continues, despite the fact that it leads to fights or arguments with close associates.
- Reduction of other activities. Patients ignore work and social interests.
- Ignoring physical dangers. Principal examples are driving a vehicle and operating heavy machinery when intoxicated.
- Ignoring health warnings. These can include ulcers, liver disease, and the well-known risk of HIV/AIDS and hepatitis, as well as suicidal ideas, mood disorders, and psychoses.
- Tolerance. Tolerance has developed when prolonged use causes the body to become accustomed to the chemical effects (especially those of alcohol, opioids, and sedatives). The patient either requires more of the substance to obtain the same effect or feels less effect from the same dose.
- Withdrawal. Sudden cessation of use causes a symptom picture that is characteristic for the specific class of substance.

So what do you say? Does Pierce meet the DSM-5 requirement for alcohol use disorder—that is, does he fulfill at least 2 of the 11 criteria above within a 12-month period? If so, which ones?

Note G

Actually, there's pretty good evidence for Pierce's alcohol use disorder, isn't there? He's been drinking heavily (if "only" beer) for several years, and at times has used more than he'd intended (he polished off the whole case of beer he received as a gift). And in the past year, he's failed to control his drinking, despite his desire to do so. His social relationships have suffered (his girlfriend has sent him packing), and he's been absent from work often enough that he's lost a coveted promotion (failure to fulfill obligations at work). He's repeatedly driven his car when intoxicated—once with disastrous consequences. That's at least five symptoms right there, and only two are required for an entry-level diagnosis of alcohol use disorder.

Step 8

Now what should we state as the level of severity for Pierce's alcohol use? Go with your gut feeling, and then compare that with the DSM-5 recommendations, which I'll discuss next. Your assessment of Pierce's severity of drinking:

☐ Mild
☐ Moderate
☐ Severe

Note H

I would judge that Pierce has a *moderate* case of alcohol use disorder. I base my seat-of-the-pants evaluation on the fact that, by my count, he's had five different problems from his drinking (so it's worse than *mild*); yet he remains employed and has not had physiological symptoms such as tolerance or withdrawal (so it's less than *severe*). And that judgment squares pretty well with DSM-5 recommendations, which are as follows: Two or three symptoms should be scored as *mild,* four or five symptoms as *moderate,* and six or more symptoms as *severe*. Anything less earns no diagnosis at all.

The two symptom rating scales—DSM-5's and my gut instinct—don't always agree so well. When they don't agree, I'll usually prefer my instincts. After all, I know the patient far better than the people who wrote the manual do. Regardless of the exact level of severity at which we peg Pierce's disorder, we can agree that his problem is pretty darned serious, and cries out for the remediation he acknowledges he needs.

Step 9

Finally, what do you tell Pierce to help him understand what's going on, what can be done, and what his outlook is?

I don't expect you to write out an entire speech, just a few notes to indicate the points you think a patient like Pierce ought to hear. Here's a leg up: In communicating our findings with patients, we should always address three sorts of information:

1. Your understanding of the patient's condition (*descriptive*)
2. Your suggestions for a way to proceed (*prescriptive*)
3. Your assessment of what's likely to lie in the future (*predictive*)

The three parts I've just stated are the bare bones of the matter; you can flesh out your speech in whatever manner suits you and seems appropriate to the individual patient. But for now, just jot down (in the margins) a few words concerning the information you'd communicate to Pierce about each of these areas.

Note I

Here's the sort of speech I'd deliver to Pierce. I have written it out, just to convey an idea as to what a patient might need to hear. However, of course, you (and I) would deliver it in as close to an off-the-cuff manner as possible. (In your interactions with a patient, it's poor form to say anything that sounds canned.)

"Thank you for your cooperation with this interview. I know it's been rough at times, but we've covered a lot of information that I think will turn out to be important for helping us understand how to proceed. Of course, this was only one session, and there's bound to be still more information that we haven't yet discussed. But I think I have enough for this initial assessment and the outline of a plan we can follow.

"Based on what you've told me, here's what I think is going on. Of course, you've experienced a serious trauma with your automobile accident and the events that came afterwards, and as a result, you've got symptoms of posttraumatic stress disorder—PTSD. But you also have a problem with alcohol, as I'm pretty sure you already suspected. I won't try to sugarcoat this: It, too, is serious and very much needs to be addressed. Then there's a third issue that I'll mention, if only to say that I cannot be sure of it right now. That's the possibility that you might also be suffering from a mood disorder. That is, even if you don't recognize it, you have some symptoms of depression. Because of the other problems—the alcohol use and the PTSD—I can't make a certain diagnosis at this time."

Next, I'd move on to discuss the approach to each of these issues. (I haven't mentioned specifics here, because clinicians will differ as to the approach.) However, I would say this:

"One of the very first things we should do is try to get a handle on your drinking, because it will be hard to address the PTSD and any other issues if you continue to rely on alcohol for support. And it's possible that once you've stopped drinking, the depressive symptoms may just fade away without much additional attention."

Notice how I've tried to couch some of this material in the most favorable light possible—by expressing optimism for the ability to understand the problem and to plan an attack on the problems. Note also that I express the outcome for the drinking problem in positive terms: " . . . once you've stopped drinking," not " . . . if you stop drinking."

And, finally, I'd give the overall prognosis, which for Pierce would be some variation on this theme:

"You've come in with two, perhaps three serious conditions—and they are distressing conditions. But here's the good news: With the right sort of treatment, and with a lot of sustained effort on your part, we should be able to make progress and arrive at a point where we have a good handle on each of them. You can have a good life, a productive career—overall, I'd expect a happy outcome.

"Now, what questions do you have for me?"

The Takeaway

What a journey we've been on with Pierce! He's begun by inappropriately trying to win us over with a gift and unearned praise; with an appropriate response, we've managed the beginnings of a solid relationship that has led to a multiple-part diagnosis and recommendations about treatment. We've made good use of the diagnostic principle "Watch for contradictory information," and managed to question apparent contradictions in Pierce's story without alienating him. We've also discussed the requirements for two diagnoses that often go hand in hand: PTSD and substance use disorder.

Here are some other topics we've touched upon: the use of small talk before a session; probing for details in a complicated drinking history; and the clinical maxim "Trust but verify." We've also discussed two methods of judging the severity of a substance use disorder—DSM-5 criteria and the clinician's "intestinal appraisal." And we've also talked briefly about the information we want to give a patient at the conclusion of our initial evaluation: descriptive, prescriptive, and predictive. Oh, yes, and—sandwiched into the middle of all this—my Rant about boundary issues.

Break Time

How often do we encounter PTSD in film and in contemporary fiction? When you consider how much of what we see and read is based on the ghastly triad of accident, sexual assault, and war, it happens pretty frequently in real life. But it occurs only rarely if at all in classical literature; it is, after all, a creation of the 20th century, first identified during World War I as a consequence of battle. To find literary representations, we cannot reach back much further than the fiction of Virginia Woolf (whose character Septimus Warren Smith in *Mrs. Dalloway* has what was then called *shell shock*) and Ernest Hemingway (whose tales about the war veteran Nick Adams were posthumously collected in a volume titled *The Nick Adams Stories*).

It's noteworthy, though we might argue all day about what it means, that both Woolf and Hemingway ended their own lives in suicide.

17

Encore—Quinn

Step 1

"It's just like the last time." Standing near the door of Quinn's apartment in the Sunny Acres Retirement Village, Quinn's sister is speaking earnestly. "And the time before that. In fact, it's been on and off, her whole adult life."

Quinn lies flat in bed, staring up at the ceiling, at the walls, even out the window—but never at the people gathered at her bedside. Her halo of grey hair radiates across the pillow; her mouth turns down at the corners; and her lips move only occasionally in a nearly silent murmur. Though what she's trying to say is hard to understand, she seems to be whispering about a coffin; perhaps she's saying she occupies one. But she only begins to speak, then drifts off without completing even one sentence.

"It's her coffin, all right," Cameron continues. "She gets totally morbid when she's this way. Talks about death—wanting to die, really. One time, maybe 15 years ago, she thought she *had* died and gone to Hell—which she richly deserved, she said, considering the enormity of her sins."

"And those were . . . ?" you ask.

"Completely in her head. I mean, the only place she ever goes is to church. But when she's in one of her spells, no one can reason with her. She just keeps crying, says she's the Evil One, and the only thing she wants is to be punished. She won't eat, can't sleep—what a nightmare!" Cameron pauses to reflect. "Of course, it's a nightmare for her, too. The doctor started her back on imipramine. She's had it on each of her previous four—no, it's five—episodes. But the last time, even that didn't work—it took ECT to snap her out of it. Since then, she's been well."

Quinn's gaze wanders around the room, never engaging with another person. Eventually it settles on her own abdomen. She plucks once or twice at her pajama top, which has crept upward a few inches. Her fingers drift over the stitch at her navel, where her appendix was removed in an emergency laparoscopic operation three nights earlier.

"Before the appendicitis, I wondered when she was going to get her depression again. I mean, it seemed about time for it—5 years almost to the week since her last episode. She's nothing if not reliable!" Cameron barks a short laugh. "She was even worse last evening. And the evening before, so the nursing staff tell me. I guess it's because none of the family's here to help her focus. And she's frightened. Though God knows, she doesn't pay us any heed when we *are* here."

As Cameron talks, Quinn becomes more active and tries to climb out of her hospital bed. However, she is too weak to do more than throw one leg across the rail.

OK, you know what's coming. I'd like a tentative (working) differential diagnosis for Quinn, with a star by the choice you consider most likely. And to make it more interesting, if the condition you award the asterisk is the same as mine, I'll include you on the "Wall of Fame" on my website (*www.jamesmorrisonmd.org*). Just email your name and what city you live in, and you'll be immortalized. (If you don't want your name used, ask to be included as "Anonymous" from your city.) Quite frankly, I'm not expecting a large number of names for my wall—though I could have it wrong.

____

____

____

____

____

Note A

Here's my tentative working differential list; I've hung stars on those I consider to be the most likely. Notice that there are two of them, because I think that more than one condition has contributed to Quinn's present state.

- ◊ Medication-induced delirium ★
- ◊ Delirium due to another medical condition ★
- ◊ Recurrent major depressive disorder
- ◊ A bipolar disorder, current episode depressed

Remember, if you starred the same diagnoses I did (anything with *delirium* in it—I'm easy!), you've earned a place on my Wall of Fame. How will I know that you actually asterisked the word *delirium*? Because I trust you to tell the truth—just as I trust what my patients tell me.

Step 2

Now that we have our working differential diagnosis, what sorts of information do we need to explore further? Here's what I'm getting at: In every initial interview, we want to obtain not just details about the present illness, but enough background information to give context to the patient's current symptoms.

Back in Chapter 1, while discussing Abby's history, we created a short list of the sorts of information that could provide direction in diagnosing a mental health patient. (For convenience, I've reprinted it below.) Please make a checkmark beside each category of information that could be important for determining our diagnosis. Do try to read and consider each line.

- ☐ Chief complaint
- ☐ History of the present illness
- ☐ Personal and social history
  - ☐ Early childhood relations
  - ☐ Family history
  - ☐ Schooling
  - ☐ Sexual and marital history
  - ☐ Employment history
  - ☐ Military experience
  - ☐ Legal issues
  - ☐ Religion
  - ☐ Leisure activities and interests
- ☐ Substance use
- ☐ Medical history and review of systems
- ☐ Mental status evaluation (MSE)

And here's one more task: What in the list above do you think we can safely ignore?

Note B

We already have quite a bit of recent history concerning Quinn's mental symptoms, and we certainly know a lot about her history of mental disorder. (Good point: We really should have tried to learn whether she's ever had an episode of mania or hypomania.) Even aside from that, there's still a lot of ground to cover. After all, we know next to nothing about her personal and social history, or her use of substances—unless we rely (too heavily, perhaps?) on Cameron's comment that "the only place she goes to is church." We'd like to know more about her medical history, and we've only scratched the surface of her MSE.

And here's my assessment of what we can safely ignore: zero. What I mean is this: Every scrap of information carries the potential for informing our decisions about diagnosis, treatment, and prognosis. Some data will be of greater value, some of less, to this enterprise, but it all goes to helping us understand this patient as an individual we need to help.

Step 3

Additional information from Cameron fills in some of the blanks in our information database.

Quinn and Cameron were born and reared in Nebraska, where their Scottish ancestors settled generations ago. ("That's the origin of her name, and mine. They're Celtic," Cameron volunteers with a hint of pride.) Their father died young of a brain tumor, leaving a young wife to cope with five children; Quinn was the youngest. She attended school through 12th grade, followed by some college. Higher education didn't seem especially fulfilling, so she drifted a bit, trying this and that, until she finally got into acting. It was mostly local stuff—a few television commercials and some dinner theater experience; once she had a small speaking role in a documentary that was being filmed in their hometown.

When Quinn was 25, she married; soon afterward, her husband was drafted into the Army. Within weeks, he was killed in a truck accident during a war games exercise—"He never even left the country," Cameron laments. That might have precipitated Quinn's first breakdown, during which she made a suicide attempt ("swallowing rat poison, actually—ugh!" Cameron comments). She was sad and withdrawn then, and she abandoned interest in her garden (flowers and vegetables), avoided her family, ate little, lost weight, and "slept most of the time." After several months of treatment that was mostly fruitless, she recovered spontaneously and went to work doing day care at a preschool. "She never remarried, never had children of her own, but she doted on the kids under her care. She'd've been a great mom," Cameron finishes up, with passion.

Cameron knows of at least two close relatives—"one of our three brothers, and an uncle on our mother's side"—who had episodes of depression. With treatment, both recovered fully.

Quinn doesn't drink. She has almost never had any physical illness, "except one July in summer stock when she came down with infectious mononucleosis." And, at last, we learn that she's never had a manic episode.

Now let's try to organize our understanding of Quinn's current mental status, following the outline just below (I've reprinted it from a Rant in Chapter 2).

- General appearance and behavior. Apparent age, race, posture, nutritional state, hygiene; clothing (neat? clean? type/fashion?); speech (clear? coherent?); activity level; mannerisms and stereotypies; eye contact; tremors; smiles.
- Mood/affect. Type of mood; lability; appropriateness (to content of thought).
- Flow of speech. Word associations (tight? loose?); rate and rhythm of speech.
- Content of thought. Phobias, obsessions–compulsions, suicidal ideas, delusions, hallucinations.
- Language. Comprehension, fluency, naming, repetition, reading, writing.
- Cognition. Orientation (person, place, time); memory (immediate, recent, remote); attention and concentration (serial sevens, counting backward); cultural information (for example, the five most recent presidents); abstract thinking (similarities, differences).
- Insight and judgment.

We already know about Quinn's general appearance (dressed in the usual hospital garb, she looks to be about her stated age of 79) and behavior (initially underactive, becoming agitated part way through the evaluation). We have only fragments of her speech. And there is so much we cannot gauge at all, due to the near-absence of cooperation from the patient. Is she oriented? Other than her concern about coffins, what is her content of thought? Even her mood is largely hidden from us, because she cannot attend well to any task presented her.

And this calls to mind an issue that we've discussed in the case of Elinor in Chapter 5, but that I would like to explore a bit further: In general, how should we assess that very important quality, attention span? The tasks DSM-5 suggests are great if you happen to carry around sets of blocks and tone-generating equipment, but we'd prefer something a bit more portable.

Just jot down one bedside test of attention you can think of, and then read Note C.

Note C

Although we sometimes tend to forget, attention is the quality we are really trying to judge in that part of the MSE where we ask patients to subtract serial sevens or spell *world* backward (two answers you may have given to the question I've posed in Step 3). However, such tests are subject to various problems. Some people are just more experienced spellers than others; some are better educated; some have greater facility with mathematical concepts and use them more frequently in their everyday lives. And when we ask for serial sevens, we tend to focus on the accuracy of the math while losing sight of how well the patient attends to the process.

Of course, you could order a full neuropsychological evaluation for Quinn. It should tell you exactly how well she can focus attention. That might take place the day after tomorrow, with a full written report sometime next week; obviously, you (and Quinn) cannot wait that long. But there's another bedside test we carry around in our heads without even realizing it, and that's what I'd like, well, to focus on.

The *months-backward test* (let's abbreviate it MBT) is simplicity itself to implement and to evaluate. First, ask the patient to recite the months of the year forward, beginning with January. Then ask the patient to do this backward, beginning with December. If the patient becomes distracted or otherwise bogs down, it is fair to supply a reminder or prompt ("What was the task again?" or "Where were we?" or, "So just before August is . . . ?"). See? No math required.

Though standards vary, most people finish the MBT within 2 minutes. Of course, if the patient accurately names all 12 months in reverse order, that's an unequivocal pass. This level of performance falls off with increasing age over 65, so that getting as far as, say, July might indicate pretty good attention span for some elderly individuals.

A 2015 article (cited in the section for this chapter in References and Suggested Reading) gives lots of details and recommends a simple grading system: 0 = Can't engage; 1 = Tries, but, even prompted, can't complete the test; 2 = The patient completes the test, though with prompts or mistakes; 3 = The patient completes the test error-free in 30 seconds or less (for a patient under 65 years of age) or 60 seconds (65 and over).

One additional caveat: If the MBT catches on in your institution, other interviewers may use it with your patient before you get the chance. If that's the case, performance may benefit from the effect of practice, and you will have to adjust your standards accordingly. Or use a different test.

Step 4

Because she cannot engage enough to name *any* month, let alone a string of them in either direction, Quinn would score zero on the MBT. That gives us the final piece of information we need to evaluate someone for delirium, which (at last) can be briefly defined as a neurocognitive disorder in which the patient's orientation to the environment *and* ability to focus attention (or shift it) are compromised. And here are the diagnostic requirements as applied to Quinn:

- A disturbance in attention *and* awareness. Quinn's ability to focus and maintain her attention is impaired: She falls asleep during the interview, and her gaze wanders. Her reduced awareness presents as disorientation (she appears to think she's in the morgue, being prepared for her coffin).
- Brief duration with fluctuating severity. Quinn has been ill only a few days, and the severity of her symptoms changes from time to time; she has the classic pattern of worsening in the evening—called *sundowning.*
- At least one other cognitive impairment. Besides the disturbed attention and orientation, choices for additional impairments include memory, orientation, language, perception, and visual–spatial abilities. Quinn would seem to qualify for a couple of these.
- Not due to coma or another neurocognitive disorder (such as worsening dementia). Quinn has no such history.
- Evidence of etiology. Finally, there must be evidence from history, physical examination, or lab testing that the symptoms are due to another medical condition or to substance use (or some of each). Keep reading.

Rant

Delirium presents a significant violation of the diagnostic mantra I've been pushing throughout this book. That is, other than another neurocognitive disorder (specifically, an evolving dementia), there are no other exclusion disorders to consider; the duration required is brief, rather than the minimal one that is true for most other disorders; and there is no requirement that it cause distress or disability.

So we now think we have identified delirium as the likely etiology of Quinn's symptoms. But what has caused the delirium? Actually, let's begin with this: What are the various possible causes for *any* instance of delirium? Please make a list of as many generic causes for delirium as you can think of.

Note D

Delirium symptoms *usually* arise somewhere outside the head. Although there are a number of possible causes to consider (see the list below), delirium usually occurs when several etiologies and precipitating factors gang up on the patient.

- Intoxication or withdrawal of substances of abuse
- Prescribed or over-the-counter medications (especially drugs that have anticholinergic effects, such as antiparkinsonian agents and antidepressants)
- Infectious diseases: infections of the bloodstream (septicemia) or urinary tract; HIV/AIDS; any infectious disease with high fever
- Endocrine disorders: Cushing's disease, hyperthyroidism, diabetes (hypo- and hyperglycemia), adrenal insufficiency (Addison's disease), inappropriate antidiuretic hormone secretion)
- Acute blood loss (shock)
- Metabolic disorders (liver and kidney disease), malnutrition, hypoxia (as with chronic obstructive lung disease)
- Toxicity (various poisons)
- Postoperative states
- Other medical conditions, such as systemic lupus erythematosus
- Vitamin deficiency: niacin (pellagra), thiamine (Wernicke's syndrome)
- And conditions arising from within the brain itself: abscess, tumors, seizures, head trauma, bleeding into the brain, meningitis, encephalitis

In addition to these specific etiologies, several general factors increase the likelihood that a patient will experience a delirium:

- Advanced age*
- Preexisting cognitive impairment
- Surgical procedures
- Impaired vision

It's so tempting, isn't it, to go with the diagnostic principle that the best predictor of future behavior is past behavior? Tempting, and so often right. But in Quinn's case, it's just plain wrong. And that's because there's another, preempting principle: Recent history beats ancient history. When the two principles are competing, I'll usually go with the latter.

Step 5

Now, very simply, how do we pull Quinn's diagnosis together? Don't overthink this one; a couple of entries will do. But then do also consider the possible specifiers for delirium: acute versus persistent, and hyperactive versus hypoactive versus mixed.

____

____

Note E

Here's the bottom line: A diagnosis of delirium needs to consider all possible contributors. That means a separate line for each possible factor. In Quinn's case, we can identify two for sure.

◊ [Antidepressant]-induced delirium, acute, hypoactive
◊ [Anesthetic]-induced delirium, acute, hypoactive

And to that I'd add, for the sake of keeping it firmly in mind:

◊ History of major depressive disorder, recurrent

Rant

With two reports published that year, 1995 was a great time for studying delirium in depressed patients. One of these reported that 6% of depressed inpatients were actually experiencing a delirium; in the second, the rate was 42%. (The difference is largely explained by the fact that the second study was limited to people age 60 and over.) In any case, the absolute numbers of patients who were misdiagnosed with depression is striking—and worrisome. Clearly, many of the clinicians involved had not been considering the safety principle of the diagnostic hierarchy.

Of course, the situation may have gotten better in the past two decades, but I'll bet there's still

*I have found that a clinician's operational definition of this factor tends to increase with passing years.

a lot of room for improvement. A principal difficulty with Quinn's diagnosis is that her symptoms are similar to those she's suffered off and on for years—but due to a different cause completely. We might well have been taken in by expectations based on previous experience.

Two other issues can complicate the assessment of delirium. One is the fact that it may coexist with depression; this was the finding of a 2009 study of general hospital patients age 70 and over, in 5% of whom the two conditions overlapped. The other confounding issue is that some patients may experience depression *after* a delirium. This relationship was documented in a survey from 2009 (another great year!) of five studies that reported this sequence of diagnoses in a mean of 31% of patients.

The Takeaway

Quinn has given us the opportunity to note (once again) that we should always adhere to our script for the full initial interview, even when the diagnosis seems obvious. Each of the major ingredients we need to include—chief complaint, history of the present illness, personal and social history, medical history, family history, MSE—makes a potentially important contribution to the quality of the final product.

It isn't often that we encounter a "clash of the Titans" as it applies to diagnostic principles, but here is such a case: The principle that the best predictor of future behavior is past behavior doesn't always pan out. Sometimes the principle that recent history beats ancient history fills the bill better.

We've also explored the meaning of the term *attention span,* its significance in the evaluation of a patient, and the methods we can use to evaluate it at the bedside—this time, the MBT comes up roses. In a Rant, I've considered the interactions (and confusions) of depressive disorder versus delirium.

Quinn has also given us the opportunity to discuss the possible causes of delirium. And finally, you've had a chance to make your mark on my Wall of Fame. If you haven't succeeded, don't feel bad; let it serve as a reminder that the pull of the past is a powerful force that sometimes keeps us diagnosing the same old thing, even when circumstances have changed.

Break Time

If you pay close attention, you'll find interviews going on around you 24/7. For example, listen to the style used by interviewers on your favorite radio or television (or podcast) news source. You'll have a fascinating opportunity to hear how news professionals ask questions. Usually they won't allow as much time for free speech as I might like (of course, they must move on quickly to develop the story of the moment). Too often, they deploy multiple questions before allowing an answer, and they may not pursue issues with logical follow-ups. So evaluate news interviewers with a critical ear, and consider carefully before adopting any elements of their style as your own.

18

Nil by Mouth—Randolph

Step 1

"I hope you can help me, but I don't see how." Somewhat uncertainly, moving slowly as befits a man of his apparent years, Randolph enters the room and sits on the edge of his chair.

"I certainly hope so, too," you reply. "Tell me what seems to be the matter."

"First, I have to know that you'll never reveal any of this—not to anyone." He pauses and fixes you with a penetrating gaze.

In this moment, you must commit yourself to a course of action. What should it be? Simple reassurance, perhaps, but do you first need a frank discussion about the limits of confidentiality? If so, what should be the content? Are there some loopholes that you need to point out and explain? Please outline in a few words what you'd say.

General statement of reassurance: ______________________________

Loophole 1: ______________________________

Loophole 2: ______________________________

Note A

As caring clinicians, our instinct is to soothe patients with comforting words about how safe they are, whatever they choose to tell. But an unwavering adherence to that instinct would be misleading, even a tad dishonest, because the promise contains an escape hatch that we need to disclose. And that, rooted in the well-known 1976 *Tarasoff* decision in California, is the duty to protect any person who is identified as a possible target of threats a patient reveals during an interview. To justify breaking confidentiality, the danger must be imminent; to fulfill our duty, we must tell someone who is in a position to affect the outcome—for example, the intended victim or a law enforcement agency.

We also have a duty to protect patients from any actions they might direct against themselves—threats or even veiled suggestions that they might make an attempt on their own lives. So I'd respond to Randolph's challenge with a statement that contains these three elements:

> "[1] Anything you say will never leave this office; you can rest assured of complete confidentiality. The only possible exceptions would be these: if it became apparent that you were [2] planning to harm yourself or [3] planning to harm another person. Then, of course, the law would require me to do what's necessary to keep you and other people safe."

The compelling logic of a statement similar to this one will almost always encourage patients to go on with their stories, in all their revealing and sometimes terrible detail.

Step 2

After a few moments of reflection, Randolph begins his story.

> "Last Thursday, my wife and I were eating breakfast. We've been married for over 40 years, and I've always felt that we had a close and loving relationship. Of course, our two daughters are grown and out of the house, with families of their own. I'm a professor of climate science at a university down state. I've been retired for several years—though I still do some consulting work—so I was in no hurry to get up from the table. But I could see that Elaine was fidgeting about something, so I put down my newspaper and asked, 'What's up?'
>
> "The following day, she told me, she was flying to San Francisco for a 3-day weekend. She was meeting a friend, who was attending a conference for work.
>
> "I was a little surprised—Ellie had never done anything like that before—and I sort of blurted out, 'Oh, that's nice. Who is she?' And she looked straight at me and said, 'Randy, it isn't a girlfriend.' "

Randolph breaks off his narrative and sits twisting his fingers. His eyes redden and his gaze turns away, then downward.

How do you respond to the storm you can see is about to break? Choose the box for each of the following that you'd pursue—and check all that apply:

- ☐ Try to forestall tearfulness with a lecture about emotional control.
- ☐ Offer something reassuring, like "I know just how you feel."
- ☐ Point out the things the patient has cause to be grateful for.
- ☐ Haul out the Kleenex.
- ☐ Take shelter and wait till the storm blows over.
- ☐ Acknowledge the patient's right to have feelings, and try to draw them out.

Rant

Randolph is older, maybe by quite a lot, than the average patient mental health care providers typically encounter. At first he speaks very slowly, and there is a lot of detail to cover. This is pretty typical of older people, who have had many life experiences and who may, especially if depressed, require more time than usual to express everything they have to say. For a younger interviewer, the combination can be a problematic drain on time and patience. The solution, of course, lies solely with the interviewer, who must learn to adapt to the needs of patients whose concerns lie on the far horizon of most young clinicians.

Note B

Let's first acknowledge that none of the five Step 2 choices is truly sufficient. But one is just plain wrong, and I wouldn't bother with a couple of the others, either.

Patient emotionality makes some clinicians feel uncomfortable. Sometimes that may be due to youthful inexperience; or perhaps it's because the clinicians cannot control the situation, and that gives them a sense of vulnerability. On the other hand, some clinicians welcome tears as an opportunity not only to tap into a patient's emotional state, but also to flush away inhibitions that may be filtering out important content of thought.

Enough theorizing; it's time for action. But, in fact, not a lot of action on your part is necessary. What you do need is a dollop each of three T's: tolerance, time, and tissues.

It's probably pretty obvious that trying to force control on someone in whom you'd like to encourage frankness of expression is usually the wrong course to take. So the first choice in the list in Step 2 is the thumbs-down loser. Of course, tolerance for tears can be a heavy lift; as mental health clinicians, we naturally want to fix things, and this is one that we cannot directly address. The clichés people commonly use to try to provide comfort ("It's OK," "It'll be all right," "I know how you feel") are likely to be either wrong (you both know that it *isn't* OK) or banal. So you should probably avoid the next two choices, too.

Mostly we're forced to sit back and wait it out. That's one reason clinicians keep boxes of facial tissues at the ready. Offering one carries the recognition that you've noticed the problem and would like to help—and that you realize it will take the patient a bit of time (usually brief) to fight through the tears and restore the flow of information. And that's what's OK. If I feel the need to say something, or if the patient hesitates or otherwise seems to need reassurance, then I'll make a short speech of this sort: "Everyone gets overwhelmed by emotion sometimes. Just take your time, and when you're ready, tell me about it."

Step 3

"Just take a moment," you say, "and in your own time, tell me what happened next." And in a minute or two, Randolph does.

"Well, I knew that Ellie'd had an email relationship with Gregory, an old friend of hers from way back in high school. They'd reconnected at their 50th reunion last year. But I didn't realize that they had been, um, that closely connected." Randolph looks up and actually smiles a little. "I asked her, 'Is this going to be a romantic weekend?', and when she said 'Yes,' I didn't comment further—didn't want to have an argument."

When Randolph pauses, you repeat, "You didn't want an argument." After a moment, Randolph nods and says, "Let me explain the situation more fully.

"You see, four or five years ago, I was having severe trouble with urination. My doctor diagnosed it as an overgrown prostate and recommended an operation. He told me there was a chance that I could become impotent, though he claimed that didn't usually happen. After a lot of soul searching, and a full, frank discussion with Ellie, I decided to have the surgery. It went very well; I had no trouble with incontinence, the other complication that sometimes occurs. But I'm one of those who have been left with a complete inability to achieve an erection."

Randolph pauses, then chuckles. "It taught me this: Impotence is a concept much more satisfactory as metaphor than as medical fact."

Randolph's revelation about his sexual difficulty poses a conundrum. Now, with two important narrative threads to pursue, which do you follow up—the main issue of his marital relationship, or the erectile dysfunction? Check your preference:

- ☐ Marital issues
- ☐ Erectile dysfunction

Note C

I'm afraid I've posed something of a false forced choice. When you come right down to it, it doesn't makes a lot of difference whether you continue with the main thread of your questioning, or divert to the other issue of the sexual side of Randolph's relationship with his wife. That is, it doesn't matter *if* you remember eventually to explore them both. (Here's a good spot to make a quick note to yourself, as a reminder that you need to come back to the issue later on.) What I would do in this circumstance is to let the patient decide. That is, simply supply something nondirective, and prepare to listen.

Step 4

We'll use the underlined portions of the last paragraph later.

You elect to stay nondirective and say, "Tell me some more." Randolph shifts uncomfortably in his chair, then leans forward.

"So that's the background. Gregory apparently was going to a meeting for work, and had invited her to meet him there. She'd pay her own airfare; he didn't want any extra bills or credit card statements that might tip off his wife. They'd spend evenings together. And nights. So considering my own health history, I thought I understood her when she told me, 'It's just something I need to do. It's only for the weekend, and then—nothing. He has a good marriage, and so do I. Neither of us wants anything further.'

"And I can fully comprehend her thinking," Randolph explains with a sigh. "Throughout my adult life, I've been cursed with the ability to appreciate the other person's point of view, almost no matter how different it might be from my own. This situation certainly comports with that paradigm! So I offered to take her to her plane, and she said, 'Thank you, that would be lovely.' On Friday, at the airport dropoff, I got her bag from the trunk of the car, we kissed, and I watched as she walked—a little hesitantly, I thought, though that might have been my wishful imagination—through the sliding door.

"The rest of the weekend is sort of a blur. I did some work, read the newspaper online—*very* thoroughly, I might add—drank coffee, but ate next to nothing. I just didn't feel hungry. She called Friday afternoon and again on Saturday to tell me what she was doing—going to museums, mainly, while Gregory was attending meetings. She told me she loved me, and was looking forward to seeing me.

"After we hung up, I cried." And, indeed, a tear escapes now and runs down the side of Randolph's nose. "But I kept on with my work. Got quite a lot accomplished, actually. I had a drink—one glass of wine, is all—with George, my next-door neighbor, who came over Friday evening to discuss the agenda for our next neighborhood association meeting; he's president this year."

On Saturday, he again drank a single glass of wine. Throughout that weekend, Randolph slept soundly, as he has done since. He says that he's continued to concentrate "pretty well" on his work. He denies feeling despondent ("Just, you know, deeply perplexed?") and insists that he is "certainly not" suicidal.

"When she returned, I met her at the airport," Randolph continues. "She hugged and kissed me, with real fervor, I thought. And we didn't say anything more about her trip. And in the days since, we've ignored it completely. Not a word has come out of her mouth. I suppose I didn't ask her for more information because I was afraid of what she might say. But I still think about it—a lot—and that's why I came in today. To see what *you* might think about it, about someone who still loves and reveres his spouse, after what's happened."

A few more questions reveal that Randolph has had no history of alcohol or drug use, and his medical history, apart from the prostate operation, has been unremarkable.

At that point, you switch to the elucidation of his erectile difficulties, which began immediately after his operation 4 years ago. Ever since, he's been completely unable to have normal intercourse. They've tried Viagra ("Total bust"), injections ("Quite frankly, it was a little too gross for either of us"), and a pump ("It totally removed romance from the equation. By mutual consent, we gave it up"). "I just resigned myself to a love life of cuddles and nothing more; I thought that was Elaine's conclusion, too. Neither one of us had ever strayed before, not in 40 years of marriage."

That's a lot of information, most of which we will use to good effect later on. For right now, let's just focus on the information about Randolph's sexual incapacity. Because it is so personal, and usually a matter of strict privacy, a person's sexuality can be difficult for clinicians to delve into. Using pretty much just the last paragraph—and especially the underlined sections—please think of some general questions (beyond my favorite, "Tell me more about that") that you think might be asked to elicit this type of information. I've left room for seven, but you might think of still more.

Note D

Here are some of the questions that should be on anyone's list in the pursuit of this sort of information:

"When did the incapacity start?"
"Is it total or partial?"
"What has been your partner's response—and overall attitude?"
"What have you done, on your own and as a couple, to try to ameliorate the impotence—pills, injections, mechanical devices?"
"Have any of these been successful?"
"Have either you or your partner had previous outside relationships?"
"Have you ever attempted to have sex with partners outside of marriage?"

Step 5

And so, after this markedly different sort of history, I'd like you to prepare a deeply traditional differential diagnosis. Please remember: I like to include anything that seems conceivable.

Note E

Here's my differential diagnosis for Randolph.

- ◊ Substance/medication-induced depressive disorder
- ◊ Depressive disorder due to another medical condition
- ◊ Major depressive disorder
- ◊ Any anxiety disorder
- ◊ Acute stress disorder (ASD) or posttraumatic stress disorder (PTSD)
- ◊ Adjustment disorder with depressed mood
- ◊ Erectile disorder
- ◊ Personality disorder
- ◊ Relationship distress with spouse
- ◊ No mental disorder

Did you include all of these? Did you list anything different?

Step 6

Of course, you know what's coming next: Please explain why almost none of the Note E choices fit Randolph's history and presentation. The winnowing process should leave us with one clear winner. You can just jot down a note or two beside each of the possibilities in the differential diagnosis, but I'm going to give my reasoning in full in Note F.

Note F

We'll keep things tidy by marching down the list in Note E, from the top.

Focusing on the tears and other indicators of depressed affect, you've likely concentrated on mood disorders for your differential diagnosis. Of course, you've included substances and medical conditions as possible sources, because you've absorbed too much nagging in the earlier chapters of this book to expect anything different. And also, of course, you just about as quickly ruled them out due to lack of evidence. But you are dead right *always* to be alert for these etiologies—for nearly any psychopathology under the sun. In response to his difficulty, Randolph did drink—two glasses of wine over a 3-day weekend. Hardly the stuff of alcohol use disorder.

When we hear *depression*, our next thought is typically *major depressive disorder*. (Make that major depressive *episode*, because we must of course always include a depressive episode of a bipolar disorder.) But for Randolph, happily, we can quickly rule out each of these. Yes, he looks sad, and he hadn't eaten much the whole weekend, but he doesn't have a single additional inclusion symptom of depression. That is, he's slept well; he's continued to be interested in, and to concentrate well on, work; he's had normal energy levels; he doesn't appear to have agitated or slowed-down motor activity; and certainly he's had no thoughts of worthlessness, death wishes, or suicidal ideas. He even seems to have maintained his wry sense of humor. There's also the major consideration of duration: Other than a hypomanic episode (which Randolph surely doesn't have), there isn't a mood condition in DSM-5 that we could diagnose with a duration as brief as 5 days.

Randolph does express some anxiety, but it's attached to a specific event, and it hasn't led to fear or avoidance. That rules out a specific phobia. He denies having panic attacks. He has ruminated about his wife's weekend with another man, but not about other issues; brooding over multiple issues, coupled with a minimum 6-month history, would be necessary for generalized anxiety disorder.

What about a trauma- or stressor-related disorder? Both PTSD and ASD explicitly require that the patient be exposed to actual (or threatened) death, serious physical injury, or sexual violence. DSM-5 mentions a whole lot of ways in which one of these could occur; learning that your spouse has been involved in an extramarital sexual liaison doesn't make the list.

Also included in the DSM-5 chapter on trauma- and stressor-related disorders are the adjustment disorders, but these require that the patient experience either an extraordinary degree of distress (that is, distress more intense than the stressor itself would seem to warrant) or impairment of social, job, or personal functioning. Obviously, those requirements force us to reject an adjustment disorder as our diagnosis of choice for Randolph. Sure, he's upset, but to an unusual degree? I wouldn't say so.

Erectile disorder? Well, for sure, Randolph has had erectile *dysfunction* that has completely disabled his sexual activity for many months; we infer that it has caused him plenty of distress. But the DSM-5 criteria for erectile *disorder* require that this failure not be explained by other mental disorders, substance use, or another medical condition. Aha! That last bit rules out the erectile disorder diagnosis: Randolph's difficulty is the by-product of surgery. However, we'd probably want to note in our written case summary the fact that he has had erectile dysfunction.

The effects of any personality disorder we'd expect to encounter throughout Randolph's life, not just at this one point. Of course, we cannot rule one out—but I think we can agree that with our available information, it would be an appalling stretch to attribute his current condition to a personality disorder.

The penultimate possibility, a relationship problem, is tempting, in part because it seems so evident. However, several issues get in the way. For one thing, DSM-5 states pretty clearly that affective, behavioral, or cognitive functioning must be impaired as a result—and although Randolph spent an unhappy weekend, his overall functioning has been pretty darned good. In DSM-5's examples of relationship problems, chronicity is prominent—but it is not at all the case with Randolph and Elaine. To be sure, since her return home they have skirted the issue, but their marriage has not been overwhelmed by the sort of difficulty a serious relationship problem might suggest, such as withdrawal, persistent conflict, or overinvolvement.

In addition to all the foregoing discarded diagnoses, Randolph isn't psychotic, doesn't dissociate, complains of no somatic symptoms, and hasn't experienced difficulties with sleep or impulse control. Although he didn't eat much the weekend Elaine was away, he comes nowhere near meeting criteria for any eating disorder. He certainly has no symptoms of a cognitive disorder. I think that runs us pretty well through the possibilities so distant that we haven't even bothered to include them in the differential diagnosis.

Of course Randolph is unhappy, but would you say that his distress is disproportionate to the provocation? I wouldn't. Would you say that his functioning is in some way impaired? Nope to that, too: He spent that difficult weekend continuing to work; he sent and read emails; and he visited with his friend George. He's felt distressed enough to make an appointment with a mental health clinician, but far from evidence of impairment, I'd call that a rather appropriate coping strategy. Buried in its introduction (which practically nobody reads), DSM-5 states that a predictable response to a common stressful event doesn't meet the definition of a mental disorder. In this, I agree completely with DSM-5. *Mirabile dictu!*

So our discussion has finally come down to a subject that seldom gets discussed: the patient with no mental disorder. Of course, we've reached this point only after ruling out everything else in the diagnostic manuals, and it's been a prolonged, picky process. Quite frankly, this end point is discouraged by the fact that in the United States, we usually pay for medical conditions through an insurance system that requires a diagnosis *other* than the absence of mental disorder. I've spoken with many clinicians who bemoan having to devise diagnoses that will pass muster for insurance purposes, even when a patient has no actual diagnosable disorder that any insurance will cover. A typical example might be an invented depressive condition in one partner to justify insurance claims for couple therapy. The diagnostic principle to invoke is this: Be careful in assessing data that are generated during a crisis—they can be unreliable.

Rant

Mental health patients who have no diagnosable disorder aren't often reported, but the condition, if we can call it that, is likely in the several-percent range. (One study of outpatients from The Netherlands reported it to be 14%.) And yet ICD-10 and DSM-5 haven't even provided a convenient term to use when it does occur. In fact, the DSM-IV term, *no mental disorder,* has been discarded, replaced in DSM-5 by this convoluted horror: "Z03.89 Encounter for observation for other suspected disease and conditions ruled out." Try squeezing *that* onto an insurance form.

The Takeaway

A diagnosis of no mental illness isn't unique, but it is pretty unusual. Or do we simply not think of it often enough? Randolph's story also provides the opportunity to consider how we offer reassurances about confidentiality and the exceptions we must always state (in the case of potential danger to self or to others). We've mentioned the problem that younger interviewers sometimes have in working with older patients, who may take quite a lot of time to tell their stories. We've also suggested how to proceed when a history contains multiple strands of information, both of which are important. And we've considered the various ways we could respond to a patient who displays emotionality while being interviewed. We've reviewed the questions we might want to ask of someone who is having sexual problems, especially impotence. Finally, there's the diagnostic principle of being wary of data that are generated during a crisis. Simply put, they are often unreliable.

Break Time

Who in the room has read *Anna Karenina*? Could I see a show of hands? (That's what I thought.) But I suspect that most readers are familiar with Tolstoy's first sentence, one of the most famous ever written. It begins, "All happy families are alike . . . " The fame of that sentiment is due, of course, to the fact that it serves as portal to his signature observation: " . . . each unhappy family is unhappy in its own way."* (You in the front row—you can put your hand down now.)

But let us put aside the widely acknowledged complexity of troubled families, while we focus instead on the happy ones and ask, "Really? There's only one way for a family to be happy?"

Traditional wedding vows, which we've experienced countless times in personally witnessed wedding ceremonies and in the course of film and television dramas, actually maintain a more realistic perspective. As the (for the moment) happy couple and their seconds gather at the altar, the person officiating invokes not a vision of blissful homogeneity, but shades of grey—not wealth versus poverty, but a sliding scale of treasure that ranges from richer to poorer; not in sickness *or* in health, but both and either, depending on what medical issues may come calling. According to the vows, then, marital bliss, with its ups and downs, is analog, not digital.

In fact, divorce is the marital state (if that's not an oxymoron) that is absolute. It's on or it's off (there's no such thing as a little bit divorced)—except perhaps when we read about two people who have married one another for the second time, which may be the topper to Samuel Johnson's observation about second marriages representing "the triumph of hope over experience."

What the marriage vows get wrong is the bit about "forsaking all others." With nearly half of American married adults admitting to affairs (sure, men are more likely than women to wander, but substantial numbers of both genders stray), that promise might be more nearly accurate if it read " . . . forsaking nearly all others, most of the time." Although nearly a fifth of divorces are attributed to infidelity, the majority of transgressing couples do not end their marriages. Or, if they

*An 2016 editorial in *JAMA Psychiatry* pointed out that unhappy families also tend to have risk factors in common.

do, their search for severance stems from other reasons. In fact, many couples endure all manner of issues of health, wealth, and strife—sometimes including serial philandering—and soldier on in, if not happiness exactly, a simulacrum of contentment.

As clinicians, it isn't our responsibility to sit in judgment (*contra* Dr. Krakower, the elderly psychiatrist who, at their initial appointment, advises Carmella to divorce Tony Soprano). Rather, our job is to provide a steadying hand when patients stumble along one of what must be many paths to "love, honor, and cherish."

For people like Randolph, spousal warfare—surely, hidden meaning lurks in the anagrammatic relationship of *marital* and *martial*?—has served to clear the air toward an armistice in which peace, and perhaps even a measure of serenity, can abide.

And now, dearly beloved, Break Time is over, and we return to our regularly scheduled programming. You may kiss the bride.

19

Ghost in the Machine—Siobhán

Step 1

A small, slight woman, Siobhán is carefully dressed in a style that seems older than her stated age of 33. Her husband, Bobby—she's requested that he accompany her into the room—sits quietly by as she starts right in to tell her story.

That tale begins with voices that she hears when no one else can. When they commenced, perhaps a year ago, they spoke to her in tones so hushed that she couldn't quite make out what they were saying. But after a few weeks they became louder—"bolder," she says—"and then they depressed me, so that I could hardly work."

At times her speech seems a bit pressured. But now, without showing any particular emotion, she pauses and looks expectantly at you.

Hmm. At this point, with a pause in the flow of information, some sort of encouragement may be called for. How do you respond? Or does it matter?

- ☐ Just wait it out; you can tolerate a little silence!
- ☐ Ask her more about the voices.
- ☐ Pursue the depression.
- ☐ Say something nondirective, such as "Just go ahead."
- ☐ Anything else?

Note A

Let's acknowledge that, this early in the interview, there are probably a number of issues yet to uncover. Right now, I'd probably smile and nod my head—the classic nonverbal, nondirective encouragement, of the sort we've discussed way back in Chapter 5 in the case of Elinor. After all, the main thing you want to express is your interest and sympathy, so that the patient will keep on with her story. But I'd make a careful note to myself to pursue in great detail whichever of these two important points she doesn't elaborate now. I know, we've already talked about the importance of free speech. But the concept is important enough, and so often ignored, that I tend to revisit it—again and again.

Step 2

"Wow," you say. "That's a lot of stuff. Please tell me more."

Maybe a month or 6 weeks after she started hearing voices, Siobhán became "continuously depressed," and her appetite plummeted to such an extent that she lost 10 pounds in a 2-month period. Almost every morning, she would awaken hours before it was time to get up. Lying sleepless in the dark, she'd become so badly frightened that she'd entertain thoughts of ending her life. "But I was so rattled by it all, so terrified, that I lost all my concentration; I couldn't have made a suicide plan to save myself," she says. At this, she begins to cry.

Because of the depression, she was hospitalized for a week. There, she'd been given an antidepressant, "which I was smart enough not to swallow. I'm pretty sure it was just part of the plan to get rid of me, so someone else could have the bed. But after a few days, they got their way anyhow—I checked myself out and went home." Although some of the depressive symptoms had eased a bit, they'd never really gone away. "I think this is just the way I was meant to feel," she says.

Siobhán pauses for a moment, apparently lost in thought. Then she spontaneously begins to reminisce about her childhood. She was born in Germany, where her father had been stationed in the (U.S.) Army. During a leave spent touring Ireland, he'd met and soon married a local girl. They'd produced three children; Siobhán is the oldest.

She remembers her childhood as a happy one. She denies ever being sexually or physically abused; just the thought causes her to shudder. She finished high school in Alabama, where her parents lived after her father retired from the military. She never considered college, but worked at a succession of clerical jobs, leaving each only at the prospect of better pay. She was married at age 25; she and her husband now have a 5-year-old daughter. The only relevant family history she knows is that a great-grandmother "had a mental illness that lasted most of her life—I don't know what they said it was."

After stating that her physical health is good, and denying that she drinks or uses other substances (Bobby nods agreement at this), she pauses again and gazes off into the distance.

Wow, indeed! So much to explore. Right now, we're dying to know more about her apparent hallucinations. How would you build a conversational bridge back to that topic? And why are bridges important, anyway? If you need a reminder, you can refer back to Elinor's case (page 58).

Note B

Using a bridge helps to maintain the perception that you are having a conversation, as opposed to running what could feel like an interrogation. In short, I'd want to avoid making Siobhán feel that she's being jerked around for the purpose of extracting information; rather, I'd want her to think that her interviewer is someone with whom she can relax and feel safe.

In this case, the bridge I'd use would be to repeat back some of her own words about the voices. Something on the order of "Earlier, you said . . . "

You can use just about anything that's gone before (names, places, anecdotes, emotions—this door is wide open) to ease your patient into another topic. And, as we've noted in discussing the case of Elinor, if you cannot find a convenient bridge, acknowledge that you are changing directions in your interview: "Now I'd like to ask something a little different . . . "

So I'd prompt Siobhán with this open-ended but directive—no, that's not a contradiction (refer back to the Chapter 5 discussion)—request: "A bit ago, you mentioned hearing voices. I wonder if you could tell me more about that."

Step 3

In response to your request, Siobhán will relate more of her story. But eventually, she'll run down, or lose the thread of her narrative, or start repeating herself. And then you'll have to start digging for details.

Any time we probe for information, there are specific issues to cover. These will vary, depending on the symptoms we are pursuing and other issues specific to the particular patient. Rather than asking you to come up with a flock of specific questions, I thought I'd write down what she says about the auditory hallucinations, and then ask you to figure out the questions that would have elicited the recorded facts. As I've done in several previous chapters, I've underlined and numbered passages that should give you hints. Ready? Here goes.

> Over a year ago,[1] Siobhán gradually became aware that her computer was trying to communicate with her—verbally! At first the voices spoke in hushed tones, and she couldn't quite make out what they were saying. But as the weeks went by, they became louder—"bolder,"[2] as she expressed it. Often there were two—sometimes even more—voices having conversations[3] with one another, about her. Although she didn't recognize any of the voices, she could tell that both men and women[4] were included among them. ("But it's not just me *thinking* I hear voices—they're real people[5] . . . real *something*.")
>
> In the beginning, the voices only bothered her at work ("That's where my computer is, so of course it would start there," she says, with a confident nod of her head); later, they began to accompany her home. Then she might hear them at any time, day or night,[6] perhaps coming from under the table or behind the refrigerator.[7] Once they even followed her into the bathroom, where they made rude comments while she was "doing, well, whatever." In fact, the voices commented on many of her actions[8]—her typing skills, the fact that she chews gum (which Bobby hates), what she was having for lunch. That's how she knows they were not just her own thoughts, spoken aloud:[9] "It's nothing like the sort of thing *I* would say—they aren't even very polite." However, she doesn't think they ever tell her what to do.[10]
>
> Once, she described these voices to a fellow worker, who advised her not to tell anyone else, lest she be fired. She has tried various tactics to make them go away.[11] But humming didn't work; neither did playing music through earbuds from her phone. "Once, when I was sure I was alone, I tried talking back, but that only egged them on. I never tried *that* again."

So, using the underlined bits above if you wish, what questions do we need to ask when probing for this sort of information?

____

____

____

____

____

____

____

____

____

Note C

Here are the principal probing questions we'd need to ask Siobhán to learn more about her auditory hallucinations:

> "When did they start?"
> "How often do they occur?"
> "When do you notice them?"
> "Are they male or female?"
> "Do you recognize them? Whose voices are they?"
> "Where do they seem to come from—inside your head or somewhere external?"
> "How loud are they? How distinct are they?"
> "What do they say?"
> "Do they give orders? To do what? Do you obey?"
> "Could they be your own thoughts? Or your imagination?
> "What has been your reaction?"

Of course, the probes we'd use to explore other symptoms will differ in their details, though not in their broad outlines: the *who, what, where, when, how,* and sometimes *why*—all of them familiar to those who read newspaper stories and thrillers.

Rant

In order to probe effectively, you need to know something about the disorder or group of disorders (psychoses, mood disorders, anxiety disorders) under consideration. Of course, any beginning mental health professional won't know enough and may forget to ask important questions. When I was a student, I could practice on patients who were hospitalized. I found that I'd have to make multiple trips to speak with them before I'd get anything like a complete picture. I learned that there's nothing like reinterviewing the same patient, sometimes several times, to help you remember the main features of a mental disorder. You probably won't memorize the complete criteria for each disorder; with over 100 criteria sets in the manuals, that would be a pretty heavy lift. What you do need at your fingertips are the main features, so that they will be in your thoughts when it comes to constructing your differential diagnoses.

Step 4

As we've discussed in earlier chapters (most recently in the case of Norman in Chapter 14), when evaluating psychosis, we need to determine whether DSM-5's A criterion for schizophrenia has been met. That criterion comprises five sorts of symptoms; what are they again? (This is one of the rare criteria for *anything* that we might as well memorize, since it is so basic and we need it so often; if you need a refresher, review the Chapter 2 material on page 26.) And in Step 2 above, we've gotten a hint that Siobhán has one of these types of symptoms that *isn't* hallucinations. Which one is it? And how do we investigate further?

Note D

To review, any patient with schizophrenia must first have two (or more) of the following symptoms, and at least one of the two symptoms must be hallucinations, delusions, or disorganized speech:

- Hallucinations
- Delusions
- Disorganized speech
- Disorganized behavior
- Negative symptoms (such as apathy and flat affect)

We've already established that Siobhán has had hallucinations. And in Step 2 she's mentioned, almost in passing, that the nurses at the hospital had joined in some sort of plot against her. That certainly sounds like a delusion, but to say for sure, we'd need further information. To get it, I'd use another bridge, one that reaches back to her previous comment—something like this: "A few minutes ago, I thought you mentioned the staff wanting to get rid of you. Could you talk more about that?"

Step 5

And Siobhán gladly crosses the bridge to tell us the following:

> During that first hospitalization, the hints were pretty vague: A glance here, a gesture there from staff members seemed to signify that she wasn't welcome. After she

"escaped from the hospital" and returned home, she continued to hear vague echoes of the voices, "like ghosts that whispered to me from my computer when I was all alone." It was then she began to feel—no, she *knew*—that someone was "putting listening devices" into her home, and that she was being followed by investigators (sometimes in cars or even by helicopter), who observed her and reported on her activities. When the voices told her that she must either divorce her husband or kill herself, she became badly frightened and agreed to another evaluation. By this time, she was so distressed she couldn't work; she was readmitted to the hospital.

"Not that it was such a bad idea, suicide," she says as she reaches for yet another tissue. "I've felt so miserable, death would be heaven by comparison."

Now she believes that her tormentors have followed her to the hospital; furthermore, they may have recruited some of the nursing staff to join the plot against her. Yet she scores a perfect 30 on the Mini-Mental State Exam.

And here is that spot in our program where, as the emcee, I ask *you* to write out a differential diagnosis. As usual, I've left some lines below for you to fill in.

____

____

____

____

____

____

____

Note E

Here's my take on Siobhán's differential diagnosis:

◊ Psychotic (or mood) disorder due to another medical condition
◊ Substance/medication-induced psychotic (or mood) disorder
◊ Mood disorder
◊ Schizophreniform disorder
◊ Schizophrenia
◊ Schizoaffective disorder

Step 6

And now, please, I'd like you to state your best diagnosis. That will involve a critical appraisal of the differential diagnosis, which I hope you will also do. Work through the list to nail down your best choice.

Note F

Here is my differential diagnosis, annotated:

- ◊ Psychotic (or mood) disorder due to another medical condition. By her own testimony, validated by her husband, Siobhán has apparently been given a clean medical bill of physical health.
- ◊ Substance/medication-induced psychotic (or mood) disorder. She and Bobby aver that she neither drinks nor uses drugs. Of course, she has been prescribed some psychotropic medications, but we know of none that might explain both severe mood disorder and psychotic features. (And she has refused to take at least some of these medications.)
- ◊ Mood disorder. Although I almost always consider a mood disorder, it certainly wouldn't be bipolar (Siobhán has no history of manic symptoms). She has symptoms that fully qualify for major depressive disorder (which can be accompanied by psychotic symptoms), but this diagnosis is ruled out if schizoaffective disorder better explains all the symptoms. Let's keep looking.
- ◊ Schizophrenia. Sure, she's been beset with both hallucinations and delusions for the better part of a year—long enough for a diagnosis of schizophrenia. But that too is overshadowed by schizoaffective disorder if the latter applies. Keep reading.
- ◊ Schizophreniform disorder. Nope, she's been ill longer than 6 months—so, despite my affection for it, we have to rule this one out too.
- ◊ Schizoaffective disorder. At last, here's where the money is. Let's break down the requirements to see how Siobhán meets them. The DSM-5 criteria for schizoaffective disorder are quite explicit, and not a little convoluted; here they are, paraphrased:

    1. During a continuous period of illness, there must be at least 2 weeks of psychosis during which there is *no* mood episode. (There may be some depressive symptoms—trouble sleeping, for example, or problems with appetite. But they must not meet the criteria for a major depressive episode during this time.) For Siobhán, the psychosis without mood episode occurred during the first few weeks that she was ill. Note that she doesn't have to meet the A criterion for psychosis during this mood-episode-free period of psychosis; she only needs to have either hallucinations or delusions. Siobhán has had hallucinations from the get-go.
    2. However, mood symptoms that meet criteria for a major depressive episode (or a manic episode) must be present for the majority of the entire duration of the patient's illness—that is, the lifetime of the illness, not just any given episode.
    3. At some time during the illness, the symptoms of mood episode must occur concurrently with the full A criterion for schizophrenia. (Briefly, this means that there must be two or more psychotic symptoms, at least one of which must be delusions, hallucinations, or disorganized thinking. Again, see Chapter 2, Note F, for a review.)

Reader, I've done my best to put these extremely confusing diagnostic criteria into plain language. Even so, I *still* find them confusing. So let's use the figure below to illustrate how Siobhán fulfills each of these requirements during the approximately 12 months* she's been ill. The relative time and symptom requirements are pretty clear when we sketch out her period of continuous illness: First, she experienced psychosis alone for several weeks, after which depression was added. The depression has continued, occupying more than half the total duration of her illness. Note that the key illustrates the DSM-5 criteria, not just Siobhán's symptoms.

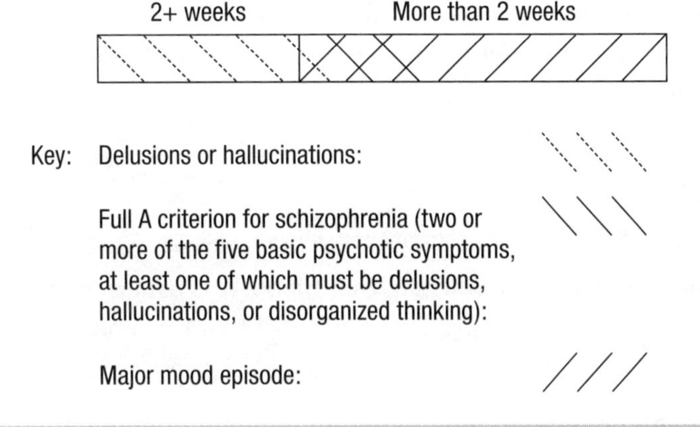

Diagram of the pattern of Siobhán's symptoms, with a key linking these to the DSM-5 criteria for schizoaffective disorder.

Step 7

And now, just to be really complete, let's consider the possible specifiers for schizoaffective disorder. They are of three sorts—*bipolar type* versus *depressive type; with catatonia;* and various specifiers for course of illness. I've listed the choices; you put an asterisk next to each of your choices.

Mood episode type:
- Bipolar type
- Depressive type

With catatonia. If the patient does not have catatonic symptoms, leave this blank; there is no *without catatonia* specifier.

*DSM-5 does not clearly state a minimum overall time requirement. However, if you use a calculator and a little logic to pick carefully through the requirements, you can deduce that just over 4 weeks is the minimum duration of time that would qualify. That is, there must be 2 weeks of *only* delusions or hallucinations, plus mood episode symptoms present for the majority of the total illness.

Course of illness (episode):

- First episode, currently in acute episode (right now, the patient meets all criteria for the diagnosis, and it is the first episode)
- First episode, currently in partial remission (there are some symptoms now, but no longer enough to fulfill the requirements for a diagnosis)
- First episode, currently in full remission (there are no symptoms of the disorder now)
- Multiple episodes, currently in acute episode (there have been one or more previous episodes interspersed with symptom remissions)
- Multiple episodes, currently in partial remission
- Multiple episodes, currently in full remission
- Continuous (the disorder is ongoing, with enough symptoms to sustain the diagnosis)
- Unspecified

Note G

Using the definitions above, we would say that Siobhán is experiencing an acute first episode of schizoaffective disorder, depressive type, and that this episode has not appreciably remitted.

The Takeaway

Siobhán's story reminds us that when we come to a fork in the road during an interview, we can follow either branch—as long as we remember later to retrace our steps to explore the other choice. This is one point where I would always make a brief "note to self" reminding me to explore the other branch.

We've discussed the use of probes, which of course will depend on how much we know about the disorder we are pursuing. (If it isn't enough, we need to be sure to reinterview the patient after boning up with a good textbook on diagnosis.) We've also stressed the importance of using bridges to move from one subject to another without making the patient feel jerked around. As I've noted before, an interview should be a conversation, not an interrogation. And, yes, I've gotten in another couple of licks about free speech and open-ended questioning. (Try to relax: We're approaching the final chapters—there can't be too many more such reminders!)

Siobhán has given us a grand excuse to review the five symptom types constituting the A criterion for schizophrenia—which are also useful to rule in schizoaffective disorder and schizophreniform disorder, and to help rule out other diagnoses of psychosis. This is an important bunch of symptoms: It's better just to go ahead and memorize it. Then we've talked about the pros and (mostly) cons of the diagnosis of schizoaffective disorder, and finished up with the specifiers to describe the course of a psychotic disorder—especially schizophrenia.

Rant

Schizoaffective disorder is a mystery in every way: It's mysterious how to make the diagnosis, and mysterious what it means. It's even a bit of a puzzle why it persists in the diagnostic manuals.

The lone clinician responsible for the seminal paper, published in 1933, was Jacob Kasanin, who was born in Russia and received his training in psychiatry in the United States. He didn't try to define schizoaffective disorder, but he did name it, and he described several patients who had both psychotic and mood symptoms.

DSM-III was the first diagnostic manual to feature actual criteria, which it included for every mental and behavioral disorder—except schizoaffective disorder. That's right: DSM-III pointedly omitted any guidelines for diagnosing this confusing condition. Since then, criteria have been included in subsequent editions of DSM, but they've changed with every new edition. Despite the ensuing confusion, this diagnosis takes precedence over other psychotic conditions—trumping, if you will, even the much better-validated schizophrenia. Popular though the diagnosis has been over the years, even today it doesn't say anything very useful about prognosis. That's one reason many clinicians disparage it.

In my opinion, some clinicians diagnose schizoaffective disorder far too freely. I'd like to avoid it completely, but some people do have a collection of symptoms that fits the definition (of the moment), and so I've discussed it. But I remain chary, and urge you to carefully examine other possibilities before making this loaded diagnosis.

Break Time

Ever think about how often homicide is the subject of dramas (stage, TV, film), as compared with suicide? The difference from reality is, well, dramatic. In 2014, over 43,000 Americans killed themselves, as compared with about 14,000 who were murdered. That's a real-life 3:1 ratio. Now let's compare that with the toll as described by an acknowledged master, William Shakespeare. In his tragedies (*Romeo and Juliet, Hamlet, Othello, Macbeth, Antony and Cleopatra, Julius Caesar, King Lear, Titus Andronicus,* and *Coriolanus,* plus the dark comedy/romance *The Winter's Tale*), a total of 64 deaths occur. Of these, 12 characters commit suicide (13 if we count Ophelia in *Hamlet,* who drowns in a murky pool under murky circumstances). At least 41 are clearly murdered.

Of course, the deaths of some Shakespearean characters are a little hard to classify. Take King Lear, for example, who succumbs to grief. Lady Montague (*Romeo and Juliet*) also dies of a broken heart, whereas Antigonus (*The Winter's Tale*) departs with the famous stage direction "Exit, pursued by a bear." Even if we disregard these anomalies, the Bard's ratio of murders to suicides is still clearly the reverse of actual experience. Of course, the world during Shakespeare's time was far more dangerous than our own—but even in contemporary films, novels (especially detective stories), and television shows, murder still wins hands down.

We can only speculate as to the reasons. There is overall greater interest in a whodunit; it is easier to depict the actions of a villain than the thoughts during a suicide; we experience a sense of satisfaction (and relief) when the murder is solved and the perpetrator is brought to justice; and once a suicide has occurred, further storytelling that involves the victim is likely to take the form of flashbacks, reducing dramatic impact.

The imbalance seems unfortunate, however, for it means that we probably pay too little attention to suicide—an almost entirely preventable conclusion to life situations for which good alternative solutions often exist.

20

Compelling Evidence—Tyler

Step 1

When Tyler gazes into a mirror, he doesn't like what he sees. Several years ago, when he was 15, he would squeeze the blackheads that had come to dot his cheeks and forehead. "I did it by the hour. Well, by the minute, maybe." His face does bear a few scars, though the cause is hard to tell.

"My mom—she's a doctor—she said I might have body dysmor—, um, dysmorphia. But I think that's just dumb." He stops talking and looks down at his hands.

"So is that why you're here?" is your next question.

"To tell the truth, I'm not even sure why I'm here, except that Mom made the appointment. I don't think I want to stay."

And, indeed, Tyler stands, picks up his backpack from the floor and slings it over his shoulder. Then he turns to leave the room.

OK, now what do you do? So many possible responses, so little time! You could:

- ☐ Keep silent and let him go on his way.
- ☐ Grab him and try to force him back into his chair.
- ☐ Shout after him that you'll call his mom for the information.
- ☐ Say, "You sound really upset. As long as you're here, perhaps you could at least tell me about that."

Do any of these appeal to you?

Note A

Of course, the laying on of hands is a total nonstarter; it would almost certainly be ineffective, and you'd be committing a minor battery upon the patient. Either saying nothing or shouting after him avoids physical contact, but neither offers much chance of rescuing the interview.

But the last choice does. It uses the well-proven technique of (temporarily) putting aside the substance of the patient's issue and focusing on the emotion behind it. Of course, we cannot be certain what Tyler is actually feeling, but it's pretty clear that he's upset. A statement to that effect carries the recognition of his unsettled state of mind, and it acknowledges his right to these feelings—whatever they are. It's a great way to proceed whenever you feel stonewalled as far as the facts are concerned.

Step 2

At the door, Tyler pauses and turns. "I'm not sure I want to tell you anything at all."

"I totally understand that," you say. "Coming here wasn't exactly your own idea. But perhaps we could just make a start, and then you can reevaluate after a couple of minutes."

"Yeah, I guess," Tyler says, and slowly returns to stand beside his chair. You wait while he shifts the backpack to his hand and finally drops it next to the chair.

"It just pisses me off, the way she criticizes," he begins. "And I stopped digging at myself last year—it was making me bleed. And none of this bothers me at all. But Mom, she thinks it's odd. And I don't want to fight her, so I'm just going along. At the bottom, it's those mental games."

"Tell me about that," you respond. Now he sits down and proceeds to relate the following story.

At age 19, Tyler is a first-year student at the local branch of the state university. Throughout the second semester, his grades have been falling, which he also attributes to "those mental games." They began during his junior year at a church-affiliated high school, when he became increasingly preoccupied with obscene thoughts about God. For no reason he could identify—"It just started out of the blue"—the thought came to him unbidden: "God sucks."

The first time it occurred, he was startled; subsequently, he became desperately upset and began to cast about for something to counteract this deeply unwelcome thought. Eventually he formulated the neutralizing thought "God does not suck ass," and for a time that seemed to do the trick. These thoughts—the unbidden blasphemy, the magical response—would interrupt him repeatedly, "even in the middle of a quiz in precalculus class."

Weeks later, he began mentally identifying each of his friends by a different, insulting, usually vulgar name. Although he never expressed these ideas aloud, he would torture himself by imagining the effect if he did. "Those thoughts terrified me, so that I then had to say the name repeatedly to myself, backward—'rekcus-tihs,' for example." He saw these mental gymnastics as a "magical effort" to ward off any chance that he would insult his friends aloud.

"It's so weird," he muses. "I feel I have to say those things in just the right way, and I'm not really that exacting sort of person at all. Otherwise, I guess you'd say I'm kinda sloppy."

Let's not be coy here. Tyler has obvious obsessional thinking and compulsive behavior. But can we establish that they meet the formal requirements for obsessive–compulsive disorder (OCD)? In the list below, I've outlined those conditions (each element is required).

Obsessions

- Repeated images, impulses, or thoughts cause distress.
- They are experienced as unwelcome and intrusive.
- The person tries to suppress, disregard, or neutralize them (perhaps with a compulsion).

Compulsions

- Repeated physical (sometimes mental) behaviors attempt to alleviate distress.
- They must be performed.
- They follow rules or respond to obsessions.
- The behaviors are unreasonable or excessive for the purpose: They are unrealistic approaches to the outcomes they seek to prevent.

So how does/doesn't Tyler fulfill each part of these definitions? You could just draw an arrow to the section in the history that supports each criterion. Or scribble some notes to yourself.

Note B

And here are my answers [in brackets] for how Tyler meets these requirements.

Obsessions

- Repeated images, impulses, or thoughts cause distress. [Tyler often has obscene thoughts that disturb him.]
- They are experienced as unwelcome and intrusive. [Tyler's thoughts are unbidden and upsetting.]
- The person tries to suppress, disregard, or neutralize them (perhaps with a compulsion). [He recites words backward.]

Compulsions

- Repeated physical (sometimes mental) behaviors attempt to alleviate distress. [Tyler repeatedly counteracts his obscene ideas with other thoughts.]
- They must be performed. [He feels he has to do so.]
- They follow rules or respond to obsessions. [Tyler is responding to an obsession, obscene ideas.]
- The behaviors are unreasonable or excessive for the purpose: They are unrealistic approaches to the outcomes they seek to prevent. [No contest.]

The bottom line: Without a doubt, Tyler fulfills baseline requirements for both obsessions and compulsions. But to determine whether he qualifies for a diagnosis of OCD, we'll need still more information.

Step 3

When Tyler traveled to Europe on vacation with his family two summers ago, he noted that he had far less difficulty with the mental games. The relative abatement continued during his final year of high school, but the problem reasserted itself at about the time he started college classes. He hadn't gone away to school—he'd received brochures from several top-flight colleges and universities, but "I think I just lost them in the mess of my room. And I kept putting it off, until the state university was the only option left. Boy, was Mom ever pissed!"

In college, he formed a new set of friends—for whom he soon created a new set of names. Although he is bright enough that he made the dean's list his first semester, by now the obsessions and compulsions are leaving him so little time for his work that he is seriously considering dropping out.

What diagnostic criterion do these paragraphs address? It is an important part of ever so many diagnoses, yet one that we too often forget to evaluate carefully. If you don't know or can't say right off the top of your head, feel free to cheat by looking in a textbook. (The very act of looking something up usually helps in remembering it.) Or you might remember that way back in Chapter 3 (page 34), we've identified a mantra for remembering the four features of any mental health diagnosis.

Note C

Yes, it is *distress!* That is, it's the "distress or disability" diagnostic criterion—the one that requires symptoms of a disorder to cause personal distress or to interfere with the person's personal, social, or occupational capabilities. (As you may recall, the full mantra is "inclusion, exclusion, duration, distress.") In the case of OCD, the behaviors must cause distress or impairment, *or* be inordinately time-consuming (operationally defined as eating up an hour or more of a typical day). Tyler's behaviors cause him distress *and* disability, *and* they consume an enormous amount of time. As we've noted previously, this requirement is an important part of many diagnoses, because it often distinguishes symptoms from the everyday thoughts and behaviors that normal humans experience from time to time. In the accompanying Rant, I've addressed it in punishing detail.

Rant

The criterion that symptoms must cause distress or disability isn't exactly ubiquitous throughout DSM-5, but it does appear in over half the various diagnoses. Many disorders that do not explicitly include this criterion strongly imply that it is there, anyway. For example, the texts for reactive attachment disorder and disinhibited social engagement disorder state that each "significantly impairs young children's abilities to relate interpersonally to adults [and/or] peers." And the text for Tourette's disorder, persistent (chronic) motor or vocal tic disorder, and provisional tic disorder says that patients "with more severe symptoms generally have more impairment in daily living." The criteria for panic disorder don't include those words, but the B criterion does include *these* words: "Persistent concern or worry

. . . " or "A significant maladaptive change in behavior . . . " Delirium "is associated with increased functional decline." And the texts for the eating and elimination disorders generally state that, depending on severity, patients may experience a spectrum of limitations, especially on social functioning.

However, a few disorders completely ignore the "D & D" requirement. The impulse-control disorders of kleptomania and pyromania, for example, may never cause distress or disability—other than for society in general or for an individual who is caught and punished. Criterion C for delusional disorder explicitly states that functioning is *not* impaired, or at least not much impaired beyond any direct impact of the delusions themselves on the patient's thinking and behavior. And of course, by definition, mild neurocognitive disorder does *not* result in functional impairment—if enough compensatory effort is put forward. All personality disorders are exempt, though personality change due to another medical condition does include the usual D & D wording.

Paraphilic disorders are a mixed bag. In sexual sadism and sexual masochism disorders, as well as in pedophilic, transvestic, and fetishistic disorders, the D & D requirement is absolute; by contrast, voyeuristic, exhibitionistic, and frotteuristic disorders include the wording as an alternative to acting upon the impulse.

Step 4

So we can now definitely include OCD in our differential diagnosis. The next step is, as usual, to consider and rule out other possible causes of obsessions and compulsions. Please write down those you think deserve at least some consideration for Tyler—as always, using the safety hierarchy.

____

____

____

____

____

____

____

____

Note D

Making the cut for my differential diagnosis for Tyler are these:

◊ Another medical disorder
◊ Substance use disorders
◊ Body dysmorphic disorder

- ◊ Excoriation (skin-picking) disorder
- ◊ Major depressive disorder
- ◊ Other anxiety disorders
- ◊ OCD
- ◊ Obsessive–compulsive personality disorder

Step 5

And now, using our differential diagnosis to suggest additional areas to explore, let's dig further into the history of Tyler's present illness.

> Other than an aversion to garden slugs and snails when he was little, Tyler denies having phobias. For years he has had anticipatory anxiety before exams, but he doesn't think it has been worse than what any of his classmates experience. He doesn't feel anxious at other times, except when he is thinking about God or his friends.
>
> Several times in the past year, Tyler has become depressed. These episodes last anywhere from 2 to 10 days and are accompanied by some initial sleep disturbance, but *no* loss of appetite or weight. He has never had manic or hypomanic episodes, delusions, or hallucinations. He admits that he has had occasional thoughts about killing himself ("I'd use a gun"), but he quickly points out that he has these ideas only during the worst of his "mental games"; they are *not* more prevalent when he is depressed. Although he volunteers that his mental games are "stupid," he feels powerless to control them.
>
> Tyler was adopted at birth, and he knows nothing of his biological parents. His father is an attorney, and his mother is a physician, "So I've never had any legal problems, and I've always been in excellent physical health," he says with a small smile. He takes no medications, and he has had no operations and no allergies. He has never abused alcohol or other substances. He has had almost no experience with dating: Although he has an abiding interest in girls, he has been afraid to try to form relationships: "I'm pretty sure I'll say something foolish and disgrace myself." Other than the presence of obvious obsessions and compulsions, his mental status evaluation (MSE) is completely normal.

Now which of the Note D disorders can we rule out? Which (if any) should we rule in? In short, what will be our best diagnosis? I think I know what you're going to say.

Note E

Because the symptoms of OCD are pretty darned blatant, this discussion may seem somewhat *pro forma*.

Obviously, on the basis of his history thus far, we can rule out substance use and other medical conditions as the cause of Tyler's symptoms (though, as ever, it pays to keep an open mind in the event that new data should emerge). We've included body dysmorphic disorder and excoriation disorder because of some historical information Tyler has given (in Step 1), though the further history seems to obviate them. He has experienced some depressive symptoms, but they appear to have developed subsequent to the onset of his OCD. Furthermore, they are not severe enough, nor do they last long enough (10 days maximum, and often shorter), to qualify for a major depressive episode. That leaves only OCD, which will be our best diagnosis.

On the other hand, later in the therapeutic relationship with Tyler, we should be vigilant for any *additional* diagnoses that might muscle their way in. There are a number of these that sometimes accompany OCD—depressive and anxiety disorders, for example, and tics, which occur in about a third of patients with OCD. Excoriation disorder and body dysmorphic disorder are also sometimes concomitant (though, as we've noted, Tyler does not currently qualify for either of these).

Step 6

Now let's tackle a question I'll bet some of you have already muttered under your breath: Why does Tyler *not* have obsessive–compulsive personality disorder? Hint: You can answer it in a single sentence.

Note F

Although DSM-5 lists eight possible criteria (four or more are required) for obsessive–compulsive personality disorder, they boil down to this: The person must show a lifelong pattern of being perfectionistic, being orderly, and manifesting a need for interpersonal and mental control. That's the single sentence I've referred to above. And just from the history we have, we know that Tyler doesn't qualify on any of these counts. That is, he doesn't appear to have a need for orderliness—far from it: His room was such a mess that he lost his college brochures, and he put off applying until he'd run out of options. Nor does he appear to feel the need for interpersonal control (he describes himself early in the interview as "just going along" with his mother). And, although he has to do his routines "in just the right way," otherwise he is "kinda sloppy," which argues against the concept of perfectionism. And—once more, with feeling—we try not to make a diagnosis of a personality disorder in the face of an active major mental disorder.

And that's the way it so often is: OCD and obsessive–compulsive personality disorder *can* occur together, but many people have one without the other.

Rant

OCD may have the longest differential diagnosis in all of DSM-5. That's because people either ruminate or perform repetitive behaviors in so many other conditions. Here's the list of disorders that must be ruled out, with relevant symptoms in parentheses.

- ◊ Another medical disorder (obsessions or compulsions, as with some autoimmune or infectious diseases)
- ◊ Autism spectrum disorder (patterns of repetitive behavior)
- ◊ Body dysmorphic disorder (excessive concern about appearance)

◊ Disruptive, impulse-control, and conduct disorders (impulses)
◊ Eating disorders, especially anorexia nervosa (ritualized eating behaviors)
◊ Excoriation disorder (frequent picking at skin)
◊ Gambling disorder (repetitive gambling)
◊ Generalized anxiety disorder (repeated worries about, well, everything)
◊ Hoarding disorder (inability to discard possessions)
◊ Illness anxiety disorder (persistent ideas of being ill)
◊ Major depressive disorder (ruminations about guilt)
◊ Obsessive–compulsive personality disorder (see Note F, above)
◊ Paraphilic disorders (repeated sexual fantasies or urges)
◊ Schizophrenia and other psychotic disorders (preoccupation with delusions)
◊ Specific phobias (repeated fears of situations or things)
◊ Stereotypic movement disorder (repetitive, non-goal-directed motions)
◊ Substance use disorders (preoccupation with using substances)
◊ Tic disorders (repeated body movements)
◊ Trichotillomania (repeated pulling out of own hair)

The Takeaway

We've started out with another lesson in combating resistance in a patient who would prefer to be sitting anywhere but in your office. We have then considered the definitions for obsessions and compulsions, and the diagnostic criteria for OCD. We've also revisited the important diagnostic component of distress and disability; quite a few DSM-5 diagnoses require the "D & D" criterion, which helps to set patients off from people who may have similar behaviors without enough disability to warrant a mental health diagnosis. And we've examined the difference between OCD and obsessive–compulsive personality disorder. Finally, we've noted that OCD has perhaps the longest differential diagnosis of any DSM-5 disorder.

Break Time

Are you a collector? (It wouldn't surprise me—most of us seem to collect *something*, even if it's only a jar full of pennies. Off and on, I've collected stamps, coins, books—even matchbooks, at one point in my extreme youth.) And is a collecting hobby anything like a mental disorder, such as hoarding or OCD?

When carefully examined, it's not even close. Collecting is neither inherently obsessional nor compulsive (the behavior is not experienced as intrusive or unwanted); it doesn't cause anxiety or distress (other than, perhaps, for the hapless collector who fails to obtain an object of overwhelming desire); and, rather than feeling driven to collect, the person embraces the desire. The aim of collecting isn't to reduce anxiety, but to increase pleasure (or pique one's curiosity or challenge one's interest).

Collectors value what they pursue for its intrinsic worth, historical interest, attractiveness, or intellectual stimulation. Hoarders, on the other hand, tend to be indiscriminate: They save everything, regardless of intrinsic or extrinsic value. Discarding anything causes them such distress that the hoarded items build up until they severely compromise living space. Collectors focus on particular classes of collectibles—dolls, toy banks, paintings, and a host of other categories limited only by availability and imagination. People with OCD see their symptoms as intrusive and (usually) try to resist; if you are a collector, you approach your hobby with enjoyment. If you have obsessive–compulsive personality characteristics, you might become so involved with organizing and perfecting your collection that its contents take a back seat to the process.

Whatever you collect, various principles can underlie its organization. Some collectors strive for an example of each possible item. For example, a Danish friend of mine is trying to collect a stamp from every country, municipality, agency, and company that has ever issued one ("ASFE—a stamp from everywhere"). Some people want only unused items; however, some (clothing collectors, for example) actually wear their treasures. Some collect only items of a certain age; others accumulate contemporary collectibles, which may have (as yet) little intrinsic worth—cat food cans, for instance?

To a few types of collecting we award special names, such as *numismatics* (coin collecting) and *philately* (stamp collecting). Less well known are terms such as *deltiology* (collecting postcards; *deltos* = a small writing tablet; the Greeks didn't use actual postcards). *Phillumeny* is the collecting of matchboxes and other match-related material. And who knew that collectors of teddy bears can claim a special name: *arctophily*?

It's been noted by others that collecting poses a challenge that entails no consequences if you don't succeed. So go right ahead and paste your stamps into just the right space in your album; fill in that missing (and valuable) Lincoln head penny from 1909; even festoon your kitchen walls with the dozens of antique cheese graters you've been accumulating in a box in the garage. As long as your kitchen and other living spaces are still available for their intended use, you're grand.

21

Character Reference—Uma

Step 1

A few days before Uma's scheduled initial interview, this note from the referring clinician arrives, clipped to half an inch or so of pages copied from her chart:

> *Uma has been my patient for the past 5 months. During that time, though at first she said I was her "savior," she has been an increasing source of disaffection and distress for me and the other people who work in my office—not to mention patients who have encountered her in the waiting room. Uma will complain to just about anyone—complain about the weather, the cramped chairs, the décor, the air conditioning, and (of course) the wait. By the time it is her turn to be seen, she has created a vortex of discontent that surrounds her and threatens to engulf our other patients. Indeed, in my opinion, she's the most personality-disordered person I've ever met.*
>
> *When you agreed to take her on, my staff cracked open a celebratory bottle of sparkling apple juice. Since she's agreed to see you, she's once again indicated that she would like to remain under our care here. But that ship has sailed.*

What's the problem with this note? (Check all that you think apply.)

- ☐ It disposes us not to like—or perhaps even to reject—the patient, even before we meet her.
- ☐ It prejudices us in favor of a diagnosis when we should be forming our own opinion.
- ☐ The clinician who wrote it may have come to a conclusion based on far too few data.
- ☐ Personality disorders are notoriously hard to treat, so should be diagnosed last.
- ☐ Symptoms of a personality disorder can cover up evidence of another, more treatable condition.
- ☐ Personality diagnoses sometimes disappear, once a major mental disorder (before DSM-5 did away with the term, we used to call them Axis I diagnoses) has been successfully treated.
- ☐ The note is too long and wordy—it needs editing.

Note A

You probably checked every one of the boxes, which is exactly what I did, too—even the bit about the length and labored syntax of the clinician's note. If anything should be clear to a reader of this workbook, it is that a complete history and full MSE are essential to making a diagnosis. Of course, no referral note can take the place of your own evaluation, though it can provide valuable context.

The other choices pretty much explain themselves. However, I do want to add a comment about how hard it can be to treat personality disorders. Notice that I said "hard to treat," not "impossible to treat." And perhaps even "hard" is inaccurate. We do know that it can take many months—perhaps a year and a half—before a patient with any personality disorder makes a lot of progress. Sticking with a difficult patient for that stretch of time can be taxing for a clinician; we prefer to see our patients improve immediately, if not sooner!

The upshot is this: When you get a referral note, be sure to take any substantive information with at least a grain of salt. And if it contains pejorative comments about the patient, better sprinkle on a second helping.

Step 2

Even before you've seen Uma, it sounds as though personality disorder is something you need to include in your diagnostic thinking. You'd like to plan the best approach to this diagnosis—either to eliminate it or to nail it down. So what should be the principal focus of your inquiry?

- ☐ Order psychological testing.
- ☐ Interview for a specific personality disorder.
- ☐ Obtain collateral information.
- ☐ Rule out major mental disorders.

Note B

To be sure, you can make an argument for any of these choices. But here's the one that's imperative: Before considering the merits of the referring clinician's impression of a personality disorder, rule out major mental disorders. Psychological testing? That's a down-the-road exercise that can augment your database, but won't accomplish what a complete history can. Collateral information? There is some already, from the referral note, but is it entirely trustworthy? However, interviewing relatives and friends who have known the patient for years will often unearth important information that might confirm, or refute, suspicions raised by the note. And, sure, if there is a personality disorder, you must determine which one—but that too should wait until you have settled the issue of other mental disorders. (Right! You know that already, but the issue is so important I have to make it explicit somewhere in this workbook.)

Step 3

From the referring clinician, you've got pages of history, including notes on office visits, physical exams, and laboratory testing. You put all this together with your own interview, yielding this story:

Uma Dunleavy is a 24-year-old single woman whose chief complaint is "I just feel scooped out inside, like a human jack-o-lantern."

The youngest of six siblings, she was born in the San Francisco Bay Area just a week before her father, a Navy retiree, died. When her mother wasn't drinking, she worked in a beauty salon; often she was absent from the home, accompanied by one of numerous husbands or occasional lovers. Uma thinks that at least two of these men may have abused her sexually when she was in elementary school, but she admits that her memories of this period in her life are "pretty sketchy." It is with clarity, however, that she recalls the physical abuse, which included beatings, kicks, scratching, and hair pulling by an older brother with whom she shared a room until she was almost 9.

Uma first consumed alcohol before she was 3, when her mother started giving her vodka so she would go to sleep. By age 14, she frequently drank beer, wine, and hard liquor, which she obtained from the older boys and men she dated. She claims that, prior to 8 months before this interview, she had no difficulties from alcohol use other than withdrawal shakiness.

She graduated from high school with her class—a testament more to her intelligence than to her diligence ("I was never a grind," she explains). Since then, she has been continuously employed, though she's moved around a bit (11 jobs in the intervening 6 years).

Her first "nervous breakdown" occurred when she was 15. When a female classmate whose popularity and poise she had greatly admired snubbed Uma in the hallway, she lost control and launched a serious assault in retribution. As a condition for remaining in school, she entered counseling and began taking Valium. Shortly afterward, she made the first of some 25 suicide attempts. About half of these have been with overdoses of various medications; the rest were by cutting her arms. Only one attempt resulted in serious harm (prolonged unconsciousness from "several" sleeping tablets); through the repeated interventions of a steadfast counselor whom she saw for 4 years, she was never hospitalized.

Most recently, Uma has worked—first as a security guard, later as a forklift operator—for a company that sells plumbing supplies. Especially during the past year, she associated with some of the warehouse workers, who introduced her to LSD. She states that during this time she would frequently "call off work sick," because she was so exhausted after a sleepless night occasioned by partying and drug use; more than once, she was threatened with dismissal. Her doctor pointed out that the LSD was causing her to have flashbacks, during which she would "see the world melt," even when she hadn't used the substance for several days. These experiences at first frightened her into swearing off the use of drugs, but as time dimmed the memory, she resumed intermittent use of LSD.

Last year, when her counselor moved out of state, Uma felt bereft: "I suddenly plunged into depression." In desperation, she called 11 different therapists before finally seeking help from a public clinic. From there, she was referred to a substance use program. In the past 8 months, she has used no drug stronger than coffee. Now rejected by the warehouse crew, she has sought new friends. In fact, she has rather suddenly entered into sexual relationships with several men; she believes two of them to be bisexual, yet she has taken no precautions as regards HIV/AIDS. "What's the difference?" she says. "You live for a while, then you die. No big deal." Not only does she feel no particular anxiety at the thought of dying; she also denies that phobias, obsessions and compulsions, and general anxiety have played much of a role (if any) in either her recent or remote history.

Without the use of substances to prop her up, she has felt increasingly "abandoned and desolate." At any imagined slight, she will fly into a rage far out of proportion to the insult; when pressed, she admits this. She has hit walls and threatened coworkers, and once she even called the police to complain that her neighbor down the hall was spying on her. "Most of the time, I realize that's foolish," she admits, "but when I'm feeling so awful, it seems everyone's on the attack. Now, without drugs, I don't even think I'm a real person any longer. I don't know who I am. I just feel all hollow. Like I said, scooped out." These periods of "feeling awful" last only a day or two at most, and she's never sought evaluation for a mood disorder. She is intelligent and generally cooperative; at her first interview, her affect seems perfectly ordinary, except when she talks about "what a waste my life's been." Then she is downcast and self-condemnatory. She denies having suicidal ideas currently. She scores 30 on the Mini-Mental State Exam.

Of course, this is the next question: What is your working differential diagnosis for Uma? And please discuss briefly each of the conditions on your list.

____

____

____

____

____

Rant

Lurking in Uma's history is the hint that she might have been abused as a child. Abuse of one sort or another has been found in the background of a good many mental conditions, including eating, dissociative, somatic symptom, and personality disorders. And even when these conditions are not the focus of inquiry, still it is important to assure ourselves that we've carefully evaluated every patient we interview for this sort of early-life experience.

Of course, most of the time our inquiries will come up dry, but when you encounter it—and you should screen for it, even when it's not presented up front—there are a number of probes you should pursue. These include the usual *when, where, what* information, as well as any information about the individual's own views on provocation, protection, and perception, both as a child and as an adult.

The screens? You can lead into physical abuse by asking whether the patient ever felt mistreated as a child, determining what disciplinary methods were used (physical punishment?), and then probing for details. For sexual abuse, you could first ask when the patient was first approached about sex.

Note C

Here is my working differential diagnosis for Uma, with brief commentary:

◊ Substance/medication-induced mental disorder. Although Uma has used LSD in the past, this does not appear to be a factor now. But it's good to keep in mind, should further information come to light.

◊ Mental disorder due to another medical condition. She's been cleared medically by the referring clinician; however, to paraphrase what a Founding Father may have said,* the price of freedom (in this case, from the effects of medical illness) is eternal vigilance.

◊ Other hallucinogen (in this case, LSD) use disorder. Of course, this certainly isn't anything very current, but, again, to note that there's a history is important—more as an alert to us, and to any successive clinicians down the road. Uma has had only a few symptoms related to LSD use disorder (as a take-home exercise, what were they?), and she hasn't used now for at least a year. So we'd list it as LSD use disorder, mild, in sustained remission.

◊ Any major mental disorder. These would include mood and anxiety disorders, evidence for which is lacking in the referral notes and from the current evaluation. I would especially underscore the possibility of a somatic symptom disorder; however, Uma's focus is on her feelings, not on her physical symptoms.

  I admit that I cheated a little here, by condensing quite a few possible conditions into one line of differential diagnosis. If you wrote down a whole flock of possibilities (major depressive disorder, for example), then go to the head of the class.

◊ Personality disorder. This comes at the bottom of the list, because treatment is hard and takes a very long time, and because a personality disorder can obscure other disorders (such as those we've just rejected!)—but it is important. Ultimately, it may turn out to be the money choice for Uma.

Step 4

After it's all done and dusted, personality disorder sits high on our list. Or rather, although it's *low* on the list, the process of elimination has floated it upward, where we have to give it serious consideration.

Patients with personality disorders have in common several features:

1. A pattern of behavior and inner experience (thoughts, feelings, sensations) that is . . .
2. . . . clearly different from the individual's culture. This pattern . . .
3. . . . includes these areas:
   - Affect *(type, intensity, lability, appropriateness)*
   - Cognition *(how the person sees and interprets self and the environment)*

*It's unclear whether Thomas Jefferson was in fact the first to say this. But he was the Big Guy, so he often gets the credit.

- Control *of impulses*
- Interpersonal relationships

Now which of these further characteristics also belongs to each and every personality disorder (check all that apply)?

- ☐ They are lasting (that is, lifelong).
- ☐ They are pervasive (they apply broadly across all areas of the patient's life).
- ☐ They are inflexible (the patient is stuck with them).
- ☐ They cause distress or impairment.
- ☐ Other disorders have been ruled out as the cause of symptoms.

Note D

If you checked all of the boxes above, you're a winner. In fact, what we've accomplished is to set down the essential features that describe any personality disorder. Now I'll appreciate it if you go back and reread Step 4; these features, taken together, are very useful when you come to analyze a patient's history for the possible presence of personality disorder. They are important enough, and they come up so often, that you should just commit them to memory.

Step 5

DSM-5 recognizes 10 named personality disorders, each with numerous distinctive features. Just to make sure we have in mind all the possibilities, here's a pretty easy exercise (really!): Match each brief description with the name of the relevant personality disorder.

1. These patients care little for social relationships; they have a restricted emotional range; and they may seem indifferent to criticism or praise. They tend to be solitary and to avoid close relationships, including sexual ones.
2. The irresponsible, often criminal behavior of these people begins in childhood or early adolescence with truancy, running away, cruelty, fighting, destructiveness, lying, stealing, and robbery. As adults they may default on debts, fail to care for dependents, fail to maintain monogamous relationships, and show no remorse for their behavior.
3. These people have trouble starting projects and making independent decisions. Easily hurt by criticism and often preoccupied with fears of abandonment, they feel helpless when alone, and miserable when relationships end. To gain favor, they may volunteer for unpleasant tasks or agree even with others who may be wrong.
4. Overly emotional, vague, and attention-seeking, these people need constant reassurance about their attractiveness. They may be self-centered and sexually seductive.
5. Such people are self-important, and they are often preoccupied with envy, fantasies of success, or ruminations about the uniqueness of their own problems. A

sense of entitlement and lack of empathy may lead them to take advantage of others. They vigorously reject criticism and need constant attention and admiration.

6. These impulsive people may make recurrent suicide threats or attempts. Affectively unstable, they often show intense, inappropriate anger. They feel empty or bored, and they frantically try to avoid abandonment. They are uncertain about who they are and unable to maintain stable interpersonal relationships.
7. These patients have such troubled interpersonal relationships that to others they appear peculiar or strange. Lacking close friends, they are uncomfortable in social situations. They may show suspiciousness, unusual perceptions or thinking, an eccentric manner of speaking, and inappropriate affect.
8. Perfectionism and rigidity characterize these people. Often workaholics, they tend to be indecisive, excessively scrupulous, and preoccupied with detail. They may insist that others do things their way. They have trouble expressing affection and they may lack generosity. They may even resist throwing away worthless objects they no longer need.
9. The behavior of others seems to confirm the expectations of these people that they will be threatened or humiliated. They can be quick to take offense and slow to forgive; they may have few confidants, question the loyalty of others, or read hidden meaning into innocent remarks.
10. These timid people are so easily wounded by criticism that they hesitate to become involved with others. They may fear the embarrassment of showing emotion or of saying things that seem foolish. They may have no close friends, and they tend to exaggerate the risks of undertaking pursuits outside their usual routines.

And here are the personality disorder choices you need to match with the possibilities above:

- Antisocial
- Avoidant
- Borderline
- Dependent
- Histrionic
- Narcissistic
- Obsessive–compulsive
- Paranoid
- Schizoid
- Schizotypal

Finally, please put a star next to the one (if any) that you think is the best match for Uma.

Note E

Here are the correct matches: 1 = Schizoid; 2 = Antisocial; 3 = Dependent; 4 = Histrionic; 5 = Narcissistic; 6 = Borderline ★; 7 = Schizotypal; 8 = Obsessive–compulsive; 9 = Paranoid; 10 = Avoidant.

Note where I've put my star; I'll bet it doesn't surprise you.

Rant

If you are especially sharp-eyed and more than a little suspicious, you might have noticed something missing from Step 5. Know what it is? Give up?

OK, it's personality change due to another medical condition. I left it out of the list for two reasons: It didn't fit into the discussion all that well, and the concept is more or less covered by the second item in my differential list in Note C. But there are instances of a change in personality caused by, for example, brain trauma, and the idea is important enough that I thought I should at least rant at you about it.

Step 6

From the brief descriptions in Step 5, I've selected borderline personality disorder (BPD) as the one that seems the best fit for Uma's history and current appearance. The final step would be to assure ourselves that she truly fulfills criteria for that diagnosis. Just below, I've put down (in abbreviated form) all the criteria that define BPD. For which of them can you find evidence in her history? You may want to underline the relevant passages from Steps 1 and 3.

1. Feels empty.
2. Struggles to avert abandonment, whether real or imagined.
3. Has disturbed identity (insecure self-image).
4. Alternates feelings of strong attachment to people with concerns about being rejected by those same people.
5. Commits impulsive actions with the potential to be self-damaging (two or more examples are required; suicide attempts don't count).
6. Has moods that are intense and unstable.
7. Under stress, has short-lived paranoid ideas or severe dissociation.
8. Has trouble controlling inappropriate anger.
9. Makes repeated attempts at suicide or self-mutilation.

Note F

With evidence for every one of the DSM-5 criteria (wow, is *that* ever unusual!—truly a textbook case), we don't need to lean very hard on the diagnostic principle: More symptoms of a given illness do increase the likelihood that it is the correct diagnosis. (DSM-5 requires only five of the nine possible symptoms for a diagnosis of BPD.)

1. Uma feels empty, as we judge from her chief complaint (feeling "scooped out inside") and her later comment that "I just feel all hollow."
2. She tried to avert abandonment by calling 11 therapists.

3. We judge her identity as disturbed from her statement that "I don't know who I am."
4. She alternates between strong attachment and rejection (based on the example from the referring clinician's letter).
5. Two examples of her impulsivity are using LSD when she didn't intend to, and having indiscriminate sex regardless of HIV risk.
6. We can deduce intense, unstable moods from her statement "I suddenly plunged into depression."
7. Short-lived paranoia is virtually defined by her claim that "when I'm feeling so awful, it seems everyone's on the attack."
8. Her anger can be inappropriate—indeed, "far out of proportion to the insult," as the history observes.
9. She's made repeated suicide attempts—some 25 of them, in fact.

Once again, *please* note: By far and away, most patients with a given personality disorder (or any other condition, for that matter) will not have all of the characteristics mentioned in the criteria. And the personalities of most patients will combine features of different personality disorders. If it's absolute certainty you crave in your profession, you might consider a career in accounting.

The Takeaway

After much huffing and puffing throughout this book about putting personality disorders at the bottom of any list of differential diagnoses, one of these has finally risen to the point of serious contention. We've pointed out the characteristics of each of the personality disorders named in DSM-5, and focused our attention on the one called *borderline*—which is probably the personality disorder diagnosis most frequently made. Although Uma has evidence of every major symptom for a diagnosis of BPD, we've discussed how rare it is to have every symptom of *anything*, and how important it is to obtain collateral information when diagnosing a personality disorder. However, Uma's case has given us the chance to mention this diagnostic principle: More symptoms of a given illness increase the likelihood that it is the correct diagnosis.

The beginning of this story has allowed us to underscore the danger of taking at face value the prejudices that may be inherent in a referral note—or, for that matter, in any other clinician's assessment of a given patient. And along the way, I've discussed (in a Rant) the importance of paying attention to any indications of childhood (or adult, for that matter) abuse, whether it be physical or sexual.

Break Time

Many composers have had mental illness. Schumann had a bipolar disorder. Schubert, who had syphilis with, perhaps, what was then called "general paresis of the insane," may eventually have died of mercury poisoning, a treatment that does kill the spirochetes that cause syphilis—but sometimes kills the patient as well. Donizetti may also have had a mental illness related to syphilis; Mussorgsky had what we today would term alcohol use disorder; Berlioz had a bipolar disorder; Bruckner had OCD; Rachmaninoff was both melancholic and phobic. Schoenberg had triskaidekaphobia, the morbid fear of the number 13; indeed, he died (of natural causes) on July 13th, 1951—a Friday, no less. But mental illness does not seem to have wormed its way into the music itself . . .

Oh, wait. We do have one candidate. It's the delirium experienced by the young artist in Berlioz's *Symphonie Fantastique*. This unnamed musician, believing that his love has rejected him, takes opium—not enough to kill him, but plenty to affect the clarity of his thinking. He imagines that he has killed his beloved. As a result, he is marched to the guillotine, where he must witness his own execution (the sound effect of the falling blade is evocative). However, most classical composers have not supplied such detailed program notes for their works. (And I am not aware that Berlioz himself was afflicted with any form of mental illness. But his wife died of alcohol-related disease; does that count?)

So various composers have had mental illness, but it has rarely seeped into the music itself. Of course, there are myriad popular songs with themes of misery, loss, and depression, even suicide. But classical music? Not so much. So far, we're missing the *Schizoaffective Symphony,* and the *Catatonia Concerto* remains to be written.

A diligent search will suss out one or two examples from grand opera. The eponymous hero of Handel's *Orlando* goes mad for love of a shepherdess, whom he imagines to be Venus; in his delirium, he kills a couple of other people, and it takes a heavy dose of magic to put this one right in the end. On the night of her wedding, the heroine of Donizetti's *Lucia di Lammermoor* loses her mind, murders her groom, sings about it (of course), and dies (also of course); in psychosis, she has achieved freedom.

And let's not forget Mad Margaret in the Gilbert and Sullivan comic operetta *Ruddigore*. To my taste, however, Margaret seems less psychotic than impulse-driven, and she calms down once she is married to her fiancé of long standing, Sir Despard Murgatroyd.

Then there was the fellow who went wooing Miss Daisy Bell on his "Bicycle Built for Two." But he was only half crazy.

22

Motion Sickness—Vincent

Step 1

Vincent enters the treatment room guided by a nurse, who says, "Look! He won't move on his own. He just goes any way I indicate. It just takes the slightest pressure on his elbow." Indeed, at the tiniest touch, Vincent moves; otherwise, he remains in place, silent and rooted to the linoleum. "It's like he's got power steering!" the nurse exclaims.

Vincent had been admitted to the hospital's secure inpatient service some weeks earlier, and he hasn't responded well to medication. Now he is about to undergo the first of a series of electroconvulsive treatments—recommended by several clinicians and sanctioned by the judge who ruled him incompetent to make his own health care decisions. That judgment was based partly on his recent history, partly on his appearance. At the hearing, conducted right here on the unit, Vincent remained almost completely mute; the only time he spoke was to repeat with partial fidelity the questions put to him. ("Do you understand what I'm saying?" the judge had intoned. After a pause, Vincent slowly mumbled, "You understand . . . I'm saying.")

But right now, he says nothing at all as, gently steered by the nurse, he shuffles across the floor to the gurney. He places one foot on the step stool next to the gurney, then withdraws it, advances again—and retreats. After the third repetition, he's finally helped to step up and lie down. "That's great!" says the nurse, patting his arm.

Vincent's response is to wrinkle his nose and draw down the corners of his mouth—a facial gesture that has become familiar over the past several weeks.

Several of Vincent's behaviors belong to a category of symptoms that's been termed *catatonia*. I've made a list of some of its typical symptoms. Would you, in a few words, describe each of these symptoms? And please put a checkmark beside each one that we've already observed (or been told about) for Vincent.

Agitation ______________________________

Catalepsy ______________________________

Echolalia ____

Echopraxia ____

Exaggerated compliance ____

Grimaces ____

Mannerisms ____

Mutism ____

Negativism ____

Posturing ____

Stereotypy ____

Stupor ____

Waxy flexibility ____

Note A

Here are brief definitions for the list of behaviors considered catatonic. The checkmarks denote those we've encountered in Vincent.

- *Agitation.* Excessive motor activity.
- *Catalepsy.* Maintaining an uncomfortable or unusual position even when told it isn't necessary.
- *Echolalia.* Inappropriate, word-for-word (or nearly) repetition of what someone else says. ✓
- *Echopraxia.* Inappropriate imitation of another's actions.
- *Exaggerated compliance.* Moving as directed by someone else, at the slightest indication. ✓
- *Grimaces.* Facial contortions that are not in response to a noxious stimulus. ✓
- *Mannerisms.* Repeated movements that seem goal-directed, though excessive in context.
- *Mutism.* Lack of (or markedly reduced) verbal output. ✓
- *Negativism.* Turning away from the examiner or resisting passive movement.
- *Posturing.* Voluntarily assuming or maintaining an uncomfortable or unusual pose.
- *Stereotypy.* Repeated movement that is not an essential part of goal-directed behavior. ✓
- *Stupor.* Markedly reduced activity; more or less the opposite of agitation.
- *Waxy flexibility.* Gentle, even resistance when an examiner tries to change the patient's position, as though bending a soft wax rod.

Step 2

Solely on the basis of the motor symptoms we've seen so far, what disorders ought you investigate for Vincent? Notice that I'm not asking for Vincent's differential diagnosis. That would imply having a lot more information about his history and symptoms than is the case right now. In short, in what conditions can we expect to encounter symptoms of catatonia?

It would be just fine for you to consult a textbook. But here's a hint: It's a lot more than just schizophrenia.

____

____

____

____

____

Note B

The word *catatonia* comes from Greek: κατά = *down*, τόνος = *tone* (as in muscle tension, not a musical note). The condition has often been equated with a diagnosis of schizophrenia, but to make that assumption would be a big mistake. That's because symptoms typical of catatonia are associated with a wide variety of medical and mental disorders. These include diverse medical conditions, including arteriovenous malformations, hyperparathyroidism, substance misuse, brain tumors, head trauma, cerebrovascular disease, encephalitis, subarachnoid hemorrhage, subdural hematoma, and tuberous sclerosis.

DSM-5 also explicitly associates catatonia with psychotic and mood disorders, though it is at least possible to find it in association with other defined conditions. Indeed, we are encouraged to attach the *catatonia specifier* any time this collection of symptoms occurs in a medical condition or in another mental disorder.

If to my Step 2 question you've only responded, "Medical conditions, mood disorders, and several psychoses," I'd say you've done pretty well.

Rant

Prior to DSM-5, when we were speaking of schizophrenia, we could apply any of four subtype designations: *catatonic, disorganized* (once referred to as *hebephrenic*), *paranoid,* and *undifferentiated.* Nearly a century of research eventually determined that these categories didn't add much to the basic diagnosis in terms of prognosis or treatment, and they were unreliable (in patients with schizophrenia, one subtype often morphed into another). So, although these terms have been identified with schizophrenia ever since Emil Kraepelin unified the concept early in the 20th century, DSM-5 has delisted them. But *catatonia* lingers as a specifier that can be used to describe quite a few classes of disorders.

Step 3

You obtain some history from Vincent's twin sister, Victoria, who knows him well. "After all, we started as womb-mates," she offers. She then explains, "Mum and Dad are in Europe, attending a conference."

Vincent and Victoria were the result of their mother's only pregnancy. Victoria has always been the dominant twin ("I know, that seems unusual for a girl"), but through their midteen years, both of them had good friends and were excellent students. She says that they led lives that were "pretty ordinary" up to their last year of high school. Then, though both continued to get good grades (Vincent scored in the top 1% of all students taking SATs that year), something began to change.

"He seemed to lose interest in his friends—who were *our* friends, actually," she tells us. "We pretty much hung with the same crowd. But part way through senior year, he started to withdraw. He stopped calling people, and mainly sat in his room reading fantasy stories and sci-fi." The summer after they graduated, she worked as a gardener at a commercial plant nursery, but he stayed home and wrote poetry—and continued to ignore their parents' warnings that he should apply to several colleges. They both started school that fall: she at an art school in another state; he at the local community college, where he majored in philosophy.

When Victoria came home for winter break, she was appalled at how her brother had changed. He'd grown a wispy beard; even in December, he wore sandals without socks; his toes were dirty, his nails ragged. He spent most of the day in his room, reading and listening to Hindi music. "When I asked why he didn't go out, he claimed that people would follow him in cars and try to dazzle him by shining their brights in his eyes. As if anyone would want to follow *Vincent!* I suggested that he must be mistaken, that he'd really seen different cars that looked the same, but he only looked at me as though I were in on 'the plot.'" She frames her disbelief in air quotes.

Victoria also learned that he hadn't studied much, and that he was probably going to fail every class, even philosophy. "He just wasn't putting in the work you need to get a grade—said it didn't matter, since he didn't need a degree. He said he really just didn't care." She pauses, and bites her lip. "At least then, he was saying *something*."

During that vacation week, whenever he did speak, "it was virtually in tongues, so that you could hardly understand him at all." Victoria had been so struck by his speech patterns that she'd recorded one of their ("super-brief") conversations. She opens the recording app on her phone and presses *Play*.

"Vincent, tell me what you're planning for next term at school."

The next voice is soft, barely audible. "I have a higher view of that, the life we live. I'd like liverwurst on rye."

Well, how would you characterize Vincent's speech in that recording? Here are some choices:

- ☐ No pathology (Hah!)
- ☐ Flight of ideas
- ☐ Loose associations
- ☐ Tangentiality
- ☐ Word salad

Note C

First, I sometimes like to include *no pathology* or some equivalent in the choices I give myself. It reminds me not to assume the absence of a logical, nonpathological explanation for an observation. However, I won't check that box for Vincent

Rather, we need to choose something that indicates a problem with his flow of speech. (The alternative wording, *flow of thought*, suggests that clinicians can read minds, which seems a little unfortunate.) Let's instead discuss the concept of *loose associations.* That's when ideas run into one another, garbling the speaker's output. It's also sometimes called *derailment,* as in the train of thought (speech!) running off the rails. Whatever we choose to call it, the words and phrases are perfectly understandable by themselves, but their meaning gets lost in a tangle. The result may signify something to the patient, but it pretty much stumps the rest of us. And that is what seems to be happening with Vincent.

There are special types of loose associations. In one type, *flight of ideas,* a word or phrase provides a launch pad for the patient's speech to take off in a direction that is slightly related to—though definitely different from—the original apparent destination. It's often associated with mania. The connection between thoughts in flight of ideas can usually be understood by an observer, but this standard doesn't seem to fit Vincent's speech sample. We sometimes call loose associations *word salad* when words are so unrelated that they don't even seem to form phrases—again, not the case here. *Tangentiality,* or *tangential speech,* is the term used when the answer you hear doesn't relate to the question asked.

In the recording made by Victoria, I'd say that Vincent was showing the tangentiality type of loose associations. Both terms qualify as examples of disorganized speech, one of the five A-group symptoms of psychosis specified by DSM-5—and that's one of the (very few) lists I've urged you to memorize. Have you? You're going to need it in a moment.

Step 4

Of course, by the time of your consultation, Vincent has become completely mute. But before that occurred, Victoria was troubled by one other piece of behavior she'd noticed.

> During that same break from school, she'd passed Vincent's door and heard him inside, apparently talking to someone. She knew he'd let his cell phone contract lapse, though she supposed he could be using the house Wi-Fi. But when she'd entered after Vincent hadn't responded to her knock, he was just sitting on the edge of his bed, staring at the floor.
>
> This time, she plays the video recording she made.
>
> "Who were you talking to?" we can hear her ask.
>
> "No one," he says. "Just forget it, OK?" But he glances away, then half turns his head, as though listening. We can see his mouth moving as he appears to whisper to someone neither she nor we can see, "Just fuck off!" No one could mistake the message of his lips.

So what do we make of this: a marked disparity between what our patient tells us, and the evidence of our senses? Is there a diagnostic principle we might want to invoke here?

Note D

Although diagnostic principles don't have the force of law, they can help us sort through the sometimes tangled strands of a patient's history. Here is a spot where we'll whip one out: Objective findings beat subjective judgment.

Of course, that guideline doesn't always hold true (we can be fooled by an optical illusion or a mirage). In this situation, however, it makes sense to pay attention to our sense of vision: Vincent strongly appears to be speaking to someone—or something. Although the conclusion isn't iron-clad, I feel reasonably confident that he is hallucinating voices, and possibly also visual images. In any event, it's important to remember and (judiciously) employ the principle that the evidence of our senses should sometimes trump what someone tells us.

Step 5

At this point, Vincent has exhibited evidence of each of the types of psychotic symptoms recognized by DSM-5—the so-called "A criteria." These are the symptoms a patient must have to gain entry to the psychosis ballpark. How many of them are there?

Right, five, and we've explicitly discussed four of the five—but, using information from both Victoria and Vincent, we've mentioned them all. So, without further prompting, can you name them all?

____

____

____

____

____

Rant

Health care services often cross paths with the law, and nowhere is this more evident than for patients affected by mental health disorders.

Although their clinical definitions do not include statements that allude to legal consequences, some disorders entail behavior that is inherently illegal. That is, a person who fulfills the criteria for kleptomania or pyromania has done something that violates the rights of others and is thereby liable to be punished by fine or imprisonment. Similar consequences attend several paraphilias—voyeuristic, exhibitionistic, frotteuristic, and especially pedophilic disorders.

Some criteria explicitly mention behaviors that are illegal everywhere. For example, the criteria for antisocial personality disorder explicitly include the wording "acts that are grounds for arrest." The criteria for conduct disorder specifically mention numerous crimes: armed robbery, extortion, conning others, forgery, mugging, purse snatching, and shoplifting. However, intermittent explosive disorder is the only DSM-5 disorder that uses the term "legal consequences" in a criterion.

And then there are those disorders that, carried to an extreme, can result in legal fallout. Sometimes, as we see in Vincent's case history, this happens because the behavior of patients imperils their own safety or that of others. In relating the histories of Liam in Chapter 12, and of Randolph in Chapter 18, we've already discussed the duty to protect patients from harming themselves. And in the discussion of Randolph, we've mentioned the *Tarasoff* rule that requires us to protect other identifiable people from a patient's actions. These two instances arise most often in the management of patients with severe mood disorders (major depressive and bipolar I), and of those with schizophrenia and other major psychotic disorders.

Other examples come to mind. Hoarding disorder, for example, can lead to complaints by neighbors and lead to forced compliance with safety and sanitation laws. Factitious disorder imposed on another may result in a battery that requires investigation and, occasionally, punishment. Rapid eye movement sleep behavior disorder sometimes results in a patient's vigorously kicking or striking a bed partner—though legal consequences are probably infrequent. And in the past few years, patients with gender dysphoria have encountered legislative and judicial challenges over the issue of bathroom access.

Finally, several categories of substance misuse are "victimless crimes" in that, whereas they concern chemicals that are not legal to sell, it is argued that their misuse harms the individual rather than society in general. These include hallucinogens, opioids, cocaine, and (in most U.S. jurisdictions, although the number is decreasing) cannabis.

With all this said, the majority (depending on how we calculate, more than 90%) of mental disorders have few or no implications at all for legal consequences. So anxiety disorders, somatic symptom disorders, dissociative disorders, and many more are free of legal risk. And yet some conditions have been used as an excuse for illegal behavior. Google legal defense and OCD, and you will find instances where people have invoked obsessions as justification for their illegal behavior. Similar findings can be obtained for dissociative identity disorder, and probably for almost any other condition you'd care to investigate.

Note E

- Hallucinations. We believe (though I admit it hasn't been proven) that Vincent has been listening—and responding—to voices; he may have had visual hallucinations as well, though that is a bit less certain. (For why I've starred this item and the next two, see below.) ★
- Delusions. From Victoria, we know that at one time Vincent had the delusion that people were following him in their cars, trying to dazzle him by turning their lights on high beam. Although we must be forever on the alert for preposterous-sounding stories that turn out to be true, this one seems nowhere nearly credible. ★
- Disorganized speech. The audio recording that Victoria made seems pretty conclusive. In Note C, we've mentioned some of the different manifestations of disorganized speech. ★
- Disorganized behavior. Sure, catatonic symptoms aren't the only possible way in

which this symptom can appear, but when you encounter in a patient like Vincent any of the behaviors we've mentioned in Note A, you can check this box. (Oops! No box.)

- Negative symptoms. DSM-5 specifically mentions lack of volition and blunted affect (though the term used there is *diminished emotional expression*). Although we haven't discussed it earlier, avolition was one of the first psychotic symptoms Vincent developed: He lost interest in his friends and made no effort to apply to colleges. By the time we meet him, he also shows no variation in his emotional range; that's called *blunting* (or *flattening*) *of affect.*

Also remember that not all of the A symptoms are created equal. In DSM-5, three of them are on the "required" list for the diagnosis of schizophrenia, schizophreniform disorder, schizoaffective disorder, and brief psychotic disorder. That is, to qualify for a diagnosis of any of these conditions, a patient must have at least one of the first three types of symptoms (I've marked each of these above with a star) on the list of A criteria for psychosis.

DSM-5 underscores the importance of these three, because they are generally considered *core positive symptoms.* That is, we should expect to find them in patients with schizophrenia. This somewhat circular argument was apparently driven by opinion, rather than by research. That doesn't make it wrong, of course—only a little less acceptable to people who like data to underpin their beliefs. That's us. And that should be DSM-5, too. Apologies for letting what should be a Rant intrude into the regular text of the workbook.

Step 6

And now the step we've all been waiting for: Please write down your differential diagnosis for Vincent, and then defend your choice for best diagnosis. I've starred mine in the list in Note F.

____

____

____

____

____

____

Note F

Here's my differential diagnosis for Vincent:

◊ Substance/medication-induced psychotic disorder
◊ Psychotic disorder due to another medical condition

◊ Mood disorder with psychotic features
◊ Schizophreniform disorder
◊ Schizoaffective disorder
◊ Schizophrenia ★

Of course, my top-of-the-list choices are nearly always the same—mental disorders caused by substance use or other medical conditions. I haven't changed my approach for Vincent, even though the best diagnosis seems so obvious.

Once I've ruled out substances and other medical conditions, I'd much rather diagnose a mood disorder with psychotic features, because that condition is more treatable and has a better prognosis than the others lower on the list. But with no clear depressive symptoms and a potful of psychotic ones, we must (reluctantly) discard it, too. The same dreary facts spell doom for schizoaffective disorder.

I try to include schizophreniform disorder as a possibility wherever I find psychotic symptoms, but that's mainly a reminder to myself about the importance of considering symptom duration. Victoria's information makes it clear that her brother has been ill for longer than the 6-month time frame for schizophreniform disorder.

And that brings us to the last disorder on the list: schizophrenia. Let's go through the requirements we've stated over and over in our mantra: "inclusion, exclusion, duration, distress."

First, the inclusion symptoms for the A criterion are present—in superabundance! That is, DSM-5 requires at least two of the symptoms we've discussed in Note E; during the course of his illness, Vincent has had them all. That reminds us of the power of this diagnostic principle: More symptoms of a given illness increase the likelihood that it is the correct diagnosis. And what could be more than *all*? However, only a tiny minority of patients with schizophrenia will come up to that mark. (Of course, the A-list symptoms also apply to schizophreniform and schizoaffective disorders, but we've already eliminated these two diagnoses.) The fact that these are *typical* features of schizophrenia also increases the likelihood of diagnosis, but by this point we're in overkill mode.

Although patients do not need to feel distressed by the psychotic symptoms of schizophrenia, there must be serious impairment of functioning in some major life area—work, study, interpersonal relationships. And this is absolutely our finding with Vincent, who hasn't gone to school, hasn't worked, and hasn't even taken good care of his physical needs (unkempt toenails, clothing inappropriate for winter weather). As regards duration, we've already noted that he's been continuously ill for more than the 6 months required for schizophrenia. Finally, we've just ruled out the competing disorders, leaving schizophrenia as our best diagnosis.

Step 7

Finally, how should we record Vincent's condition? That is, what do we add to the barebones diagnosis of schizophrenia, so that other clinicians will have the fullest possible picture of his condition? Here are a couple of very broad hints: We'll use two specifiers.

One—the episode specifier—we've already discussed for Siobhán in Chapter 19, but for the utmost convenience, I've restated the choices below. Just pick the episode specifier that's appropriate for Vincent.

- First episode, currently in acute episode (right now, the patient meets all criteria for the diagnosis, and it is the first episode)
- First episode, currently in partial remission (there are some symptoms now, but no longer enough to fulfill the requirements for a diagnosis)
- First episode, currently in full remission (there are no symptoms of the disorder now)
- Multiple episodes, currently in acute episode (there have been one or more previous episodes interspersed with symptom remissions)
- Multiple episodes, currently in partial remission
- Multiple episodes, currently in full remission
- Continuous (the disorder is ongoing, with enough symptoms to sustain the diagnosis)
- Unspecified

The other specifier has to do with recording the catatonic symptoms Vincent has displayed. I'm not even going to try to encourage you to do this on your own; just go on to Note G.

Note G

Here's how we'll record Vincent's condition:

◊ F20.9 Schizophrenia, first episode, currently in acute episode
◊ F06.1 Catatonia associated with schizophrenia

DSM-5 says that the phrase *with catatonia* should be appended to the diagnosis of schizophrenia. But that doesn't create any space for the code number, which is important to the folks in the record room. And, it seems to me that including catatonia twice in the diagnosis is a waste of ink. So I've done it this way. Clinician's prerogative.

The Takeaway

This chapter has been a romp for diagnostic principles: More symptoms increase the chances of diagnosis; typical features increase the likelihood of diagnosis; and objective findings beat subjective opinions. We've also listed and defined the symptoms typical of catatonia (and, in the end, discussed how to indicate them as a specifier in a final diagnosis). In between these bookends, we've mentioned (again) the symptoms included in the A criterion for schizophrenia and some other psychotic disorders.

Break Time

The other day I encountered a kid wearing a T-shirt that bore an image of *The Scream*, by Norwegian painter Edvard Munch. Although Munch appears to have had no particular disorder in mind (though at times he drank heavily and feared madness), it caused me to wonder what that iconic screamer might have been thinking. (Note the resemblance to the *Home Alone* poster image of Macaulay Culkin—but we know why he was upset.)

The T-shirt started me thinking about other works of visual art that portray mental health issues. Largely, they have to do with mood disorders and psychoses. With a few keystrokes, you can find any of these images (and many more) on the Internet. Here I mention just a few:

Dating from about 1494, *The Extraction of the Stone of Madness* by Hieronymus Bosch shows a patient being relieved of the supposed source of his malady by clinicians who, from the looks of their headgear, may themselves be mad.

Melencolia I (1514) depicts the troubled mind of its artist, Albrecht Dürer. You can find a ton of descriptive material to help you interpret this powerful, iconic image.

The Madhouse is the eighth and final painting in the series *The Rake's Progress* by William Hogarth; it is notable in part for showing how people of fashion would visit asylums as entertainment in the first half of the 18th century.

The so-called "Black Paintings" of Francisco de Goya depict the artist's fear of becoming insane and his increasingly morbid view of life. *Saturn Devouring His Son* is probably the best known of these works. Goya also created a couple of paintings on the subject of insanity: *Yard with Lunatics* (1794) and, some 20 years later, *The Madhouse.* (Goya's own illness remains shrouded in mystery: he may have had Ménière's disease, though a form of encephalitis has also been suggested.)

Vincent van Gogh was his own best subject; some of his self-portraits show him with his face bandaged after he cut off his own ear in a fit of madness that may have been caused by temporal lobe epilepsy, heavy absinthe drinking, and depression (possibly bipolar).

The diagnosis of Louis Wain is similarly indeterminate. On the tail of a successful career as painter and illustrator (lots of cats, many of them anthropomorphic), Wain became psychotic in his 60s and spent his final 15 years in mental institutions. There he drew cats in varying stages of fragmentation—though not, contrary to the opinion of some writers, in proportion to the severity of his psychotic state. Other writers have suggested that his psychosis could have been related to the parasite *Toxoplasma gondii,* which cats can shed in their feces.

I've mentioned only a small sampling of what you can find when you browse for art and the mental disorder of your choice.

23

Role of the Dice—Whitney

Step 1

"I definitely need some help with this." Her back ramrod straight, Whitney sits on the edge of her chair and nervously fingers her iPhone. She's hooked her cane over one arm of the chair.

"Look," she continues. "I've read the book, I've done the research online. I know what makes a problem gambler. Let *me* take *you* through it." Stifling a yawn, one by one she ticks off the points on nail-bitten fingers.

"First, and the main reason I came in, is that I don't do anything other than gamble. I mean, with my spare time. Of course I do my job at work. Otherwise, I wouldn't have the money to put in play. And I have plenty of time for placing bets, ever since my boyfriend left—he said he couldn't take any more lies about how much I've lost. Last year I borrowed money from my parents to help with the rent, but now *they've* said 'nevermore,' so I sponge off whatever friends I have left for something to eat. One of them made this video last week and emailed it to me."

She taps the screen of her phone a couple of times and pushes it toward you across the corner of the desk. The image is unmistakably of Whitney, perched between two machines in a casino. Like a slow metronome, she swivels back and forth, mechanically pressing the *Bet* button of first one, then the other; she shows no facial expression whatsoever. "Does this look like I'm having a good time? But whenever I try to stop—I've joined and quit Gamblers Anonymous so many times I have them on speed dial—I just feel cranky."

She retrieves her phone and spreads her fingers wide apart. "I think I'm up to five symptoms so far. I could go on, but it's too depressing. I mean, for well over a year, this's been my life!"

So the first thing I'd like you to do is to verify that Whitney's own diagnosis is fully warranted. As with nearly every DSM-5 disorder, that means you need to check on the four issues of the mantra: "inclusion, exclusion, duration, distress."

1. Does she fulfill a list of required inclusion symptoms?
2. Are there any exclusion disorders we need to consider?
3. Has the duration been sufficient for inclusion?
4. Has she experienced significant distress or impaired functioning (or have those around her noticed that she has been impaired)?

Let's start off with the inclusion symptoms for gambling disorder. Briefly stated, in a 1-year period, the person must have many instances of at least four of the following. The individual . . .

- Places more money at risk to get the same thrill.
- Has tried to cut down or stop gambling.
- Is restless or irritable when trying to limit gambling.
- Is preoccupied with thoughts about gambling.
- Gambles when feeling distressed.
- Returns to try to get even after a losing session of gambling.
- Lies about the extent of gambling.
- Gambles to the point of losing friends, family, jobs, or other opportunities.
- Needs financial assistance from other people due to gambling.

Now put an asterisk beside each of the behaviors above that you've noted for Whitney.

Note A

The phrase *inclusion symptoms* usually signifies a list of behaviors typical of the disorder in question. When a certain number of these—not all, but usually close to half—must be present, we say that the requirement is *polythetic* (from Greek: *many + placed, arranged*). Indeed, Whitney's specific problems with gambling (those you should have marked with an asterisk) include repeatedly trying to quit, lying to her boyfriend (which has led to the rupture of their relationship), relying on friends and family for support, and feeling irritable when trying to control her addiction. And those five symptoms (four are enough) are just the issues she mentions spontaneously, without any pestering on your part. In a longer interview, we might learn that she's experienced even more of these behaviors. Also, note that the inclusion symptoms must be both persistent and recurring; from the history she gives, that would certainly seem to be the case. Clearly, she meets this important criterion for gambling disorder.

Step 2

Let's not prolong the suspense; we'll take the remaining three parts of the mantra together. Here they are as applied to gambling disorder:

- Exclusion. Most mental diagnoses require that we rule out several other disorders. Gambling disorder lists only one—the behavior must not be explainable as an episode of mania.

- Duration. Although DSM-5 doesn't require any minimum duration, it does state that the symptoms must bunch together within a 12-month time frame.
- Distress or disability. In a Rant in Chapter 20 when discussing Tyler (page 228), I've previously noted that relatively few DSM-5 disorders do *not* include such a requirement.

So how would you evaluate Whitney on each of these three criteria?

Note B

Here is how we'd round off the requirements for a diagnosis of gambling disorder for Whitney:

- Exclusion. Well, as responsible clinicians, at some point we should directly ask Whitney a question about possible symptoms of mania—but from what she has related so far, a manic episode would seem to be pretty far-fetched.
- Duration. All the behaviors Whitney has described appear to have occurred within the past year or so, though of course they might have begun even earlier.
- Distress or disability. And her experiences with gambling have led both to clinically important distress and to social impairment.

And so, yes! We can in fact justify the diagnosis of gambling disorder; so far, we cannot specify whether to call it episodic or persistent. We'll also wait just a bit to discuss the severity of her addiction.

Step 3

Whitney seems to have given us her diagnosis on a silver platter. But wait a moment: When that happens, what should be our immediate response? We should ____________________

____

Note C

My answer would be some variation of "Look under the platter; something might be stuck there." Or perhaps you said, "Check for additional disorders." Either formulation would be just about perfect.

Let's think some more about what other problems might underlie or accompany her gambling disorder. One of my diagnostic principles is this: Because they are nearly ubiquitous, always consider mood disorders—specifically, some type of depression. And when we scrutinize the Step 1 material for Whitney, we do find hints in her expression of persistent irritability and low mood. That's only a straw in the wind, but it's one we ought to pursue. For that, we'll have to investigate further.

Step 4

Among other bits of data concerning mood, you'd like to know how Whitney's feeling right now. So how do you ask someone about current mood? Or does it even matter what question you use? In the list of possibilities below, check those you think could work well:

- ☐ Directly ask about a specific feeling ("Have you been feeling depressed?"). Or would this be considered "leading the witness"?
- ☐ Ask something open-ended that gives the patient an opportunity to express feelings: "Tell me about your mood now," or "How have you been feeling generally?"
- ☐ Carefully observe the patient's facial expression and body language for signs of depression or other mood states.
- ☐ Express sympathy for the patient's situation.
- ☐ Give the patient a checklist to fill out.

Note D

Actual studies (unhappily, precious few have investigated the act of interviewing with any scientific rigor) suggest that something open-ended will probably serve best when you are trying to probe for emotional state. Indeed, Cox and colleagues, in one of a series of articles in the *British Journal of Psychiatry* way back in the 1980s, reported that open-ended questions provide the best way to start prospecting for feelings. Such questions yield the greatest amount of information about emotions, and they give the patient scope for bringing up other related facts that you might not think to ask about in a more structured, closed-ended sort of way. Here are a couple of examples:

"Can you describe how you've been feeling about all this?"
"Tell me about your mood right now."

Cox et al. found that in addition to open-ended questions, several other techniques can help complete the picture of a patient's emotional state. One is simple: Just stay out of the way. That is, what they called "a low level of interviewer talk" encourages patients to divulge their feelings. Expressions of sympathy are also helpful; so are direct requests for feelings. In fact, for an initial interview, I'd endorse any of the Step 4 choices except the last one—the checklist. Checklist depression rating scales (like the Zung Self-Rating Depression Scale and the Beck Depression Inventory–II) are great for tracking a person's emotional status from one time to the next, but they do put a paperwork barrier between you and the patient. I don't recommend them as the first step for an initial interview.

Step 5

So in response to your open-ended request, "Please tell me more about how your life has been," you learn the following.

Whitney begins, "I have so much to be happy about—good job, friends, a lovely family. Well, Mom lives in California, but we talk on the phone a lot. And text. I keep asking myself, 'What's so awful in my life that, over and over, I keep wishing I could just end it all?'"

This aspect of Whitney's tale of woe seems to have begun not long before she started in her new job—designing software for a commodities trading company that's based half a continent away.

Whitney is obviously bright, and she seems well informed. She certainly is articulate. "Maybe it was the threat of change, that I started to feel so burdened every day. And tired: I crawl through the work day, and collapse, often without eating anything. I'm achy all over, and I just feel so sad all day."

She goes on to say that nearly every day, for weeks, she has felt despondent and increasingly useless. "It's horrible! I force myself to do my job, but I don't seem to accomplish anything, and now I truly don't care if it gets done or not. And I just can't imagine things will ever improve."

Indeed, she says that she cannot focus on her work "or much of anything else"—though she does still gamble, which "lets my mind off the leash, at least for a time." Although she used to sleep long and heavily, she's suffered lately from insomnia. "Not all the time—maybe when I'm most worried about things. Well, that's nearly always." She yawns again, hugely. Behind dark glasses, her eyes are hooded and afraid.

"I've lost so much weight." She tugs her sleeve down toward her wrist, perhaps to conceal even from herself how bony she's become. Her hand shakes as she reaches out for the tissue box. Soon a soggy stalagmite of discarded tissues has claimed the tabletop.

"What can I do?" she cries. "For the first time in my life, I just feel so desperate."

Now what does this all of this add up to? Specifically, at this time, can you diagnose:

- ☐ A mood disorder?
- ☐ A mood episode?
- ☐ Or maybe neither of these? And if this is the case, then why?

(Hint: Think about the mantra.)

Rant

Why do I keep banging on about this issue of mood symptoms versus a mood diagnosis? It's because I think it is just too darned easy—I've seen it *way* too frequently—for clinicians to count numbers of symptoms and then abandon the hunt in the belief that they've done their job. Although keeping in mind the exact criteria for the different disorders can be difficult (well, OK, impossible, save perhaps for the odd savant), we should be able to remember that durable diagnostic mantra. And we'll also need to know the inclusion requirements for a major depressive episode; they're the same as for major depressive disorder. Note that at least one of the first two in the Note E list must be present for either major depressive episode or disorder.

Note E

Whitney has fielded a pretty impressive collection of mood symptoms for inclusion. If you count them up (and I hope you did), you'll find more than enough for a major depressive episode. As for duration, by her own account, these symptoms have lasted "for weeks." And they have certainly led to distress *and* to disability for adequate performance of her job. Here is my full accounting of the inclusion symptoms, with a note in brackets on how each applies to Whitney:

- Low mood, majority of time. [Yes for Whitney.]
- Loss of interest in things formerly enjoyed, majority of time. [Unsure; need more information.]
- Fatigue. [Yes for Whitney.]
- Trouble concentrating or thinking. [Whitney cannot focus.]
- Problems with sleep—too little or too much. [Whitney reports insomnia.]
- Motor agitation or retardation almost every day. [Not noted for Whitney.]
- Feeling worthless or guilty beyond reason. [Not noted for Whitney.]
- Change in appetite and/or weight, up or down. [Whitney has lost weight.]
- Alarming, repeated thoughts of death or committing suicide. [Whitney wishes she could "end it all."]

But you can't afford to stop your queries there. That's because, as with most other diagnoses, you still need to exclude other causes of depressive symptoms. And that is why I would check the third box in the Step 5 checklist.

In the case of major depressive episode *or* disorder, we need to rule out two competing etiologies: other medical conditions and substance use disorders. And to accomplish that, we'll need more information.

Rant

Most diagnoses include a criterion for excluding other, competing disorders. (Gambling disorder and major depression, both under consideration for Whitney, fall into this category.) However, there are a few mental disorders that include no such requirement. Presumably, then, we could diagnose these conditions along with just about any other diagnosis.

Some of these we can quite readily understand. For example, there's no a priori reason to think that a person with intellectual disability couldn't fall victim to mood, anxiety, or psychotic disorders—indeed, to pretty much the full spectrum of other mental and behavioral disorders described in the manuals. The same might be said for someone who has any of several sleep disorders, including narcolepsy, obstructive sleep apnea hypopnea, and circadian rhythm sleep–wake disorders. And here are a few other conditions that could theoretically coexist with nearly anything else: disinhibited social engagement disorder, anorexia nervosa, gender dysphoria, conduct disorder, and all substance use disorders.

For other diagnoses, the lack of an exclusion criterion may be a little harder to rationalize. I'd especially complain about somatic symptom disorder (but then I *always* complain about that diagnosis, which DSM-5 defines so loosely). And why are rule-outs included for antisocial, schizoid, schizotypal, and paranoid personality disorders, but not for the other personality disorders—histrionic, dependent, narcissistic, avoidant, obsessive–compulsive, and borderline? Why for all the paraphilias *except* fetishistic disorder? Maybe DSM-5.1 will provide some clarity.

Step 6

I'm afraid that Whitney may be an unreliable informant; something is still missing from her narrative. Of course, you'd love to have a source for collateral information, but in the moment, how can you encourage candor in a person who may be reluctant to give fully accurate information, even to a clinician? Are there a few words that might help encourage her to come clean? Here are the elements I'd want you to include:

- The importance of telling all, even the embarrassing bits
- The effect of leaving stuff out
- What to do if the patient simply feels unable to talk about something sensitive

Now try writing down a short speech that includes these elements. It will turn out to be one you'll use over and over throughout your career.

____

____

Note F

To approach this thorny issue, I'd make a rather impassioned plea for openness, something like this:

> "I need to know everything, even if it's embarrassing. Look, you probably can't tell me anything that I haven't heard before; you're not going to shock me. So please be frank with me. And if I ask something you feel you simply cannot disclose fully, just tell me that you'd like to put off that discussion temporarily. The absolute *worst* thing for us would be if you told me something that isn't true. That would only confuse me. And it could even harm you."

Step 7

With a somewhat elaborate lead-in similar to the one presented just above, you finally obtain this vital information:

> Whitney sighs. "OK, here's what really happened. About a year ago, I was standing on a ladder, trying to hang Christmas lights along the roofline of my parents' house. I slipped off the top of the ladder and landed butt-first on the sidewalk. From the hor-

rible sound it made—never mind the pain!—I knew right away I'd done something pretty awful."

Whitney had sustained a fracture of her right hip. It was stable and nondisplaced, so it didn't require surgery, but for several weeks she was in bed. Afterward, she could only get around by using a walker and generous amounts of oxycodone. After a month, her doctor thought she'd gone through her pain medication too quickly, and would only give her enough for a week at a time. "It hurt pretty bad, so in desperation, I bought some on the street. Then, to shorten a boring story, I found that heroin worked faster."

As she tells this story, her eyes again fill with tears. "It was amazingly inexpensive. In monetary terms, I mean. From there, it was a gradual slip and a slide into constant heroin use, which turned out to be a lot more costly in every other way."

Even before any of this, Whitney would drink when she was rolling dice. "It helped me to feel strong and capable. What a laugh! Maybe the drinking helped make the use of drugs seem OK. Who knows?" She shrugs as she adds another sodden tissue to the pile.

Now she's been using heroin for several months, despite repeated attempts to wean herself. "It's so cheap I haven't resorted to criminal means to get drugs—I haven't stolen anything and I haven't sold myself, not that anyone's offering to buy." (With dismay, she taps an emaciated arm.) But she has to use heroin at least a couple of times every day. And several times she's driven her car when she's been high—"In this town, you can't go anywhere without driving."

With her hip knitting nicely, according to the doctor, she repeatedly tried to cut back, but discovered that she couldn't. "Every time I've tried to stop using, it's been cold turkey, and always too awful to bear. Withdrawal symptoms were the flu on steroids; I mean, horrible joint pains! And throwing up till there was nothing left but my stomach lining. Which I tried to heave up, too." Afterward, she craved the drug even more. "When I started waking up with the desire to use, I knew I was really, really hooked."

Today so far, she hasn't used at all. "It's a terrific struggle, but I'm determined I won't backslide, no matter how strong the urge becomes. I know that for sure!" As she speaks, you notice the hairs standing up all along her arm.

Now, at last, we can try for a differential diagnosis. And, when all's said and done, you should be able to identify *four* best diagnoses. OK, because there's more than one, let's call them *better diagnoses*—and put a star after each one of them.

____

____

____

____

____

____

____

Note G

A simple listing doesn't go nearly far enough. So I'll start with the differential list (and stars for the better diagnoses); then, over the next couple of Steps and Notes, I'll offer some explanations.

◊ Opioid withdrawal ★
◊ Opioid use disorder ★
◊ Opioid-induced depressive disorder ★
◊ Gambling disorder ★
◊ Depressive disorder due to another medical condition
◊ Major depressive disorder
◊ A bipolar disorder, current episode depressed
◊ Persistent depressive disorder (dysthymia)

In Note B, we've already validated Whitney's diagnosis of gambling disorder, so now let's discuss opioid withdrawal. We'll take it next because it most immediately threatens her health and well-being. It could even cause her to step away from treatment.

Whitney has used prescription opioids and heroin recently and frequently. She stopped about 24 hours ago, and this has led to considerable distress. This sequence satisfies the DSM-5 duration and distress/disability criteria for heroin withdrawal. The symptom inclusion requirements she has experienced include dysphoric mood, aching muscles, runny nose, insomnia, and yawning. At the very end of the Step 7 narration, we've noticed piloerection, and if we'd asked her to remove her dark glasses, we might have discovered dilated pupils. However, with so many other symptoms and signs—only three are required—do we really have to subject her to this indignity? (I can think of responses pro and con.) Finally, though we've already ascertained that she doesn't drink actively now, we should review the other substances of abuse to assure ourselves that heroin is the only likely candidate for her withdrawal disorder.

That's one diagnosis down—or, rather, two: We've already got gambling disorder safely tucked under our belts.

Step 8

Now let's pursue the issue of opioid use disorder. We'll use the same list of 11 criteria that apply to all substances. I've abbreviated them below; if you want to review them in greater detail, go back and reread the case of Pierce in Chapter 16 (Step 7, page 189). At least 2 of the following symptoms are required within a 12-month period.

- Using more
- Control issues
- Time investment
- Craving
- Shirking obligations
- Worsening social or interpersonal relations
- Reduction of other activities

- Ignoring physical dangers
- Ignoring health warnings
- Tolerance
- Withdrawal

For which ones can you find evidence in Whitney's Step 7 information?

Note H

The symptoms underlined below are the ones I've identified from Step 7.

Of course, Whitney has suffered withdrawal, and she's taken more than she intended over a very considerable period of time. She awakens craving heroin. From our information, it isn't clear whether Whitney has realized that drug use is in part the cause of her mood disorder; apparently nobody's told her that, so we shouldn't include the factor of ignoring a health warning in our evidence for opioid use disorder, even though she has gone right on using despite the depressive symptoms. In any event, there's more than sufficient evidence for opioid use disorder (only 2 of the 11 symptoms listed above are required). As far as severity is concerned, I'm going to exert my clinician's prerogative and call it *moderate*, regardless of the exact number of symptoms we can come up with.

Three "better diagnoses" down, one to go.

Step 9

This brings us to mood disorder. In Note E, while trying to make a case for Whitney's experiencing a major depressive episode, we've gotten hung up on the exclusion criteria. Now let's take a different approach and try to find evidence that would allow us to rule *in* a substance/medication-induced depressive disorder. Here are the requirements:

Inclusion

- Depressed mood (or significant loss of interest/pleasure in all, or nearly all, activities) must be prominent.
- The suspected substance must be known for its ability to cause these symptoms.
- The symptoms must start during or shortly after substance use begins.

Exclusion

- We would reject the diagnosis of a substance-related disorder if the symptoms in question (here, depressive) *started before* the drug use.
- Or if they *continued long after* (at least a month after) drug use stopped.
- Or if there was a prior history of the condition that was *not* drug-induced.

Duration

- DSM-5's only requirement here is that the symptoms be "persistent." Interpret that as you will; I think it means the problem has existed longer that a few days—probably weeks or even months.

Distress

- The substance-induced condition causes clinically important impairment or distress.

Now, using this outline, check through the information in Steps 5 and 7 to determine whether you can make a case for opioid-induced depressive disorder.

Note I

Marching briskly through the four categories of the mantra, we can make the following determinations. Whitney easily fulfills the inclusion criteria, inasmuch as her mood has been prominently depressed ever since she began the heavy use of opioids—which are known to cause depressive symptoms. We infer (from Step 5 information) that she's had no previous episode of depression, and we've already noted that the symptoms began after, not before, the onset of heavy drug use (that's the Step 9 exclusion criterion dealt with). Her depressive symptoms have persisted for several weeks at least, certainly long enough to satisfy us of the duration criterion. And surely no one will dispute her degree of distress.

Now we can finally state that opioid use is a good candidate for the cause of Whitney's depressive symptoms. And that is where we will leave it. If after she's been off all substances for a substantial period of time (weeks or months), we find that her mood disorder has continued unabated, we will have to reassess this part of her diagnosis. For, of course, patients who have substance use disorders can and do have independent mood disorders—and just about any other condition known.

By the way, if ever you need to consider a differential diagnosis for, say, anxiety symptoms or psychosis (or sleep–wake problems or a bunch of other symptoms) that could be caused by substance use, you can use the same basic procedure I've outlined in Step 9. Just plug in *anxiety* or *psychosis* (or whatever) each time I've written *depression* above.

Step 10

Uh-oh, there's still one more item: Justify the severity rating you'd attach to her gambling disorder.

Note J (Whew!)

DSM-5 recommends the following severity levels for gambling disorder: Four or five of the Step 1 symptoms indicate *mild*, six or seven *moderate*, and eight or nine *severe*. Of course, fewer than four equate to no diagnosis at all. Thus the severity requirements for gambling disorder are quite a bit more stringent than for the substance use disorders.

However, if you've rated Whitney as having a moderate gambling disorder, I'm not going to sit you on a stool in the corner, despite the fact that we've identified only a few symptoms. These severity guidelines are only recommendations. We shouldn't let them shackle the patient *we* know to someone else's concept of magnitude.

The Takeaway

For Whitney, the dice have not only taken a roll, they've taken on a role: They've helped both to drive the substance use and to obscure it from our view. Indeed, they've played a very substantial part. In addition, we have stumbled on an important precept, which is to beware of the obvious diagnosis—and verify it ourselves. We've also discussed some effective ways to develop information about mood disturbances. But Whitney, by withholding information about her substance use, has shown a degree of resistance that we've tried to combat by crafting a speech that encourages candor. Along the way, we've discussed the diagnostic criteria for gambling disorder and substance/medication-induced mood disorder. And we've even trotted out the unusual word *polythetic* to describe the condition where some set number of items from a list is required for inclusion.

Break Time

You could read for a decade and never run out of books with a mental health theme (or aspects) written for—I won't say *lay readers,* because many of them appeal to professionals, too—general consumption. These are books (mostly novels and memoirs) I have not discussed in other Break Time pieces.

One Flew Over the Cuckoo's Nest, by Ken Kesey, leads my list. I've already mentioned the motion picture starring Jack Nicholson, but the novel provides lots more detail and is extremely well written and engaging.

Myriad books take alcohol use as their theme. One of the most famous, in part because it too was made years ago into an iconic motion picture, is Charles Jackson's *The Lost Weekend.* It gives a riveting account of the symptoms (and tragedy) of someone descending into what today we call alcohol use disorder.

In Dickens's *The Old Curiosity Shop,* the grandfather's pathological gambling (cards) leads to the death of Little Nell.

For such a rare condition, dissociative identity disorder (formerly multiple personality disorder) is remarkably well represented in literature. *The Three Faces of Eve,* by Corbett Thigpen and Hervey Cleckley, is probably the best known, but *Sybil,* by Flora Rheta Schreiber, also tells the story of a real person. The actual person who experienced the 16 multiple personalities described herein has been long since "outed" by her real name, whereas the actual clinician, Cornelia Wilbur, has been accused of inducing multiple personalities in a suggestible patient. With all this, it's still a highly interesting read. But appearing three years earlier was Shirley Jackson's *The Bird's Nest,* which went *Eve* one better: It tells the story of a woman with four personalities.

Girl, Interrupted is a memoir by Susanna Kaysen, who writes about her 18-month stay as a teenager in McLean Hospital, where she was diagnosed as having borderline personality disorder.

"The Yellow Wallpaper" is a classic short story by Charlotte Perkins Gilman that is often cited in lists of feminist literature. Presented as a series of entries in the diary of a young woman married to a physician, it describes the development of psychotic symptoms in someone who is subjected to the so-called "rest cure" that was for many years in vogue as a treatment for nervous conditions. I invite you to download it (it's available free from Project Gutenberg) and then try to construct your own differential diagnosis for the unnamed narrator. (Of course, you'll work on the differential diagnosis only when you're not on break.)

Mark Haddon's novel *The Curious Incident of the Dog in the Night-Time* was made into a terrific play that premiered in London before being filmed for worldwide distribution on the United Kingdom's *National Theatre Live.* But the original story is a riveting exploration of some of the symptoms of Asperger's syndrome. (Some, but by no means all, I should emphasize.)

Of Mice and Men, by John Steinbeck, depicts the heartbreaking life trajectory of a person who is affected by what today we call intellectual disability.

In *An Unquiet Mind,* Kay Redfield Jamison—a psychologist, researcher, and Johns Hopkins faculty member—recounts her own harrowing battles with bipolar disorder, a subject on which she has become a world authority.

Through the eyes of a patient, *The Passion of Alice* by Stephanie Grant tells the story of people with anorexia and bulimia nervosa being treated at an eating disorders clinic.

Sylvia Plath's beautifully written novel, *The Bell Jar,* describes the protagonist's descent into depression. Ultimately, the heroine is saved by a caring physician and a second course of electroconvulsive therapy. Plath herself, however, famously committed suicide (via gas from her oven) a month after her book was published in the United Kingdom.

The editor of *The Atlantic,* Scott Stossel, in *My Age of Anxiety* recounts his own experiences with anxiety disorders. His various symptoms include those of panic attack, generalized anxiety disorder (even as a child), and various specific phobias (including fears of cheese and vomiting).

Finally, I recommend a trio of books about psychopathy. *The Mask of Sanity* by Hervey Cleckley is a work of nonfiction describing the classic psychopathic personality—attractive, yet cold and utterly lacking in conscience. You can download a PDF of the fifth edition (credited to Cleckley and his second wife, Emily S. Cleckley) for free (see this chapter's section in "References and Suggested Reading"). The father, Rick, in John Le Carré's *A Perfect Spy* is just such a charming con man. However, Cathy in *East of Eden* by John Steinbeck begins her lifetime of murder and other crimes when she is just a child: She burns down her house with her parents in it just before heading off to the city to become a prostitute and madam. Not so much charm.

24

Fill in the Blanks—X

Step 1

The report from the emergency room, apparently transcribed verbatim, reads:

Q: What is your name?

A: I, I . . . don't know.

Q: Can you say where you live?

A: No, I can't.

Q: How long has your memory been so poor?

A: I'm sorry, I know it sounds like a sick joke—but I don't remember.

A day earlier, "X" had been found wandering along a residential street, sometimes peering into garages, once or twice starting up a front walk. A man watering his lawn tried to engage him in conversation; then, noting the evident confusion, he called 911.

Now X denies feeling depressed or anxious; he doesn't seem to be withdrawing from alcohol or other substance use. There is no evidence of trauma; in fact, he doesn't appear physically ill at all. A neurological examination has revealed no abnormalities. He has signed the admission form with an *X*, written in a small, shaky hand. So, with no other information forthcoming—even his pockets are empty, save for a nearly depleted ChapStick and a "lucky penny"—they've called him X and admitted him to an observation room. And, of course, they've put in a call for the shrinks.

The question now is this: What should guide our mental health evaluation of X? What we need is a tentative list of conditions that can cause a major lapse of memory. I'd like you to write down your suggestions (feel free to consult texts for ideas), and then compare your efforts with mine in Note A.

___

___

____

____

____

____

____

____

____

Note A

In interviewing someone like X, we need to cover all of the possible causes of amnesia. That is, we want a list that focuses solely on the symptom of acute memory loss. We will use it from the beginning of our evaluation and constantly revise it as new information comes in. Of course, the first iteration should be the most comprehensive.

Our list for X will include the following:

- ◊ Neurocognitive disorder (NCD) due to another medical condition (especially traumatic brain injury and seizure disorders)
- ◊ Substance intoxication
- ◊ Dissociative identity disorder (DID)
- ◊ Dissociative amnesia (DA) (with or without dissociative fugue)
- ◊ Somatic symptom disorder
- ◊ Conversion disorder
- ◊ Posttraumatic stress disorder (PTSD) or acute stress disorder (ASD)
- ◊ Factitious disorder
- ◊ Malingering

As possibly comorbid, we might also consider personality disorders (especially dependent, avoidant, and borderline).

Rant

Memory is zero when we enter the world and, sometimes and tragically, zero when we exit. In between lie all the experiences, knowledge, and emotions revisited again and again that help make us the human beings we are. Cognitive scientists have studied memory, broken it down into a variety of domains, and named them. We can recall them with the help of a mnemonic—PEWS:

- Procedural memory. We use this for skills like typing, playing a musical instrument, and riding a bicycle. It allows us to repeat a sequence of behaviors without having to expend conscious effort.

- Episodic memory. This is what we use to recall events that we experience as personal history—what we were doing on 9/11, what we ate for supper last night, where we went on our last vacation. Episodic memory is always visual and always takes our personal point of view.
- Working memory. This is the short-term storing of data for active processing, often considered synonymous with attention. It's sometimes tested by asking the patient to do mental arithmetic or spell words backward.
- Semantic memory. This is what we mean when we speak of general knowledge—in short, facts and figures. Most of what we learn ends up as semantic memory, because we no longer associate everyday facts with anything concrete in our lives, such as where we were or what we were doing when the learning took place.

Step 2

The problem with our differential list in Step 1 is that much of what's on this list can only be evaluated in people who have access to their own personal information. Testing can determine whether someone currently has this or that substance on board, but such tests are only a snapshot in time; they convey little about the *history* of substance use. We can also test for neurological deficits that might accompany, say, traumatic brain injury, but even with magnetic resonance imaging of the patient's head, we'd still be far behind the curve in terms of defining objective symptomatology.

Happily, while we've been contemplating this conundrum, X has been gradually recovering his memory—a typical course for many patients with amnesia. We now know that his name is Malcolm, and we can begin to question him about his history. So here is what we know about Malcolm (as we'll call him from now on), obtained from collateral information, from the use of many of the standard interview techniques we've discussed previously, and from the questions that we'll make explicit in Note B, where we will use the underlined parts of the following summary.

> Malcolm's return of memory begins with "flashes" that illuminate the moments just before he was taken into care by the police. Later, he experiences the sudden dawning of entire aspects of his life—where he lived, what he did for a living, his family. "That stuff unfolded before my eyes, almost like a movie," he says, his facial expression reflecting considerable astonishment.
>
> Malcolm, it develops, is a repo man. His business is to locate cars whose owners have fallen months ("Sometimes it's years") behind in their payments, and bring them in. Then the bank sells them for whatever a vehicle that's been used, and often ill used, will fetch. He describes his repossession work with some flair and real pride in a skill that approaches art: In a moment, without ever leaving the cab of his truck, he can attach the tow, winch the vehicle aboard, and drive safely away.
>
> Despite the precautions he always takes, Malcolm got into deep trouble some months earlier with a "customer" who wished to retain the use of a showcase 1987 Corvette for which he hadn't made a payment in 4 years. In fact, without informing the bank, he'd shipped it from Hawaii to Los Angeles. As Malcolm drove off with the 'Vette in custody, in his mirror he could see an irate pedestrian snapping cell phone photographs.

"Usually that would be the end of it," Malcolm remarks. "They're pissed, then they calm down a bit and make other transportation arrangements. But this guy was a real fighter—I'd stolen 'his' property, and he wanted it back. With interest!"

So began a campaign of payback, launched with harassing phone calls. The former owner ("We'll call him *Y*," Malcolm says, with a tight smile) had apparently obtained Malcolm's information, including his home address, through the business license number lettered on the tow truck. In addition to the phone calls, he began receiving abusive letters and, once, a package containing a dead squirrel.

"It wasn't exactly a horse's head in the bed," Malcolm explains, "but it looked like roadkill, and Marilyn freaked. That's my wife."

Marilyn began a campaign to move. She also said that Malcolm should change jobs. "Hey! I like where we live, and I don't know anything but driving a tow truck. But Marilyn can really apply the pressure, and I didn't know what I'd do."

Malcolm underscores that nothing like this has ever happened to him before. In fact, he's always been healthy, and has never previously been hospitalized. He doesn't use drugs; he barely even drinks. "OK, I'll have a beer after mowing the lawn, if it's hot." He's adamant that he has never sustained any head injuries or had seizures, and he hasn't ever had blackouts or other times when he couldn't remember what he'd done. "Quite frankly," he says, "I've never been—I mean, to the best of my recollection—the sort of person who worries a lot about health stuff."

Although he hadn't been threatened with death or violence, "I did feel pulled in two directions." But as he wrestled with his predicament, he started losing sleep. And appetite. "I wasn't depressed, just, y'know, stalled. I felt I sure couldn't stay where I was, and I didn't see any way that I could move forward. I was stuck in neutral, and I had to get unstuck, and I didn't know how. And that's the last thing I remember. Until now."

What are the questions we need to ask of someone who reports severe memory loss? This may seem a little unfair—we haven't covered it elsewhere. But some of it you can infer from the underlined bits above. So, write down the questions (plus any others that seem pertinent) that would serve as probes to elicit the history just given. They'll probably be a mix of closed- and open-ended questions.

Note B

How do my questions below compare with those you've derived from the underlined bits in Step 2?

"What sort of stresses have you been under?"
"Has anything like this ever occurred before?"
"Have you experienced head injuries? Seizures? Any other medical illnesses?"
"Tell me about your use of alcohol and other substances."
"Do you ever have blackouts—times where you cannot remember what you've done?"
"Has this ever occurred in the absence of using alcohol or some other substance?"
"Has anything really awful happened recently—something involving death or horrific threats?"
"Are you the sort of person who worries a lot about health issues?"

Step 3

And now which of the nine disorders we've tentatively considered in Note A are we still considering? Wait, let's do it this way: List what you would *eliminate*, and explain your rationale.

____

____

____

____

Note C

The Note B questions should allow us to discard substance intoxication as the etiology of Malcolm's dilemma. His physical health has been good, and he doesn't seem to have had extraordinary health concerns, enabling us to rule out a somatic symptom disorder such as illness anxiety disorder or somatization disorder (as defined in DSM-IV). We've also determined that his neurological exam is normal, so we can rule out NCD due to another medical condition.

What about PTSD and its sibling, ASD? Dissociation can certainly occur with them, but the traumatic event must involve the threat of death or serious injury or sexual violence. By no means do I intend to disparage the degree of stress Malcolm has experienced. However, it was apparently a result not of threats from the irate car owner, but of irreconcilable desires imposed by the demands of his job and his own and his wife's desires.

All of this leaves us still struggling with these possible diagnoses:

◊ DID
◊ DA (with or without dissociative fugue)

◊ Conversion disorder
◊ Factitious disorder
◊ Malingering

Step 4

Bit by bit, even as they conduct the initial interview, experienced clinicians chip away at the list of diagnoses they are considering. I'd like to winnow our list for Malcolm a bit further by focusing on the last three Note D possibilities, none of which have we discussed much in the course of this workbook. What reasons would you give to help eliminate them? For each one, I've included just the essential defining features, which should give you some pretty good hints.

- Conversion disorder. The patient's symptom—it could be an alteration of either sensory or voluntary motor functioning—seems clinically inconsistent with any known medical illness. And your rationale for eliminating it for Malcolm is: ____________________
- Malingering. Some patients will intentionally exaggerate or falsify cognitive symptoms to obtain funds (insurance, worker's compensation) or to avoid punishment. Suspect it when the patient has legal problems or the prospect of financial gain, tells a story that does not accord with the known facts, does not cooperate with the evaluation, or has antisocial personality disorder. You'd disregard it because: ____________________
- Factitious disorder. To present a picture of someone who is ill, injured, or impaired, the patient (or another person acting for the patient) feigns physical or mental signs or symptoms of illness, or induces an injury or disease. This behavior occurs even without evident benefits (such as financial gain, revenge, or avoiding legal responsibility). Malcolm doesn't have this one either, because: ____________________

Note D

Conversion disorder involves loss of sensory or motor function (not memory); amnesia isn't included among its symptoms. Malingering is ruled out by the absence of any external incentive (such as financial reward or avoiding punishment or other personal advantage), and by the fact that Malcolm has none of the four factors suggested in the definition we've used above. Falsification of psychological symptoms, as in factitious disorder imposed on self, can be very difficult to prove. However, Malcolm has shown no evidence of intentional deception, and his behavior *is* explained better by other disorders. Let's save that discussion for Step 5.

Rant

Malingering should always be reserved for the bottom of the differential diagnosis. Why? As a diagnosis, it is absolutely lethal. That is, it poisons our trust in the patient, whom we must regard as dishonest. To label a patient as malingering also prejudices us against doing anything effective in the way of treatment; in fact, we are likely to regard this person as untreatable. The bottom line: I would make the diagnosis of malingering only with proof, such as video or eyewitness evidence that the patient has in fact manufactured symptoms.

Step 5

Our evaluation of Malcolm's amnesia has now come down to just three possibilities—no, two actually; in DSM-5, one of them can have a specifier. I've included brief definitions.

- DID. The patient appears to have at least two discrete individual personalities, each with unique attributes of mood, perception, recall, and control of thought and behavior. There are repeated memory gaps for personal information and ordinary events that common forgetfulness cannot begin to explain.
- DA. Far beyond common forgetfulness, the patient cannot recall important personal, usually traumatic or distressing information.
- DA with dissociative fugue. In association with an episode of DA, the patient wanders in a confused state or may travel in an apparently purposeful way from home.

Quite frankly, there is a lot of confusion about the dissociative disorders. Here are some issues that can make it difficult to determine whether DID or DA is what applies to a given patient.

- The classic portrayal (as in movies or on TV) is of a patient who turns on a dime from a mild-mannered milquetoast into someone who suddenly becomes assertive, taking charge of a situation—perhaps the interview itself. In reality, this dramatic sort of switch is rarely observed.
- Experiences such as the patient's unaccountably losing possessions or acquiring something (such as a new app that suddenly appears on a smartphone) can occur in DA or in DID.
- When considering DA, we tend to think about people (like Malcolm) who have completely lost all their personal memories and are found wandering. However, most episodes tend to involve amnesia for a specific event or for a more circumscribed period of time.
- Episodes of derealization can occur in patients who have depersonalization/derealization disorder, but patients with DID can have them too.
- Dissociative fugues, where patients find themselves in a strange place without being able to recall traveling there, occur in DA *and* in DID.
- Patients with DID can present with dissociative episodes that masquerade as NCDs.
- On the other hand, a patient with DID may have what is termed a *possession* form, wherein a spirit has apparently taken over the individual's personality. The interface here is with "normal" possession, found in some cultures around the world, which are a part of religious practice and are not considered pathological.

However, there is one feature of Malcolm's history that can absolutely move us along to the correct diagnosis. And that would be: ______________________________

(OK, here's a hint: It has to do with the number of episodes he has experienced.)

Note E

If any aspect of DID is extremely clear, it is this: It involves symptoms (and signs) that occur *repeatedly* over significant stretches of a person's lifetime. Having distinct personality states, as is definitional with DID, necessarily involves multiple time frames. Another criterion for DID is that the patient must have repeated memory gaps for items of everyday functioning. However, we know from his own testimony that Malcolm has had only this one episode.

For a time, Malcolm can recall nothing of his own personal information (that's DSM-5's Criterion A), which causes him significant distress (Criterion B). Medical conditions and substance use cannot explain the symptoms (C), and we've just ruled out the other, competing conditions (D). QED, the diagnosis is DA!

Step 6

Now would you assign Malcolm the *with dissociative fugue* specifier for DA?

Note F

Well, Malcolm hasn't exactly traveled far from home, but he's been picked up wandering in a bewildered state. Technically, that qualifies him for the specifier *with dissociative fugue.* Although we could invoke it, fugue states usually involve more extensive travel than we've noted in Malcolm. Besides, the specifier doesn't really have a lot to offer in terms of prognosis or treatment. It's your call, but I probably wouldn't bother.

Step 7

> At his next appointment, Malcolm asks this question: "One of the clinicians I talked with mentioned 'defense mechanisms.' What does *that* mean?"

So here's a multiple-part question. First, how should we define *defense mechanisms*?

____

Now fill in the blanks below with the names of the defense mechanisms that are indicated by examples couched in terms of Malcolm's story. Notice that I've separated these mechanisms into two groups: the potentially harmful and the generally effective.

Potentially harmful defense mechanisms

________________ Malcolm goes into Starbucks and picks a fight with the barista.

________________ Malcolm says, "It was a horrible job anyway; I'm glad to be heading out."

________________ He says, "I've got this harassment thing under control. Another day or two, we'll be golden."

________________ (We already know how this one worked out for Malcolm.)

________________ "I'll find him, collar him, and collect a big reward for his capture."

________________ "I like what Capote said: 'Failure is the condiment that gives success its flavor.'"

________________ (Unconscious thought: "I hate that guy.") Malcolm says, "He hates me."

________________ Malcolm calls the police with the false report that the person harassing him has planted a bomb on a plane.

________________ (Malcolm thinks, "Marilyn's so hard to live with!") He says, "She's only looking out for my best interests."

________________ Malcolm "forgets" he's borrowed equipment from the office.

________________ Malcolm develops persistent low back pain. He says, "I'd've had to retire, anyway."

________________ "Some of my 'clients' are great; others are bastards. His parents were barely acquainted."

Generally effective defense mechanisms

________________ "Of course I'm upset, but at least no one's been harmed."

________________ "Next time, I'll make sure the guy is watching TV."

________________ "And just when my business was picking up, this happened. Of course, that *is* my business—picking up."

________________ "I'll get retraining for a safer job."

________________ "I'll put the job on the back burner; I've got other issues to deal with."

And here is the list of defense mechanisms that I'd like you to fit into the blanks above:

- Acting out
- Altruism
- Anticipation

- Denial
- Devaluation
- Displacement
- Dissociation
- Fantasy
- Humor
- Intellectualization
- Projection
- Reaction formation
- Repression
- Somatization
- Splitting
- Sublimation
- Suppression

Note G

Defense mechanisms is a term that denotes the (largely unconscious) psychological techniques we use in the effort to cope with our feelings.

Potentially harmful defense mechanisms

Acting out	Malcolm calls the police with the false report that the person harassing him has planted a bomb on a plane.
Denial	He says, "I've got this harassment thing under control. Another day or two, we'll be golden."
Devaluation	Malcolm says, "It was a horrible job anyway; I'm glad to be heading out."
Displacement	Malcolm goes into Starbucks and picks a fight with the barista.
Dissociation	(We already know how this one worked out for Malcolm.)
Fantasy	"I'll find him, collar him, and collect a big reward for his capture."
Intellectualization	"I like what Capote said: 'Failure is the condiment that gives success its flavor.'" (This is one intellectual tow-truck driver!)
Projection	(Unconscious thought: "I hate that guy.") Malcolm says, "He hates me."
Reaction formation	(Malcolm thinks, "Marilyn's so hard to live with!") He says, "She's only looking out for my best interests."
Repression	Malcolm "forgets" he's borrowed equipment from the office.

Somatization	Malcolm develops persistent low back pain. He says, "I'd've had to retire, anyway."
Splitting	"Some of my 'customers' are great; others are bastards. His parents were barely acquainted."

And, here are a few defense mechanisms generally considered to be effective:

Altruism	"Of course I'm upset, but at least no one's been harmed."
Anticipation	"Next time, I'll make sure the guy is watching TV."
Humor	"And just when my business was picking up, this happened. Of course, that *is* my business— picking up."
Sublimation	"I'll get retraining for a safer job."
Suppression	"I'll put this on the back burner; I've got other issues to deal with."

The Takeaway

A slow crawl through the various suggestions for X (who soon recalls that his name is Malcolm) has demonstrated how clinicians methodically work through diagnostic possibilities to settle on a best diagnosis. We've also taken a look at the symptoms of dissociation, covering some of the questions that we'd need to answer when evaluating its differential diagnosis. We've explored definitions of defense mechanisms, both helpful and potentially harmful, and given examples of each as they might relate to Malcolm's own story. Moreover, we've considered: What questions do we need to ask—*can* we ask—someone with acute amnesia? In searching for a diagnosis, we've trotted forth several conditions that our diagnostic principles recommend: mood, substance use, physical, and somatic symptom disorders. Oh, yes, and I've added yet another Rant—this time, about the perils of using the diagnosis *malingering*.

Break Time

Let us consider memory. Memory is so important, such an integral part of our daily lives, that we venerate it in song (when we can remember the words): Famous examples include "Memory" from the musical *Cats* (composed by Andrew Lloyd Webber and T. S. Eliot) and "Yesterday" by The Beatles. "It Was a Very Good Year" was composed by Ervin Drake and made famous by Frank Sinatra—but who remembers (!) that it was originally recorded by Bob Shane of The Kingston Trio? Google *memory* and *song lyrics*, and you'll find dozens of other relevant entries from sources as widely divergent as Bob Hope (his theme song was "Thanks for the Memory," composed by Ralph Rainger and Leo Robin) and Merle Haggard ("House of Memories").

The effort to be memorialized is a familiar, perhaps universal human endeavor—yet one that, save for the most exceptional of cases, is ultimately doomed to fail. We erect tombstones in a cemetery, but all they achieve are records of people who, other than those such as Mozart (who never had a tombstone) and Lincoln and a few chosen others, will be utterly forgotten within a lifespan or two.

25

In Other Words—Yasmin

Step 1

"Sorry, I'm not understanding."

These are almost the only words 17-year-old Yasmin speaks that you can understand. Since arriving from her native country several months ago, she has lived exclusively among her close relatives, never venturing beyond the hallway of the apartment they all share. What little she's learned of her new language has come from watching TV.

The regular professional interpreter employed by the mental health clinic has called in sick today, but Yasmin's cousin, who's been in this country for a decade, has offered to translate.

Is this a good idea? If not, why not? And if so, why?

Why good? ____

Why not? ____

Note A

I'm pretty sure we can agree that the world is chock-a-block with pluses and minuses, and that most issues have some of each. This would certainly be true of interpreting for a mental health patient. On the one hand, it is vitally important to get the information necessary to make a solid diagnosis. To that end, an amateur translator is probably better than none at all. However, professional interpreters know how to facilitate the exchange of information without inserting themselves into the conversation; they even know where to sit so that they don't block line-of-sight communication or interfere with the patient–clinician relationship. Too, because they are relatively anonymous, they can help draw forth material from patients who might be reluctant to reveal personal, perhaps embarrassing information to relatives and others they must interact with daily. And only someone who does this sort of work day in and day out is likely to have the experience to avoid actual mistakes in translation—errors that can potentially alter a clinician's understanding of a patient's problems.

Step 2

Today, in the absence of the professional interpreter, you have to rely on Yasmin's cousin (who prefers to use his assimilated name, Joe) to provide translation. Four of you—Yasmin, her mother, Joe, and you—all crowd into the office, with Joe perched on a folding chair. The entire conversation is a polyglot mix: The mother mainly speaks her native language; Joe speaks both; Yasmin is largely silent throughout the interview. Nonetheless, here (largely from the mother, through Joe) is what we learn:

Yasmin came to this country 6 months ago with others in her family, after they'd fled the war-torn neighborhood where she'd been born and reared. She has learned hardly anything of her new language, and spends most of her time sitting in the room she shares with a younger sister. She has almost completely ignored the other immigrants in her community; after a few initial approaches that she rebuffed, they in turn have paid her little attention.

In the family's home country, Yasmin had been a normal girl who played with dolls, loved music, and excelled in school. "She always said she wanted to be a doctor," her mother volunteers. But when she was 15, about the time the rioting heated up, she had suddenly withdrawn from the rest of the family. She also avoided seeing her friends, preferring to stay by herself in her room (which, back home, she also shared with her sister).

"She didn't seem to do anything there, just sat. Sometimes she would read, but she never talked about what she read. She just didn't seem to be interested," Joe translated from her mother. "Even if I told her she was lazy or stupid, she didn't seem to care."

"It seems she's falling into psychosis." Joe, already a naturalized citizen, has taken a course in abnormal psychology, and he's clearly soaked up the terminology. "Auntie [meaning Yasmin's mother] says she hears her talking to herself at night, when she gets up and sits in the kitchen. She says someone tries to kill her. And her face—it's always just a blank. Isn't that a negative symptom?"

Interesting observation! Just so we're sure, let's review once again the concept of negative symptoms. In particular, how do they fit into the overall picture of psychotic disorders? We've mentioned them before, but this time I thought we might obsess about them, just a little.

Let's start out with a pretty simple matching quiz. Write an N after each word or phrase that indicates a negative symptom.

1. Speech using few words
2. Visual hallucination
3. Absence of pleasure
4. Persecutory delusion
5. Poor sociability
6. Tangential speech

7. Blunted affect
8. Deliberately turning away from the interviewer
9. Low interest in most matters
10. Aggressive hostility

And now formulate a definition—but try to keep it simple and brief: Negative symptoms are those that ______________________________

Note B

In the Step 2 list, each odd-numbered choice is a negative symptom. With some application of the linguistic shoehorn, you can describe each one by using an *A* word or phrase: Alogia, Anhedonia, Asociality, Affective blunting, Avolition. And here is my rather lengthy answer to Joe.

Positive and negative symptoms are mainly matters of addition and subtraction. The hallucinations and delusions that we most commonly associate with psychosis are called *positive symptoms,* meaning things that have been added to the human characteristics we all have. On the other hand, *negative symptoms* are features that people normally have, but that in an affected patient seem to have gone missing. The DSM-5 description of negative symptoms specifically mentions *diminished emotional expression* (also known as *affective blunting*) and *avolition,* in which the person has trouble beginning or sustaining goal-directed activities. These include working for a living and sometimes even maintaining adequate personal hygiene. (Avolition is therefore associated with action, or its absence, whereas *apathy* refers to lack of interest or concern. Found in many mental disorders, apathy does not itself serve as a criterion for psychotic disorders.)

Besides avolition and affective blunting, at least three other types of behavior are considered negative symptoms. *Asociality* occurs when a person does not engage with other people and perhaps has few friends. In *alogia,* communication skills are severely affected. The person may speak some, but not much—perhaps using sentences that are short and vague, perhaps with brief statements that don't convey much content. In *anhedonia,* the patient appears unable to experience pleasure from normally agreeable stimuli, including sex.

In addition to the foregoing five negative symptoms, some writers include lethargy, whereas others specify a reduction in expressive gestures—especially of the hands—that most of us habitually (and unconsciously) use to facilitate communication. To me, however, such motor manifestations can be hard to differentiate from disorganized behavior. Whatever symptoms you include, patients will usually not report negative features as *symptoms;* strictly speaking, they are instead apparent to clinicians and other observers as *signs.*

One way to uncover these negative signs and symptoms might be to ask, "From the time you awaken, how do you spend a typical day?" Besides ascertaining the degree to which the person engages in work, has contact with other people, and enjoys hobbies and other interests, you can assess the patient's ability to give a detailed response without the aid of further prompts.

Negative symptoms tend to persist longer than do positive ones, and they are harder to treat. Indeed, antipsychotic drugs sometimes even produce an apparent increase in negative symptoms; for example, some medications may cause a blank facial expressions and stiffening of the face or of extremities. When negative symptoms endure despite treatment, they are sometimes referred to collectively as a *deficit syndrome.* A deficit syndrome worsens the prognosis in a patient who has it.

So, yes, Joe, a blank face can be a negative symptom—if it's a sustained feature of the person's general appearance. But it is only a symptom, not a disorder or diagnosis, and it certainly doesn't mean that the person has a psychotic disorder. Negative symptoms constitute only one of DSM-5's five possible A criteria for several psychotic disorders, including schizophrenia. The others are, of course, delusions ★, hallucinations ★, disorganized speech ★, and disorganized behavior. For a diagnosis of schizophrenia, the patient must have two of these five sets of symptoms, including at least one of the three I've marked here with stars. (I'm sure you've memorized this list by now. Haven't you?)

And how would I word the simple definition I've asked you for? A negative symptom indicates the absence of something that should be there—for example, a lack of drive or an affect that's too bland.

Step 3

In Step 1 for X (eventually identified as Malcolm) in Chapter 24, we've used a tentative list of possible working diagnoses to help guide our evaluation. Does it help us any with Yasmin to start thinking in terms of such a list at this point? A brief justification of your yes-or-no answer would be appropriate.

Note C

In my estimation, a tentative working diagnosis doesn't add all that much value here. That's because at this point in the interview, I'd have to write down a huge amount of what's included in the diagnostic manuals. And, quite frankly, I just don't trust the information we have so far, which is incomplete and possibly corrupted—I don't think that's too strong a word—by the fact that it comes largely filtered through relatives whose agendas could be different from Yasmin's.

Yet, I do believe that there is something fundamentally wrong. That's why, if an interim diagnosis is necessary, I'd go with *mentally ill but undiagnosed.* This is a safe way to indicate that something is wrong, while keeping your options open.

Rant

In *DSM-5 Made Easy,* I've noted the surprising variety of ways to say, "I don't know the cause of [this disorder]." (The words clinicians use include *idiopathic, essential, primary, functional, essential,* and *cryptogenic.*) Just for fun, let's broaden the scope of this inquiry: How many different ways do we have of confessing (or perhaps obfuscating) our lack of an explanation for any event or entity, whether it's clinical or not?

- By putting some kind of name to it (an *unidentified* flying object), perhaps we strive to make it seem more familiar, or at least less scary.
- We can distance ourselves by emphasizing its otherness with a term such as *foreign* or *alien.*
- Just a tinge of censure adheres to such words as *curious, odd,* and *peculiar;* a larger dollop of disapproval attends *strange, weird,* and *bizarre.*
- In a more neutral vein, we can call it *novel* or *new,* or even *extraordinary* or *anonymous.*
- On the other hand, we can deploy a positive connotation with *exotic, enigmatic,* or *virgin.*
- We can emphasize our failed attempts at unraveling it with *mysterious, puzzling, inexplicable,* and *unfathomable.*
- Or we simply reject it altogether with *abnormal* or *queer* (in the older sense) or *deviant.*
- Or we can instead try to bury our mystification under a mountain of *un's—uncharacteristic, uncharted, undetermined, undiscovered, unexplained, unexplored, unfamiliar, unfathomable, unnamed, unrecognized, unplumbed, unsounded,* and *unspecified.* Add *unidentified,* and we've come full circle.

We employ each of these terms in the service of an effort that carries with it a certain flavor of, um, *je ne sais quoi.*

Step 4

So now, with our professional interpreter off the sick list and back on the job (and Yasmin's relatives waiting safely out of earshot), let's have another go at unraveling this history.

> During the confusion of the horrific siege that preceded the eventual flight from her homeland, five combatants forced Yasmin into the back of their truck and hauled her off to an abandoned building. There, she spent an excruciating 12 hours being alternately raped and beaten by men who stopped only because they became sexually depleted. They then turned her loose, with the admonition that if ever she told anyone what had happened, all in her family would be hunted down, tortured, and killed. When she finally stumbled back home, she told her mother that she had been to a friend's house and lost track of time. After that she bathed and went to bed, where she sobbed into the small hours of the night.
>
> When she did sleep, it was with repeated awakenings from dreams that she was being assaulted all over again. Right up to the present, these dreams have recurred "almost every night"—that is, those nights when she can sleep at all. "I am always waking up, throughout the night, with feeling bad," she reports. She believes that she invited what befell her—that she was being punished for seeking an education and thereby trying to invade traditionally male territory.
>
> Since arriving in this country, if anything comes on television that relates to warfare or to her country of origin, Yasmin will quietly turn it off (or leave the room, if others complain). She has been unable to keep her mind on "anything that I read," and now she sees no future for herself or for her family. "I want only to be dead," she says, in one of the few statements she makes that require no interpretation at all.

First, we can observe that—no surprise!—using a professional translator has made a terrific difference. For one thing, it has facilitated an interview that takes place with none of Yasmin's family in the room, even the psychologically minded Joe. However pure their motivation, the presence of relatives has undoubtedly inhibited her from sharing intimate details of something she considers shameful. A professional interpreter, on the other hand, has heard similar stories from countless others and may have helped extract details without further increasing Yasmin's anxiety. That said, I'd like you now to tell me what you think about—

Wait a minute! We haven't even talked about Yasmin's mental status! Wouldn't a mental status evaluation (MSE) be pretty hard to conduct through an interpreter?

Maybe not. I think it might help to consider separately each part of the MSE. For our convenience, I've reprised them in the table below, from the list I've made in a Rant during the discussion of Brad in Chapter 2 (see page 24). For each of the six parts, check one of the three boxes to indicate that we can gather this information from observation alone, or whether you would need an interpreter. Or perhaps this part of the task is simply not possible without direct communication between you and the patient.

Conducting the Six Parts of the MSE with Yasmin

	Observation works	Interpreter needed	Cannot evaluate
General appearance and behavior	☐	☐	☐
Mood/affect	☐	☐	☐
Flow of speech	☐	☐	☐
Content of thought	☐	☐	☐
Cognition	☐	☐	☐
Insight and judgment	☐	☐	☐

Note D

To answer our question, let's consider the different parts of the MSE, one by one.

- General appearance and behavior. This is an observational issue that transcends language; you could probably judge this category pretty well from a video with the sound off.
- Mood/affect. It is easy enough to ask about mood through the interpreter; however, the quality (type) of affect is another issue that speaks every language. You can also assess lability from observation alone, but appropriateness will require the context that an interpreter must provide.
- Flow of speech. You can tell even from speech you cannot understand how spontaneously, how rapidly, and at what length the patient speaks; you'll need to ask the interpreter to help with such issues as looseness of associations.
- Content of thought. No question about this one; it requires accurate translation.
- Cognition. Whereas you might be able to gauge attention, the remainder of the cognitive exam will require interpretation.
- Insight and judgment. Both aspects of this final category will also require interpretation.

But, overall, mental status can be evaluated accurately and well, even if the MSE is filtered through a third party. What it requires from you is an extra dollop of patience.

Step 5

So here is an assessment of Yasmin's mental status.

> Face framed by her hijab, Yasmin appears even younger than her stated age of 17. She sits quietly, occasionally glancing up from her hands, which are folded and still in her lap. Her facial expression is sad and shows little variation, other than when she speaks about the assault she endured so many months ago. Then her eyes redden and fill; overall, her affect appears entirely appropriate to the content of her thought.
>
> Yasmin speaks mainly when a question is put to her, though once or twice she will say something, then pause, then interrupt the translator's efforts to reproduce her thoughts. From the translated material she offers, the flow of her thought appears linear and to the point of the discussion.
>
> She denies having either hallucinations or delusions. Her explanation for some of the behavior that occasioned this evaluation? She says that she only gets up at night to go to another room to cry, so that she won't awaken her sister with her distress. And *she* awakens because of her terrible dreams—about what happened to her, about what she imagines will be her future. "Of course I am sad," she says. "Who wouldn't be?" Although she sometimes wishes she were dead, she denies having any suicidal ideas.
>
> Yasmin admits that she is still afraid of the men who assaulted her, but she acknowledges that they cannot actually harm her—not now, although she fears she could be deported. She says that she has no actual phobias. Although at first she is puzzled by the next few questions, ultimately she also denies any obsessional thinking or compulsive behavior.
>
> To direct questioning, she is fully oriented to date, place, and person. She is only vaguely aware of political events in this country, though she can talk about the status of refugees from her own homeland. She is also aware that an Olympic competition is in progress, but cannot give details, inasmuch as she does not follow sporting events.
>
> Her insight and judgment appear unimpaired: She acknowledges that there is something wrong, and that she needs help, though she cannot imagine that any will be forthcoming.

Now, utilizing all of what we have learned, what would be your diagnosis? Differential diagnosis, please, with your best effort at a best diagnosis (signify it with a star):

____

____

____

____

____

Note E

◊ Mood or psychotic or anxiety disorder due to another medical condition
◊ Substance-induced mood or psychotic or anxiety disorder
◊ Major depressive disorder
◊ Posttraumatic stress disorder (PTSD) ★
◊ Psychotic disorder such as schizophrenia

And the winner is . . . not psychosis after all, but PTSD. We can verify this conclusion by going through the PTSD criteria, one by one. You might remember that in discussing the case of Pierce in Chapter 16, we've dreamed up a clever mnemonic for the precipitant and four classes of required symptoms:

- Stressor
- Physiological symptoms
- Avoidance symptoms
- Intrusion symptoms
- Negative ideas (thoughts and emotions)

So let's now consider how these apply to Yasmin.

- Was there a horrendous stressor in which she was directly exposed to threats of death, severe injury, or violent sexual assault? You bet! In fact, all three types are relevant, and they have happened to her personally, not just to someone she knows.
- She has at least a couple of physiological symptoms signifying increased arousal and reactivity: She sleeps poorly and has trouble with concentration.
- She avoids anything that reminds her of the attack, including TV or video material related to warfare and her country of origin.
- Has the stressor resulted in intrusion symptoms? Again, yes: She has recurrent dreams that cause her to get out of bed and sit in the kitchen.
- She also has plenty of negative emotions and thoughts, including persistent feelings of shame and guilt, refusal to participate in activities with others, and the wish that she were dead. (Note that these negative responses are *not* the same as the negative symptoms that we identify for patients with psychosis.)

All of this has lasted far longer than the 1-month minimum, has caused obvious and clinically important distress, and does not appear to be the result of a medical condition or substance use. Yep, we've addressed all four parts of our diagnostic mantra: "inclusion, exclusion, duration, distress." And if you wish, you can flip back (page 187) to the chart we've used when discussing Pierce to identify all the components of a PTSD diagnosis.

However, did you write down that Yasmin could have a mood disorder as well? I hope so. Though the vignette doesn't adequately explore this, clinicians who frequently treat PTSD say that many (perhaps most) such patients have accompanying mood disorder.

Going forward, then, we must be careful to evaluate Yasmin for major depressive or persistent depressive disorder.

Rant

How unusual is it to have multiple diagnoses? Not to put too fine a point on it, pretty darned common. The National Comorbidity Survey Replication study of over 9,000 English-speaking adults in the United States found a 12-month prevalence of 26% for any of these types of disorders: mood, anxiety, substance use, and impulse disorders. Of these individuals, 45% had two or more diagnoses; 23% had three or more. (The data on non-mood-related psychotic disorders were considered too few for accurate assessment.)

The Takeaway

In considering the story of Yasmin, we have observed the value of using a professional interpreter for an initial interview, rather than a relative or friend, for someone with limited skills in our shared language. We've discussed the meaning of negative symptoms of schizophrenia and other psychotic disorders, and we've once again talked about the symptoms of PTSD. (In passing, we've also noted the connection of the trauma- and stressor-related disorders to major depression.) We've also found an opportunity to (briefly) employ the term *undiagnosed* in confronting complicated diagnostic problems. I've expanded on that term in a Rant, and briefly rant about the frequency of multiple diagnoses in mental health patients.

Break Time

When Yasmin and her family were fleeing from home, monuments to mental health were undoubtedly far from their thoughts. But when *we* travel—in our armchairs or otherwise—we might keep in mind some of the potential destinations that harbor a rich mental health history.

For so many reasons, where better to start than London, site of the Bethlem (or St. Mary Bethlehem) Royal Hospital, founded in the mid-13th century as an institution that collected alms to care for the needy. Probably the longest-serving mental health facility in the world, it has been associated with care of the mentally ill as far back as the early 15th century, and possibly years earlier. In the beginning, it wasn't exactly a happy refuge, however: Inmates were treated largely as prisoners, and those deemed dangerous (or who deeply disturbed other people) were kept in chains. (The term *bedlam*, meaning a scene of confusion and commotion, was derived from Bethlem several hundred years later.)

It was in Paris, in the late 18th century, that the chains were eventually struck from the limbs of the mentally ill. That brave step was the work of a hospital superintendent named Jean-Baptiste Pussin, originally a tanner of hides who subsequently joined the staff of l'Hôpital Bicêtre and worked his way up to become the administrator of a mental ward. (Even back then, I don't think his was a typical career path for a mental health professional.)

Pussin instituted such practices as keeping records (!) and treating the patients with relative consideration—methods eventually observed by visiting physician Philippe Pinel. However, only *after* Pinel left did Pussin order that chains no longer be used to restrain patients (straitjackets were still permitted). Once Pinel became superintendent of l'Hôpital Pitié-Salpêtrière, he asked Pussin to join him in Paris; subsequently, the shackling of mental patients was prohibited there too. Although Pinel always credited Pussin (and Madame Pussin, who also played a role in promoting the humane treatment of mental patients), Pinel's is the name we celebrate today for striking the chains from the mentally ill. Whoever promised life would be fair?

Half a century later, the Salpêtrière was also the site of the female ward that housed together patients with epilepsy and what was then called hysteria . There, the patients with hysteria began to imitate the seizures of the patients with epilepsy—a phenomenon that so fascinated neurologist Jean-Martin Charcot that he wrote papers about these symptoms. This attention initiated a worldwide epidemic of so-called *grand hysterie,* in which people with hysteria developed pseudoseizures that became more and more elaborate as they were passed by imitation from one person to the next. (After Charcot died, interest in grand hysteria declined, and the whole edifice of grand hysteria quickly collapsed.)

We have miles to go before we sleep. In Germany we should visit Dresden, Leipzig, Heidelberg, and Munich—each at one time or another the workplace of Emil Kraepelin, who founded modern scientific psychiatry. In 1883, at the tender age of 27, Kraepelin published the first edition of the seminal textbook that placed psychiatry in the family of medical specialties. It was he who sparked the rise of descriptive psychiatry, based on the analysis of data from mental patients, to determine patterns of illness (syndromes) as distinguished from merely classifying symptoms.

Then on to Rome, where Ugo Cerletti devised electroconvulsive therapy, the first effective somatic treatment for sufferers from some mood and psychotic disorders. And of course, how complete could any tour be that bypassed Vienna? There we can kneel at the shrine of Sigmund Freud, who famously created psychoanalysis (and whose theories of psychological causation of mental illness Kraepelin rejected).

Let's finally stop in St. Louis, Missouri, where over 40 years ago, the psychiatry faculty at Washington University School of Medicine published an article that collected definitions and criteria for major mental disorders. That document provided the basis for DSM-III, which has evolved through subsequent editions to become the standard for mental disorder diagnosis everywhere in the world. (Personal note: The first author of that seminal article was my late brother-in-law, John Feighner.)

26

Goodbye and Good Luck—Zander

Step 1

"I want to be up-front and clear about this—I'm only seeing you this once. That w-w-work for you?" Bespectacled and a little prim, your would-be "one-time-only" patient sits down with an air of easy authority and crosses his legs. His chin slightly raised, he regards you with a steady gaze.

Whoa! A challenge thrown down in the first moments of a clinical encounter! Your response to that would be . . .

- ☐ Saying, "Fine, what's your issue?"
- ☐ Replying, "No, I don't work that way."
- ☐ Trying to negotiate a compromise.
- ☐ Well, doing something else. Any suggestions?

Note A

Of course, you need to structure your own clinical practice so it's comfortable for you, but you must also consider the well-being of your patients. Here's how I'd approach these issues.

Let's begin with the low-hanging fruit. I suspect we can agree that the second option—a flat-out "No, I don't work that way"—would be exactly the wrong way to go. What would such an approach gain? If the patient stays anyway, it will probably be with some fear and resentment; right from the start, you'd be playing catch-up in the rapport department. (Keep in mind the truism "No one ever wins an argument with a patient.") And if your patient gets up and departs, you're left to wonder what the original problem might have been. Maybe something interesting; perhaps something you could have helped with. So that choice is out.

But the remaining choices could occasion mild disagreement. OK, perhaps you want to do a little negotiating ("Let's just wait and see what we discover in our first meeting"). What's the harm? Maybe none at all, but I don't think I'd bother with any sort of equivocation, no matter how strongly I might feel that time can change the course of any clinical relationship. Honestly, it isn't that big a deal. If you have the time (and, hey, if the patient leaves in a huff, you'll have quite a lot of it to kill!), and if the patient seems in need of help and thinks that a single session with you can provide it, I'd just say "Yes." After some of the clinical facts are in, *then* might be the time for negotiation.

Step 2

Alexander ("When I was 3, 'Zander' was the b-b-best I could do with my own name, and it just sort of stuck") settles into his chair and relates this story.

"I was halfway through my third year in college when disaster struck. I know, that sounds a bit dramatic, but it sure is how I experienced it at the time."

You smile and nod as encouragement, and he continues.

"I'd been feeling a little down, well, pretty b-b-blue, actually, for most of that spring. My concentration had suffered; I'd failed to turn in a couple of papers; and my advisor'd told me I was on the cusp of being asked to take a leave of absence. I was majoring in biology." Zander closes his eyes and clenches his fists on the word "biology," but manages to pronounce it cleanly.*

"Then—almost overnight, it seemed—everything changed. I began awakening each morning—earlier and earlier, I might add—feeling rested, renewed. I had a real zest for living. I'd spring out of bed, throw on some clothes, maybe go for a brisk run around the campus, and then sit down to 12 or 14 hours of productive work.

"Suddenly I *loved* my schoolwork, couldn't wait to get at it, almost couldn't work long enough. I got those papers done, aced a couple of exams, and made an appointment to talk to my department chair about some ideas I had for improving the course offerings."

Zander pauses to take a folded page of notes from his shirt pocket. "After that, I'm a little fuzzy on the details. What I think I remember is rather different from what I've been told—by several people I trust."

For a moment, he reads over his notes, then sighs and continues. "The next thing I remember clearly was when I woke up in a jail cell. Seems the professor had disagreed with some of my ideas, and I took a swing at him. Then I sort of destroyed his office." Zander pauses again to shake his head and take some deep breaths.

"The next day, the judge sent me to an inpatient unit, where they kept me for a couple of weeks. They started me on lithium and, pretty quickly, things returned to normal. I was released; I apologized to the professor; he was very gracious, said he understood I had a problem, and even let me return to class. The doctor told me that because of the risk of recurrence, I'd have to be on the drug for a long time—maybe all my life. But, after a few months, I just gradually stopped taking it. Little by little, I weaned myself off and—nothing happened! And I've been pretty normal ever since."

"Great!" you enthuse. "So you've been well for, let's see, the last . . . "

"Almost 13 years!" Zander's pride is palpable. "I feel I've defeated a real enemy. In fact, after the first few months off the drug, I've never really thought much about having cyclothymia—until just recently."

---

*To facilitate reading, during the balance of this account I've not recorded Zander's stuttering, though it continues pretty much unabated.

Wait a minute! We know *that* diagnosis isn't right, don't we?

Don't we? And what gives us that knowledge? Maybe your response could take the form of a list of all the disorders you can think of that involve an upswing of mood. Yes, and please add a brief discussion as to what makes these disorders different from one another.

Note B

Here's what I'd include in a first-pass differential diagnosis for Zander, followed by some brief arguments.

- ◊ Bipolar disorder due to another medical condition
- ◊ Substance/medication-induced bipolar disorder
- ◊ Bipolar I disorder
- ◊ Bipolar II disorder
- ◊ Cyclothymic disorder

First, let's tackle Zander's own suggestion. I'm afraid that he, or someone, has misunderstood—or perhaps not bothered to read—the DSM-5 criteria, which would completely disallow a diagnosis of cyclothymia for his particular collection of symptoms. We know that cyclothymic disorder (its formal name) is relatively mild and involves both highs and lows of mood, but it must last for at least 2 years, during which the mood swings are present at least half the time. We don't get the sense of any such duration from Zander, and we certainly wouldn't regard the experience he related as especially mild. Perhaps whoever suggested cyclothymia to Zander was trying to make him feel better by downplaying the seriousness of his condition. If so, it wasn't an especially thoughtful gift.

As we move *up* the differential list for a change, bipolar II disorder is also relatively mild. However, any time there's been an upswing of mood so extreme that it either requires hospitalization or includes psychotic symptoms, we must diagnose a manic episode, and bipolar II is no longer a possibility.

What about bipolar I? For sure, Zander's mood upswings have been severe enough to qualify; his brief history also seems to fit pretty well the requirements for bipolar I. His illness apparently began years ago with an episode of major depression. Having a major depressive episode isn't required for bipolar I, though it is for bipolar II. (Of course, these are somewhat artificial distinctions; it is highly likely that all three of these named disorders exist on a continuum marked by fuzzy borders. Nonetheless, these are the rules by which we must play the bipolar disorder diagnosis game.)

I'd like to focus attention on one other aspect of Zander's history: the rapid recovery he apparently made with lithium. That isn't rock-solid evidence of a bipolar disorder (much information can get lost in the mists of time or distorted with retelling), but having a typical response to treatment can sometimes provide support for a diagnosis. The response of manic symptoms to lithium is the best example I can think of in support of this diagnostic principle.

Zander's history does contain an oddity, however, and that is his continuing good health ever since that initial depression followed by a manic episode. For more than a decade, without benefit of any prophylactic measure such as lithium, he's remained completely asymptomatic. That isn't unheard of, of course (perhaps 10% of patients who have had one manic episode never have another), but it is unusual. In fact, it should serve as a spur to search diligently for other etiologies of his lone mood swing—principally, substance/medication use and other medical conditions.

I'd suggest that we don't yet have enough information to rule out either of those two possibilities. And although I always consider those two, here they appear high on the list for importance, but rather low on any list for the probability that they caused Zander's manic symptoms. So, with less than an hour to work, we should focus on what seems the most likely diagnosis. We won't exactly discard other causations, but for right now we'll put them to the side, leaving bipolar I disorder by far the most likely diagnosis for Zander.

Rant

An underappreciated issue is how a patient's longitudinal history can outweigh the cross-sectional appearance in determining diagnosis. That is, the course of an illness over a lifetime can relay diagnostic information that may be determinative. Take the case of a patient with psychosis. The presence of delusions and hallucinations only tells us that this person, well, has psychosis. That the symptoms began years ago and have continued without complete recovery suggests that the diagnosis may belong in the realm of schizophrenia and its cousins. Another patient—one who has episodes of psychosis that last a few months, separated by spells of complete return to good health—may have an illness that is more properly grouped with the mood disorders.

Step 3

Even though you are under the gun to make a diagnosis by the end of the hour, let's carve out a moment to consider how to approach someone with a physical characteristic such as Zander's stutter. You could:

- ☐ Ask about it during the initial interview.
- ☐ Ignore it for now, with a mental note to explore it later.
- ☐ Acknowledge it only if the patient is the one who brings up the subject.

Note C

Of course, there appears to be quite a lot on Zander's plate (and on yours!) right now, so it might seem disruptive to bring up his obvious stammer. However, if at all possible, now—during the first interview—is the time to pursue a physical issue that a new patient might present with. For one thing, it's a bit more graceful to ask about potentially embarrassing issues in the context of gathering initial information than it would be later on. Here's another, perhaps more substantive justification: Obvious physical conditions that make a person stand out—especially anything that may have been present during the developmental years—may have helped form that individual's understanding of what kind of a place the world is, how accepting (or threatening) the environment is, and how supportive its other inhabitants are. This argument holds for any visual or hearing impairment, a skeletal deformity, a prosthesis, a limp, or any other physical issue that could conceivably produce special challenges during the formative years.

Of course, I'd be less likely to follow this general rule scrupulously in the case of someone I was likely to encounter only once. For Zander, I might just decide to check the second box in the list above and move on. But to follow up on these matters when they first appear is useful general advice.

Step 4

You've decided to ask about the stutter right now. I won't fault you; I'm curious too.

> Zander appears a little startled to be speaking about his stuttering, but he responds with this information. From about the age of 5 through the first few grades of school, it was noticeable enough that other kids teased him. Then his parents sent him to speech therapy, which actually reduced the frequency and intensity of the problem. Although the stutter is still present, especially when he is under stress, it really doesn't trouble him today. No, he's never had the experience of feeling compelled to utter sounds or words—"No one's ever suggested I had Tourette's," he volunteers.
>
> "Besides, that's got nothing to do with why I'm here. But I *am* here because of something in my past history, something I need to keep very private. I mean, my employer, my family—*nobody* must know! Right?"

Zander has asked a question that has to do with clinician ethics. To answer it, let's first ask: What are the core ethical principles that any health care provider should follow? Below, I've listed four that are so commonly mentioned and described that they are generally accepted and (mostly) not controversial. I'd like you to associate each term with the appropriate definition-example, which I've stated still further below. (You shouldn't infer relative importance from the order in which I've listed these principles and rules.)

The four principles

1. Autonomy. ____
2. Beneficence. ____

3. Nonmaleficence. ____
4. Justice. ____

Definition–examples

a. As clinicians, we should act in the best interests of others. *Before recommending treatment for Zander, you carefully determine that the diagnosis is correct and that the proffered treatment is known to be effective in preventing future episodes.*
b. Individuals have the right to make rational, personal life decisions. *Years ago, Zander was advised that he should continue to take lithium to prevent future (likely) episodes of bipolar disorder. He discontinued the medication anyway.*
c. Benefits and burdens should be distributed equitably across society; people should be treated fairly. *You would recommend the same course of action for anyone with Zander's diagnosis and other risk factors, regardless of race, religion, gender, sexual preference, or income level.*
d. We should avoid doing harm. *You carefully enquire as to Zander's overall health, especially his kidney functioning, and caution him not to initiate a low salt diet, which could unintentionally elevate lithium levels.*

Note D

Here are the four ethical principles discussed in Step 4, with my answers to the matching test I've presented there.

1. Autonomy. _b_
2. Beneficence. _a_
3. Nonmaleficence. _d_
4. Justice. _c_

Several additional rules and professional values either derive from the four principles listed above or exist independently of them:

5. We should always tell the truth.
6. If we make a promise, we should keep it (trustworthiness).
7. We should protect each individual's privacy; we should not disclose what others tell us in confidence.
8. We should maintain collegiality (our duty to our health care colleagues).
9. We should obtain informed consent before proceeding with treatment (or a research protocol).

Some rules are "relatively absolute" (let's just agree to tolerate that oxymoron):

10. We should never state a professional opinion about anyone for whom we have not conducted a personal examination (for example, a political figure), and we should

state an opinion about someone we have treated only when given permission by the individual. We've encountered this one previously, in the guise of the Goldwater rule (see Chapter 14's Break Time, page 161).

11. We should not have sexual contact with any patient, ever.
12. We should always report child abuse.
13. We should protect others from whatever injury our patients could cause.

Several of these rules may seem a little stark, so let's discuss some in just a bit more detail.

Early in training, clinicians are likely to encounter the ancient admonition "First, do no harm," by which we mean *nonmaleficence* (item 3, above). Harm can come from a variety of directions—if we are ignorant about the effects of what we do (or fail to do) for a patient; if we are reckless or ill considered in determining our actions; or if we simply neglect to pay the required attention to our own behavior and its effects.

The flip side of nonmaleficence is, of course, *beneficence* (item 2). That's the obligation we all have as health care professionals to provide benefit to others. (It's not the same as *benevolence*, which is the disposition we have to do good, as opposed to the good things themselves that we do.) As we seek to help others, we must balance the supposed benefits of our actions against the possible harm that they could cause instead. This is only one of many ways in which ethical principles can conflict with one another. Indeed, instances where two or more principles conflict with one another supply most of the cases that ethicists address.

Principles and rules sometimes collide, especially when confidentiality (7) is involved. For example, it may take a back seat to the rule of reporting child abuse (12). Another often-cited example occurs should we learn that harm is about to befall someone whom we can identify. This is the well-known 1976 *Tarasoff* decision of the California Supreme Court, which mandates that we take steps to warn and protect that individual (item 13), even if it means divulging something that a patient has told us in confidence. The court's summary statement has often been repeated: "The protective privilege ends where the public peril begins." Most jurisdictions in the United States have adopted some form of what's variously called the *Tarasoff* duty, principle, or warning. I've mentioned *Tarasoff* in connection with the case of Randolph in Chapter 18.

You can find plenty of other examples of colliding principles. Often cited is the conflict of beneficence (2) with autonomy (1) in the case of, say, an adult patient who for religious reasons rejects a potentially life-saving medical procedure. Another is to question the justice of spending hundreds of thousands on a heart transplant to benefit one person (2) when the same money could inoculate thousands of individuals against a potentially lethal infectious disease (4).

Step 5

You assure Zander that, in the absence of any threat that he plans to harm himself or someone else, you are committed to maintain the confidentiality of the information he is about to impart.

Seemingly a little more comfortable, Zander settles into his chair. "I was pretty sure that'd be your response," he says with a smile, "but I wanted to hear it with my own ears. So now I need you to get me another prescription for lithium. Enough to last 9 months."

"But you haven't taken it for a decade!" you exclaim, somewhat taken aback. "Why should you—?" He waves the question away and interrupts; his stammer has nearly disappeared as he relates more of his story.

Zander is a climate scientist; next month he is scheduled to depart for Antarctica. He will winter over, spending 9 months studying the ice pack. He wants the lithium as "a hedge against unlikely disaster."

"For months," he points out, "we'll have no access to the full range of mental health treatment. Sure, I think the chances are extremely good that I won't have another episode of, well, whatever you say it was. But what if I do? All hell could break loose."

Without appropriate medication, he could require restraint, even seclusion. Those facilities, that expertise, wouldn't be available until spring, many months away. "During that interval, I could create quite a lot of havoc, if what I've been told is right." He goes on to recite a brief history of medical emergencies that have entailed evacuation from Antarctica. More than a few have involved some risk to the pilots who have flown to the rescue through winter weather conditions.

The bottom line is this: Zander feels that he cannot disclose his previous illness to his employers. "For sure, that would be the end of my participation in the project." So he's depending on you to facilitate a prescription for prophylactic medication.

So now what are your ethical responsibilities to the patient? To the expedition? To Zander's family? Even to the pilots who might be called upon to fly a dangerous emergency mission? Which of the following actions that you could take, *should* you take? And what would justify them? There are no pat answers here; these are issues you will have to figure out for yourself. But I encourage you to choose a course of action by indicating yes (Y) or no (N) in the list below, and to write down your justification for it, based on the principles/rules/professional values presented in Note D.

- ☐ Should you advise Zander to disclose his history and concerns with his prospective employers?

  Y/N Citing principles: ____________________
- ☐ May you ethically provide (or facilitate the obtaining of) a prescription for lithium, knowing that he probably will not take it now, but wants to have it with him as a hedge against the possible onset of an episode of bipolar I disorder?

  Y/N Citing principles: ____________________
- ☐ Do you have a duty to break confidentiality and warn Zander's employers yourself?

  Y/N Citing principles: ____________________
- ☐ On the other hand, should you perhaps simply deny Zander's request and send him on his way with empty hands?

  Y/N Citing principles: ____________________

Note E

Let's say that Zander comes clean, in effect, with his prospective employers. That would resolve someone's major dilemma—yours. You would then be relieved of any decision to violate his autonomy (1) and confidence (7). His candor would promote truth telling (5) and reduce potential harm to others as well as to Zander himself (3). Problem solved, except that from what he has already said, Zander is highly unlikely to go this route.

Should you (may you) advise Zander to take lithium with him to his job in Antarctica? Or even facilitate his obtaining it? On the one hand, you would thereby be respecting Zander's autonomy (1); he is an adult who is currently able to think rationally about his choices, and hence able to decide what is best for his own health care. Helping him obtain a prescription for lithium would improve his chances of surviving the possible recurrence of a manic episode, should one develop while he is deployed. If we assume that he will go to Antarctica anyway, regardless of your advice, then you've moved the needle a little toward his own safety, and possibly that of the anonymous pilots (to whom, we should note, you owe no actual ethical duty). Thus you would be addressing the core ethical principles of autonomy (1) and beneficence (2).

However, suppose that in the dead of the Antarctic winter, Zander becomes seriously ill despite the use of medication and requires medical evacuation. Then haven't you helped put him in danger, in effect violating the principle of nonmaleficence (3)? He might not even realize that he is becoming ill, and what a mess that would be! And haven't you also abetted his deception, violating the professional value of always telling the truth (5)? Then there are the pilots who might have to extract him—they've been endangered. (On the other hand, you wouldn't know which individual pilots to warn; this is what they get paid to do, and they enter into their contracts freely, knowing that there could be risk.)

OK, suppose you blow the whistle and notify Zander's employers. This would have several consequences, none of them good. Without the twin justifications of immediacy and an identified target of threat (as mentioned in the *Tarasoff* decision), you'd be violating Zander's confidence (7). At the same time, wouldn't you also be violating your duty to your health care colleagues (8) by potentially increasing distrust in all of those who are sworn to protect the confidentiality of patients? (Unfortunately, whether or not you warn Zander's employers, you risk a decrease in the public's confidence in the mental health professions, which could result in decreased willingness of other prospective patients to seek help.)

On the other hand (I've lost count, but I think we're now somewhere north of three hands), if you simply deny Zander's request, you've once again solved your own problem (sort of), leaving Zander's unaddressed. That's not what we clinicians are paid to do. In fact, wouldn't you be abandoning him to struggle—autonomously (1), to be sure, but alone—with the balance of beneficence versus nonmaleficence?

None of the decisions we could make is without flaws; as noted above, that's the essence of the ethical dilemma. What we choose to do will depend on a lot of different factors, including our own perceptions (as clinicians) of the world. I have decided which of the choices I would make; have you?

Rant

There is a great deal of information available in books and online concerning many, many aspects of health care ethics. However, some situations—like Zander's—add details more complicated than textbooks tend to address. Then you may need to seek advice from an ethicist or an ethics committee, such as you'll find at many health care schools and other facilities. The consultation can be enormously helpful in sorting out competing principles, duties, and rules, especially if your personal moral views conflict with a patient's needs or desires. It's worked for me.

Step 6

Finally, whatever you work out with Zander, this is your last meeting with him, and you need to summarize. I realize it is also your *only* meeting with him, but still treat him as you would any other patient. What elements do you want to include in these last few moments with this patient? There should be three elements. If you need a hint, refer back to our discussion of Pierce (page 191).

____

____

Note F

At the close of an evaluation, whether or not there's to be ongoing treatment, I like to include three main parts: a *précis,* or summary of the interview with my findings; a *recommendation* for future steps to be taken; and a message of hope for the future (modified *prognosis*). Of course, for someone you have had in treatment for an extended period, the first part would be modified to include a review of what has been done and its effects. In the case of Pierce in Chapter 16, we've encapsulated these three parts as *descriptive, prescriptive,* and *predictive.*

Step 7

And now, along the lines we've just discussed, what might you say to Zander?

Précis: ______________________________________

Plan: ______________________________________

Prognosis: ______________________________________

Note G

Fleshed out just a bit, here's the message I'd try to communicate to Zander:

"Based on what you've told me, years ago you probably had an episode of mania—it's what clinicians call bipolar I disorder. Although you haven't had a recurrence in all these years, that may just be your extraordinarily good luck; there's still a pretty good chance you could have a recurrence—either another manic attack or an episode of what could be very severe depression (or either of these, followed rapidly by the other)—at some time in the future. If that should ever happen, you'd need to deal with it very quickly. But bipolar I disorder is a condition that we know a lot about, and for which we've developed good methods for treatment. It therefore carries an excellent prognosis for full recovery.

"However, as you yourself have said, that recurrent episode could come while you are deployed in Antarctica, without adequate facilities or even possibly medication to treat you. Just as you thought even before this consultation, this means that special steps should be taken to help protect you, as well as those around you."

Then I would summarize whatever recommendations I've decided upon, as we've discussed in Note E. And as he's heading out the door, I would be sure to offer Zander my help again, whenever he might want or need it.

The Takeaway

There's a lot to process in this final case, but the greatest part of it has to do with determining an ethical approach to a patient with needs and goals that conflict with one another—and potentially with those of other people. Of course, this is a situation that affects many of our patients (and it certainly affects us as clinicians), but it's one that we too seldom confront explicitly. In getting to the kernel of this conundrum, we've discussed the difficulties of acceding to (or rejecting) a patient's demands prior to being seen, as well as the issue of dealing with a patient's obvious physical conditions. We've also discussed the differential diagnosis of bipolar symptoms, including bipolar I, bipolar II, and cyclothymic disorders. In addition, we've noted that ethical dilemmas arise when principles conflict with one another. At the end, we've talked a bit about the arts of closure and of sharing our findings with the patient. We've also had a view of what it's like to be a biomedical ethicist: It involves parsing the many competing issues driving our decisions that can potentially affect patients and those around them. Along the way, we've mentioned a diagnostic principle that is occasionally useful: Previous typical treatment response increases the likelihood that this disorder is once again responsible for a patient's symptoms.

Break Time

As I write, rain is falling in Oregon. This will come as no surprise to anyone who lives in the lush Pacific Northwest, which has an abundance of the stuff. We Oregonians (and Washingtonians and British Columbians) are inured to rainfall; we relish it; we celebrate it. Rain here tends to be relatively light—some of my neighbors, without intended irony, refer to it as "dry rain"—but the region makes up for a relative dearth of cloudbursts with longish periods of sustained drizzle.

However, even in regions distant from the Promised Land, rain has had a long-standing relationship with depression. Perhaps that's in part due to the physical similarity of raindrops to teardrops. Consider, for example, Malvina Reynolds's ballad "What Have They Done to the Rain?", wherein "rain keeps falling like helpless tears." Then that ever-popular ballad of disappointment, "Stormy Weather," begins with these lines: "Don't know why/There's no sun up in the sky . . . " And of course, seasonal affective disorder is an altogether real form of major depression in which spirits tend to droop during the winter months, when for some people there just aren't enough photons around to sustain a positive mood. Even aside from mood, cold causes chronic pain to feel worse, as with arthritis and chilblains.

The Santa Ana winds that blow in from the Southern California desert are featured in the crime novels Ross McDonald and Raymond Chandler set in Los Angeles and environs. Sometimes called *devil winds,* they are reputed to drive people to extremes of anxiety and behavior, perhaps even madness.

In the extreme north, long winter months with little sun exposure foster the tradition of cabin fever. Sam McGee, who "was from Tennessee, where the cotton blooms and blows," died in the throes of delirium during the course of one Arctic winter. His nameless companion—the narrator of the Robert Service poem "The Cremation of Sam McGee"—went mad trying to find a venue where he could cremate Sam. In the same tradition are prairie madness and *piblokto,* the latter a culture-bound (Inuit) syndrome of dissociation that could be related to an excess of vitamin A. (If, indeed, it exists at all—they're still debating it in the pages of the journal *Arctic Anthropology* and the magazine *Up Here.*)

Flooding from rivers that have escaped their banks has been associated with depression and anxiety disorders. And then there's the risk of posttraumatic stress disorder (PTSD) for anyone who has experienced the trauma of a horrendous, one-off weather-related catastrophe, such as a hurricane or a forest fire.

Perhaps you have other examples of weather-related disturbance of mind. I'd love to hear about them. But right now, I'm heading outdoors to soak up a little liquid sunshine.

Appendix—Tables

These three tables summarize the main material covered in the 26 chapters of this workbook. The "Page" column in each table lists the page numbers in one of my earlier books where the issues/techniques, principles, or diagnoses listed in the table are discussed. For Table 1, the book referred to is *The First Interview,* fourth edition; for Table 2, it's *Diagnosis Made Easier,* second edition; and for Table 3, it's *DSM-5 Made Easy.* The letters in the column heads to the right of the "Page" column stand for the names of the patients discussed in the present book: A for Abby in Chapter 1, B for Brad in Chapter 2, C for Candice in Chapter 3, and so forth.

Table 1. Interviewing Issues and Techniques

Issue/technique	Page	A	B	C	D	E	F	G	H	I	J	K	L	M	N	O	P	Q	R	S	T	U	V	W	X	Y	Z
Chief complaint	18		×																								
Free speech	20	×			×		×	×			×									×							
Time management	23									×																	
Seating arrangements	10								×																		
Small talk	12																×										
Sample openings	14				×											×	×										
Nondirective questions	16					×													×								
Open-ended questions	17	×				×		×	×	×		×	×							×				×	×		
Closed-ended questions	18									×	×	×		×											×		
Areas of clinical interest	22											×				×											
Rapport	26				×			×																			
Using patient's language	31							×																			
Boundaries and ethics	32										×				×		×										×
Addressing the patient	32													×													
Informed consent	192									×																	
Nonverbal encouragements	37					×		×																			
Verbal encouragements	38				×	×		×																			
Offering reassurance	40																		×								
Confronting the patient	60		×					×									×										
History of present episode	42				×											×											
Vegetative symptoms	43												×														
Definition of psychosis	161		×					×																		×	
Qualities of mood	128					×																					
Definition of depressive episode	164			×																							

Consequences of illness	45			×																							
Stressors	48					×													×							×	
Previous episodes	50			×			×											×									×
Previous treatment	51																	×									×
Eliciting feelings	64																				×			×			
Encouraging candor	224																							×			
Taking notes	13								×										×								
Onset/sequence of symptoms	47						×																				
Probing for details	57				×							×					×			×				×	×		
Use of interpreter	227																									×	
Emotional patient	70			×															×								
Defense mechanisms	69			×																					×		
Childhood history	74		×								×																
Legal history	80																×						×				
Medical history	84						×		×							×											
Review of systems	86								×																		
Family history	87		×								×					×											
Personality traits/disorders	89																					×					
Suicidal ideas/behavior	96	×					×						×									×					
Severity of suicide attempt	99	×											×														
Violence history	101								×																		
Safety of patient and clinician	219						×		×						×												
Substance use history	104						×										×					×		×			
Sexual history	108																		×								
Abuse—sexual and physical	76																					×					

(*continued*)

Table 1. Interviewing Issues and Techniques *(continued)*

Issue/technique	Page	A	B	C	D	E	F	G	H	I	J	K	L	M	N	O	P	Q	R	S	T	U	V	W	X	Y	Z
Transitions (bridges)	120					×														×							
MSE—general appearance	124		×													×							×			×	
MSE—affect/mood	128	×	×			×			×	×						×										×	
MSE—flow of speech	131	×	×													×							×			×	
MSE—content of thought	137		×						×							×										×	
Negative symptoms	291		×																				×			×	
MSE—sensorium	149		×			×				×						×		×								×	
MSE—insight and judgment	157		×							×						×										×	
Art of closure	187																										×
Differential diagnosis	238	×	×	×	×	×	×	×	×	×	×	×	×	×	×	×	×	×	×	×	×	×	×	×	×	×	×
Use of informants	191		×	×					×		×			×	×							×	×				
Coping with resistance	200															×					×						
Lying patient	213																×										
Hostile patient	215								×							×											
Confidentiality	192																										×
Older patient	221												×	×													
Vague, rambling patient	210										×			×													
Potential violence	218								×						×												
Pt. with disability or disfigurement	84																										×
Control—time is short	116										×			×													
Sharing findings with patient	251																×										×
Sharing findings with others	258															×											
The writeup	261				×											×											

Table 2. Diagnostic Principles

Principle	Page	A	B	C	D	E	F	G	H	I	J	K	L	M	N	O	P	Q	R	S	T	U	V	W	X	Y	Z
Safety hierarchy for diff. dx.	16		×			×			×												×						
Family history as a guide	30		×								×																
Physical causes of mental symptoms	16	×							×																×		
Somatic symptom disorder	112					×										×									×		
Substance use as cause	17	×					×						×		×										×		
Consider mood disorders	122	×										D	×	×			×			×				×	×		
History beats current appearance	25			×																							
Recent history beats ancient	26						×				×							×									
Collateral beats patient's history	27		×								×																
Signs beat symptoms	28												×														
Be wary crisis-generated data	29																		×								
Objective beats subjective	29			×																			×				
Use Occam's razor	30													×		×											
Horses, not zebras	32											×															
Watch for contradictory data	37																×										
Past behavior predicts best	47																	×									
More symptoms ↑ likelihood of dx.	50				×																	×	×				
Typical feat. ↑ dx.	50																						×				
Typical tx. response ↑ dx.	50																										×
If unsure, use *undiagnosed*	51									×																×	
Consider no mental dx.	53							×											×								
Multiple dx. if one won't do	62															×	×							×			
Avoid pers. disorder in acute illness	62	×						×				×				×	×				×	×					
Multiple dx.—order of listing	65				×							×				×											
Use decision trees	19				×																						

Here, I've stated in full the diagnostic principles that are abbreviated in Table 2:

- Arrange your differential diagnosis according to a safety hierarchy.
- Use family history as a guide.
- Physical disorders can cause or worsen mental symptoms.
- Consider (often!) somatic symptom disorder.
- Substance use can cause many disparate types of symptoms.
- *Always* consider mood disorders.
- History beats current appearance when information sources conflict.
- Recent history beats ancient history.
- Collateral information sometimes beats the patient's own history.
- Signs beat symptoms.
- Be wary of crisis-generated data.
- Objective findings beat subjective judgment.
- Use Occam's razor: Choose the simplest explanation.
- Horses are more common than zebras; prefer the more frequently encountered diagnosis.
- Be alert for contradictory information.
- The best predictor of future behavior is past behavior.
- More symptoms of a given illness increase the likelihood that it is the correct diagnosis.
- Typical features of a disorder increase its likelihood; atypical symptoms suggest that you keep looking.
- Previous typical response to treatment for a disorder increases the likelihood that it is responsible again.
- Use the word *undiagnosed* whenever you cannot be sure of your diagnosis.
- Consider the possibility that this patient should be given no mental diagnosis at all.
- When a single diagnosis cannot explain all the symptoms, consider multiple diagnoses.
- Avoid personality disorder diagnoses when your patient is acutely ill with a major mental disorder.
- Arrange multiple diagnoses to list first the one that is most urgent, treatable, or specific. Whenever possible, list them chronologically, too.

A point that isn't a principle:

- Use decision trees.

Table 3. Diagnoses Covered by Chapter

Diagnosis	Page	A	B	C	D	E	F	G	H	I	J	K	L	M	N	O	P	Q	R	S	T	U	V	W	X	Y	Z
Intellectual disability	20									×																	
Autism spectrum disorder	26									D																	
ADHD	33																										
Tourette's	39																										
Schizophrenia	64		D					D	D	D					D					D			×				
Delusional disorder	82							×	D																		
Schizophreniform disorder	75		×					D	D	D					D					D			D				
Schizoaffective disorder	88	D	D					D												×			D				
Brief psychotic disorder	80														D												
Substance/med.-induced psychotic disorder	93		D					D	D						×					D						D	
Psychotic disorder due to AMC	97		D					D	×						D					D			D			D	
Catatonia specifier	100																						D				
Bipolar I disorder	129	D		D					D		×		D			D								D			×
Bipolar II disorder	135			×							D																D
Cyclothymic disorder	143			D																							D
Bipolar disorder due to AMC	153																										D
Substance/med.-induced bipolar disorder	151					D					D																D
Disruptive mood dysregulation disorder	149																										
Major depressive disorder	122	×		D		D	D			D	D	D	×	D	D	×	D	D	D	D	D			D		D	
Atypical depression	160												×														
Persistent depressive disorder (dysthymia)	138	D											D			D	D							D			
Premenstrual dysphoric disorder	146	D																									

(*continued*)

Note. ×, best diagnosis in this vignette; D, included in differential diagnosis; ADHD, attention-deficit/hyperactivity disorder; AMC, another medical condition; GAD, generalized anxiety disorder; OCD, obsessive–compulsive disorder; PTSD, posttraumatic stress disorder; ASD, acute stress disorder; DID, dissociative identity disorder; DA, dissociative amnesia; REM, rapid eye movement; NCD, neurocognitive disorder; TBI, traumatic brain injury; PD, personality disorder.

Table 3. Diagnoses Covered by Chapter *(continued)*

Diagnosis	Page	A	B	C	D	E	F	G	H	I	J	K	L	M	N	O	P	Q	R	S	T	U	V	W	X	Y	Z
Depressive disorder due to AMC	153	D		D		D	D					D	D	D		D			D	D				D		D	
Substance/med.-induced depressive dis.	151	D		D			×			D		D	D	D		D	D	D	D	D				×		D	
Separation anxiety disorder	188										×																
Selective mutism	187																										
Specific phobia	182				×	D													D		D						
Social anxiety disorder	185				D																						
Panic disorder	176				×	D					D				D				D								
Agoraphobia	179				D																						
GAD	191				D	D	D												D								
Substance/med.-induced anxiety disorder	193				D	D									×												
Anxiety disorder due to AMC	195				D	D																					
OCD	200				D																×						
Body dysmorphic disorder	204																				D						
Hoarding disorder	207																										
Trichotillomania	210																										
Excoriation disorder	212																				D						
OCD due to AMC	215																										
Substance/medication-induced OCD	214																										
PTSD	219					D											×		D						D	×	
ASD	224																		D								
Adjustment disorder	228	D		D		×	D									D											
DID	245																								D		
DA	239																								×		
Depersonalization/derealization disorder	237																								D		
Somatic symptom disorder	251					D						D				×									D		

Illness anxiety disorder	260															D											
Conversion disorder	262															D									D		
Psychol. factors affecting other med. conds.	266																										
Factitious disorder	268															D									D		
Anorexia nervosa	277											×															
Bulimia nervosa	281											×															
Binge-eating disorder	284											D															
Insomnia disorder	299																										
Hypersomnolence disorder	309																										
Narcolepsy	313																										
Obstructive sleep apnea hypopnea	318																										
Central sleep apnea	318																										
Sleep-related hypoventilation	321																										
Circadian rhythm sleep–wake disorder	323																										
Sleepwalking	331																										
Sleep terror	333																										
Nightmare disorder	340																										
REM sleep behavior disorder	343																										
Restless legs syndrome	336																										
Substance/med.-induced sleep disorder	346																										
Delayed ejaculation	359																										
Erectile disorder	355																		D								
Female orgasmic disorder	368																										
Female sexual int./arousal disorder	362																										

(*continued*)

Note. ×, best diagnosis in this vignette; D, included in differential diagnosis; ADHD, attention-deficit/hyperactivity disorder; AMC, another medical condition; GAD, generalized anxiety disorder; OCD, obsessive–compulsive disorder; PTSD, posttraumatic stress disorder; ASD, acute stress disorder; DID, dissociative identity disorder; DA, dissociative amnesia; REM, rapid eye movement; NCD, neurocognitive disorder; TBI, traumatic brain injury; PD, personality disorder.

Table 3. Diagnoses Covered by Chapter *(continued)*

Diagnosis	Page	A	B	C	D	E	F	G	H	I	J	K	L	M	N	O	P	Q	R	S	T	U	V	W	X	Y	Z
Genito-pelvic pain/penetration disorder	364																										
Male hypoactive sexual desire disorder	352																										
Premature ejaculation	357																										
Substance/med.-induced sexual dysfunction	370																										
Gender dysphoria	372																										
Oppositional defiant disorder	380																										
Intermittent explosive disorder	384								D																		
Conduct disorder	381																										
Pyromania	387																										
Kleptomania	390																										
Alcohol use disorder	397															×	×										
Alcohol intoxication	412															D									D		
Alcohol withdrawal	406															D											
Caffeine intoxication	416																										
Caffeine withdrawal	418																										
Cannabis use disorder	421																										
Cannabis intoxication	421											D															
Hallucinogen use disorder	428																					D					
Hallucinogen intoxication	428																										
Inhalant use disorder	436																										
Inhalant intoxication	436																										
Opioid use disorder	440																							×			
Opioid intoxication	440																										
Opioid withdrawal	443																							×			
Sedative/hypnotic/anxiolytic use disorder	446																										

Sedative/hypnotic/anxiolytic intoxication	446																										
Sedative/hypnotic/anxiolytic withdrawal	448																										
Stimulant use disorder	453																										
Stimulant intoxication	453								D																		
Stimulant withdrawal	457											D															
Tobacco use disorder	462						×																				
Tobacco withdrawal	462						×					D															
Gambling disorder	470																							×			
Delirium	477									D								×									
NCD due to AMC	518																										
NCD due to Alzheimer's	498												D	×													
Frontotemporal NCD	512																										
NCD with Lewy bodies	504																										
NCD due to TBI	508									D				D											D		
Vascular NCD	516																										
NCD due to HIV infection	519																										
NCD due to prion disease	519																										
NCD due to Parkinson's	519																										
NCD due to Huntington's	519																										
Substance/medication-induced NCD	522													D													
Personality disorder/traits	528	D		D		D	D		D			D				D	D		D		D	×			D		
Paranoid PD	533							D																			
Schizoid PD	535																										
Schizotypal PD	538																										

(*continued*)

Note. ×, best diagnosis in this vignette; D, included in differential diagnosis; ADHD, attention-deficit/hyperactivity disorder; AMC, another medical condition; GAD, generalized anxiety disorder; OCD, obsessive–compulsive disorder; PTSD, posttraumatic stress disorder; ASD, acute stress disorder; DID, dissociative identity disorder; DA, dissociative amnesia; REM, rapid eye movement; NCD, neurocognitive disorder; TBI, traumatic brain injury; PD, personality disorder.

Table 3. Diagnoses Covered by Chapter *(continued)*

Diagnosis	Page	A	B	C	D	E	F	G	H	I	J	K	L	M	N	O	P	Q	R	S	T	U	V	W	X	Y	Z
Antisocial PD	541								D																		
Borderline PD	545															D						×					
Histrionic PD	548															D											
Narcissistic PD	550																										
Avoidant PD	553																										
Dependent PD	556																										
Obsessive–compulsive PD	558																				D						
Personality change due to AMC	560																					D					
Voyeuristic disorder	586																										
Exhibitionistic disorder	567																										
Frotteuristic disorder	571																										
Sexual masochism disorder	578																										
Sexual sadism disorder	580																										
Pedophilic disorder	574																										
Fetishistic disorder	569																										
Transvestic disorder	583																										
Malingering	599															D									D		
Uncomplicated bereavement	590					D							D														
Relationship distress with spouse/partner	589					D													D								
No mental illness	600							D											×								
Undiagnosed	600									D																	

Note. ×, best diagnosis in this vignette; D, included in differential diagnosis; ADHD, attention-deficit/hyperactivity disorder; AMC, another medical condition; GAD, generalized anxiety disorder; OCD, obsessive–compulsive disorder; PTSD, posttraumatic stress disorder; ASD, acute stress disorder; DID, dissociative identity disorder; DA, dissociative amnesia; REM, rapid eye movement; NCD, neurocognitive disorder; TBI, traumatic brain injury; PD, personality disorder.

References and Suggested Reading

Unless a specific website is given, "[Free]" at the end of an entry means that a reference is free for downloading via the U.S. National Library of Medicine's PubMed database (see the Introduction to this workbook).

General Texts

Black DW, Andreasen NJ. *Introductory textbook of psychiatry.* 6th edition. Arlington, VA: American Psychiatric Publishing, 2014.

Sadock BJ, Sadock VA, Ruiz P. *Kaplan & Sadock's comprehensive textbook of psychiatry.* 10th edition. Philadelphia: Wolters Kluwer, 2017.

Chapter 1 (Abby)

Lichstein PR. The medical interview. In Walker HK, Hall WD, Hurst JW, editors. *Clinical methods: The history, physical, and laboratory examinations.* 3rd edition. Boston: Butterworths, 1990. [Free]

Nordgaard J, Sass LA, Parnas J. The psychiatric interview: Validity, structure, and subjectivity. *European Archives of Psychiatry and Clinical Neuroscience* 2013; 263:353–364. [Free]

Rutter M, Cox A. Psychiatric interviewing techniques. I. Methods and measures. *British Journal of Psychiatry* 1981; 138:273–282.

Wittenborn AK, Rahmandad H, Rick J, Hosseinichimeh N. Depression as a systemic syndrome: Mapping the feedback loops of major depressive disorder. *Psychological Medicine* 2016; 46:551–562. [Free]

Chapter 2 (Brad)

Arciniegas DB. Psychosis. *Continuum* 2015; 21(3):715–736. [Free]

Bhavsar V, Maccabe JH, Hatch SL, Hotopf M, Boydell J, McGuire P. Subclinical psychotic experiences and subsequent contact with mental health services. *BJPsych Open* 2017; 3:64–70. [Free]

Marchesi C, Paini M, Ruju L, Rosi L, Turrini G, Maggini C. Predictors of the evolution towards schizophrenia or mood disorder in patients with schizophreniform disorder. *Schizophrenia Research* 2007; 97:1–5.

Chapter 3 (Candice)

Beers C. *A mind that found itself.* London, Longmans, Green, 1908. [Free download at *www.gutenberg.org/ebooks/11962*]

Muneer A. The neurobiology of bipolar disorder: An integrated approach. *Chonnam Medical Journal* 2016; 52:18–37. [Free]

Muneer A. Mixed states in bipolar disorder: Etiology, pathogenesis and treatment. *Chonnam Medical Journal* 2017; 53:1–13. [Free]

Chapter 4 (Douglas)

Crocq MA. A history of anxiety: From Hippocrates to DSM. *Dialogues in Clinical Neuroscience* 2015; 17:319–325. [Free]

Locke AB, Kirst N, Shultz CC. Diagnosis and management of generalized anxiety disorder and panic disorder in adults. *American Family Physician* 2015; 91:617–624. [Free]

Marewski JN, Gigerenzer G. Heuristic decision making in medicine. *Dialogues in Clinical Neuroscience* 2012; 14:77–89. [Free]

Morgan RD, Olson KR, Krueger RM, Schellenberg RP, Jackson TT. Do the DSM decision trees improve diagnostic ability? *Journal of Clinical Psychology* 2000; 56:73–88.

Song YY, Lu Y. Decision tree methods: Applications for classification and prediction. *Shanghai Archives of Psychiatry* 2015; 27:130–135. [Free]

Chapter 5 (Elinor)

Casey P, Doherty A. Adjustment disorder: Implications for ICD-11 and DSM-5. *British Journal of Psychiatry* 2012; 201:90–92. [Free]

Jäger M, Burger D, Becker T, Frasch K. Diagnosis of adjustment disorder: Reliability of its clinical use and long-term stability. *Psychopathology* 2012; 45:305–309.

Sabin JE, Daniels N. Seeking legitimacy for DSM-5: The bereavement exception as an example of failed process. *AMA Journal of Ethics* 2017; 19:192–198. [Free]

Tang B, Liu X, Liu Y, Xue C, Zhang L. A meta-analysis of risk factors for depression in adults and children after natural disasters. *BMC Public Health* 2014; 14:623–635. [Free]

Chapter 6 (Fritz)

Edwards SJ, Sachmann MD. No-suicide contracts, no-suicide agreements, and no-suicide assurances. *Crisis* 2010; 31:290–302.

Evins AE, Cather C, Laffer A. Treatment of tobacco use disorders in smokers with serious mental illness: Toward clinical best practices. *Harvard Review of Psychiatry* 2015; 23:90–98.

Foster DW, Langdon KJ, Schmidt NB, Zvolensky M. Smoking processes, panic, and depressive symptoms among treatment-seeking smokers. *Substance Use & Misuse* 2015; 50:394–402. [Free]

Chapter 7 (Gloria)

Lindner R. *The fifty-minute hour: A collection of true psychoanalytic tales.* New York: Rinehart, 1955.

Sim LA, Lebow J, Billings M. Eating disorders in adolescents with a history of obesity. *Pediatrics* 2013; 132:e1026–e1030. [Free at *http://pediatrics.aappublications.org/content/pediatrics/132/4/e1026.full.pdf*]

Chapter 8 (Hank)

Cowin L, Davies R, Estall G, Berlin T, Fitzgerald M, Hoot S. De-escalating aggression and violence in the mental health setting. *International Journal of Mental Health Nursing* 2003; 12:64–73.

Distasio CA. Violence in health care: Institutional strategies to cope with the phenomenon. *Health Care Supervisor* 1994; 12:1–34.

Faulkner LR, Grimm NR, McFarland BH, Bloom JD. Threats and assaults against psychiatrists. *Bulletin of the American Academy of Psychiatry and the Law* 1990; 18:37–46.

Hagerty BB. When your child is a psychopath. *The Atlantic* 2017 June; 78–87. [Free at *www.theatlantic.com/magazine/archive/2017/06/when-your-child-is-a-psychopath/524502*]

Riskin A, Erez A, Foulk TA, Kugelman A, Gover A, Shoris I, et al. The impact of rudeness on medical team performance: A randomized trial. *Pediatrics* 2015; 136:487–495. [Free]

Riskin A, Erez A, Foulk TA, Riskin-Geuz KS, Ziv A, Sela R, et al. Rudeness and medical team performance. *Pediatrics* 2017; 139(2):e20162305.

Schmidt HG, van Gog T, Schuit SCE, Van den Berge K, Van Daele PLA, Bueving H, et al. Do patients' disruptive behaviours influence the accuracy of a doctor's diagnosis?: A randomised experiment. *BMJ Quality & Safety* 2016; 26:19–23.

Stewart JB. *Blind eye: How the medical establishment let a doctor get away with murder.* New York: Simon & Schuster, 1999.

Swanson JW, McGinty EE, Fazel S, Mays VM. Mental illness and reduction of gun violence and suicide: Bringing epidemiologic research to policy. *Annals of Epidemiology* 2015; 366–376. [Free]

Chapter 9 (Inez)

Bertelli MO, Munir K, Harris J, Salvador-Carulla L. "Intellectual developmental disorders": reflections on the international consensus document for redefining "mental retardation-intellectual disability" in ICD-11. *Advances in Mental Health and Intellectual Disabilities* 2016; 10:36–58. [Free]

Carlson L. Research ethics and intellectual disability: Broadening the debates. *Yale Journal of Biology and Medicine* 2013; 86:303–314.

Carroll Chapman SL, Wu LT. Substance abuse among individuals with intellectual disabilities. *Research in Developmental Disabilities* 2012; 33:1147–1156.

Harris JC. New terminology for mental retardation in DSM-5 and ICD-11. *Current Opinion in Psychiatry* 2013; 26:260–262.

Ludi E, Ballard ED, Greenbaum R, Pao M, Bridge J, Reynolds W, et al. Suicide risk in youth with intellectual disabilities: The challenges of screening. *Journal of Developmental and Behavioral Pediatrics* 2012; 33:431–440. [Free]

Munir KM. The co-occurrence of mental disorders in children and adolescents with intellectual disability/intellectual developmental disorder. *Current Opinion in Psychiatry* 2016; 29:95–102. [Free]

Chapter 10 (Julio)

Best films involving psychologists/psychiatrists/therapists. [Free at *www.imdb.com/list/ls008570084*]

McCormick U, Murray B, McNew B. Diagnosis and treatment of patients with bipolar disorder: A review for advanced practice nurses. *Journal of the American Association of Nurse Practitioners* 2015; 27:530–542. [Free]

These 10 movie therapists might damage you worse than you were. [Free at *http://whatculture.com/film/10-movie-therapists-that-would-damage-you-worse-than-before*]

What films can teach us about therapeutic ethics. [Free at *www.zurinstitute.com/movies_clinicalupdate.html*]

Chapter 11 (Kylie)

Lavender JM, Wonderlich SA, Engel SG, Gordon KH, Kaye WH, Mitchell JE. Dimensions of emotion dysregulation in anorexia nervosa and bulimia nervosa: A conceptual review of the empirical literature. *Clinical Psychology Review* 2015; 40:111–122. [Free]

Lindner R. *The fifty-minute hour: A collection of true psychoanalytic tales.* New York: Rinehart, 1955.

Morrison J. *When psychological problems mask medical disorders.* 2nd edition. New York: Guilford Press, 2015.

Walsh BT. The enigmatic persistence of anorexia nervosa. *American Journal of Psychiatry* 2013; 170:477–484. [Free]

Chapter 12 (Liam)

Berman AI, Silverman MM. Suicide risk assessment and risk formulation. Part II: Suicide risk formulation and the determination of levels of risk. *Suicide and Life-Threatening Behavior* 2014; 44:432–443.

Buzuk G, Lojko D, Owecki M, Ruchala M, Rybakowski J. Depression with atypical features in various kinds of affective disorders. *Psychiatria Polska* 2016; 50:827–838. [Free]

Pitman AL, Osborn DPJ, Rantell K, King MB. Bereavement by suicide as a risk factor for suicide attempt: A cross-sectional national UK-wide study of 3432 young bereaved adults. *BMJ Open* 2016; 6:e009948. [Free]

Sachs-Ericsson N, Selby E, Corsentino E, Collins N, Sawyer K, Hames J, et al. Depressed older patients with the atypical features of interpersonal rejection sensitivity and reversed-vegetative symptoms are similar to younger atypical patients. *American Journal of Geriatric Psychiatry* 2012; 20:622–634. [Free]

Turecki G, Brent DA. Suicide and suicidal behaviour. *Lancet* 2016; 387:1227–1239. [Free]

Zero Suicide in Health and Behavioral Health Care. [Free at *www.zerosuicide.sprc.org*]

Chapter 13 (Melissa)

Amer A, Fischer H. "Don't call me 'Mom'": How parents want to be greeted by their pediatrician. *Clinical Pediatrics* 2009; 48:720–722.

Berisha V, Wang S, LaCross A, Liss J. Tracking discourse complexity preceding Alzheimer's disease diagnosis: A case study comparing the press conferences of Presidents Ronald Reagan and George Herbert Walker Bush. *Journal of Alzheimer's Disease* 2015; 45:959–963.

Berisha V, Wang S, LaCross A, Liss J, Garcia-Filion P. Longitudinal changes in linguistic complexity among professional football players. *Brain and Language* 2017; 169:57–63.

Frank C, Forbes RF. A patient's experience in dementia care: Using the "lived experience" to improve care. *Canadian Family Physician* 2017; 63:22–26. [Free]

Gallaway PJ, Miyake H, Buchowski MS, Shimada M, Yoshitake Y, Kim AS, et al. Physical activity: A viable way to reduce the risks of mild cognitive impairment, Alzheimer's disease, and vascular dementia in older adults. *Brain Sciences* 2017; 7(2):22. [Free]

Le X, Lancashire I, Hirst G, Jokel R. Longitudinal detection of dementia through lexical and syntactic changes in writing: A case study of three British novelists. *Literary and Linguistic Computing* 2011; 26:435–461. [Free]

Macfarlane S, O'Connor D. Managing behavioural and psychological symptoms in dementia. *Australian Prescriber* 2016; 39:123–125. [Free]

Makoul G, Zick A, Green M. An evidence-based perspective on greetings in medical encounters. *Archives of Internal Medicine* 2007; 167:1172–1176.

Saunders L. Diagnosing with Dickens. *The New York Times Magazine* 2006 December 17. [Free at *www.nytimes.com/2006/12/17/magazine/17wwln_diagnosis.t.html*]

Chapter 14 (Norman)

Davidson JRT, Connor KM, Swartz M. Mental illness in U.S. Presidents between 1776 and 1974: A review of biographical sources. *Journal of Nervous and Mental Disease* 2006; 194:47–51.

Hoch E, Bonnetn U, Thomasius R, Ganzer F, Havemann-Reinecke U, Preuss UW. Risks associated with the non-medicinal use of cannabis. *Deutsches Arzteblatt International* 2015; 112:271–278. [Free]

Kroll J, Pouncey C. The ethics of APA's Goldwater rule. *Journal of the American Academy of Psychiatry and the Law* 2016; 44:226–235. [Free]

Murray RM, Quigley H, Quattrone D, Englund A, Di Forti M. Traditional marijuana, high-potency cannabis and synthetic cannabinoids: Increasing risk for psychosis. *World Psychiatry* 2016; 15:195–204. [Free]

Pies, RW. Deconstructing and reconstructing the "Goldwater rule." *Psychiatric Times* 2016 October 7. [Free at *www.psychiatrictimes.com/blogs/deconstructing-and-reconstructing-goldwater-rule*]

Rabin RA, George TP. Cannabis and psychosis: Understanding the smoke signals. *Lancet Psychiatry* 2016; 3:909–910. [Free]

Chapter 15 (Olivia)

Creed F, Guthrie E. Techniques for interviewing the somatising patient. *British Journal of Psychiatry* 1993; 162:467–471.

Feighner JP, Robins E, Guze SB, Woodruff RA Jr, Winokur G, Muñoz R. Diagnostic criteria for use in psychiatric research. *Archives of General Psychiatry* 1972; 26:57–63.

Haller H, Cramer H, Lauche R, Dobos G. Somatoform disorders and medically unexplained symptoms in primary care. *Deutsches Arzteblatt International* 2015; 112:279–287.

Perley MJ, Guze SB. Hysteria—the stability and usefulness of clinical criteria—a quantitative study based on a follow-up period of six to eight years in 39 patients. *New England Journal of Medicine* 1962; 266:421–426.

Yates GP, Feldman MD. Factitious disorder: A systematic review of 455 cases in the professional literature. *General Hospital Psychiatry* 2016; 41:20–28. [Free]

Chapter 16 (Pierce)

Bisson JI, Cosgrove S, Lewis C, Robert NP. Post-traumatic stress disorder. *British Medical Journal* 2015; 351:h6161. [Free]

Gabbard GO, Nadelson C. Professional boundaries in the physician–patient relationship. *Journal of the American Medical Association* 1995; 273:1445–1449.

Gradus JL. Prevalence and prognosis of stress disorders: A review of the epidemiologic literature. *Clinical Epidemiology* 2017; 9:251–260. [Free]

Lancaster CL, Teeters JB, Gros DF, Back SE. Posttraumatic stress disorder: Overview of evidence-based assessment and treatment. *Journal of Clinical Medicine* 2016; 5(11): E105. [Free]

Pai A, Suris AM, North CS. Posttraumatic stress disorder in the DSM-5: Controversy, change, and conceptual considerations. *Behavioral Sciences (Basel)* 2017; 7(1):E7.

Chapter 17 (Quinn)

Davydow DS. Symptoms of depression and anxiety after delirium. *Psychosomatics* 2009; 50:309–316.

Farrell KR, Ganzini L. Misdiagnosing delirium as depression in medically ill elderly patients. *Archives of Internal Medicine* 1995; 155:2459–2464.

Givens JL, Jones RN, Inouye SK. The overlap syndrome of depression and delirium in older hospitalized patients. *Journal of the American Geriatric Society* 2009; 57:1347–1353.

Inouye SK, Westendorp RG, Saczynski JS. Delirium in elderly people. *Lancet* 2014; 383:911–922. [Free]

Meagher D, O'Regan N, Ryan D, Connolly W, Boland E, O'Caoimhe R, et al. Frequency of delirium and subsyndromal delirium in an adult acute hospital population. *British Journal of Psychiatry* 2014; 205:478–485.

Meagher J, Leonard M, Donoghue L, O'Regan N, Timmons S, Exton C, et al. Months backward test: A review of its use in clinical studies. *World Journal of Psychiatry* 2015; 5:305–314.

Nicholas LM, Lindsey BA. Delirium presenting with symptoms of depression. *Psychosomatics* 1995; 36:471–479.

Chapter 18 (Randolph)

Blazer DG. Techniques for communicating with your elderly patient. *Geriatrics* 1978; 33(11):79–84.

Blazer DG. Psychiatry and the oldest old. *American Journal of Psychiatry* 2000; 157:1915–1924.

Brent DA, Melhem NM, Wilcox HC. Violent offending and suicidal behavior have common familial risk factors: A rejoinder to Tolstoy. *JAMA Psychiatry* 2016; 73:1005–1007.

De Figueiredo JM, Boerstler H, O'Connell L. Conditions not attributable to a mental disorder: An epidemiological study of family problems. *American Journal of Psychiatry* 1991; 148:780–783.

Singh A. Covert treatment in psychiatry: Do no harm, true, but also dare to care. *Mens Sana Monographs* 2008; 6:81–109. [Free]

Spinhoven P, Van Der Does AJ. Conditions not attributable to a mental disorder in Dutch psychiatric out-patients. *Psychological Medicine* 1999; 29:213–220.

Chapter 19 (Siobhán)

Bergsholm P. Is schizophrenia disappearing? The rise and fall of the diagnosis of functional psychoses: An essay. *BMC Psychiatry* 2016; 16:387–396. [Free]

Kasanin J. The acute schizoaffective psychoses. 1933. *American Journal of Psychiatry* 1954; 151 (Suppl. 6):144–154.

Madre M, Canales-Rodríguez EJ, Ortiz-Gil J, Murru A, Torrent C, Bramon E, et al. Neuropsychological and neuroimaging underpinnings of schizoaffective disorder: A systematic review. *Acta Psychiatrica Scandinavica* 2016; 134:16–30.

Rink L, Pagel T, Franklin J, Baethge C. Characteristics and heterogeneity of schizoaffective disorder compared with unipolar depression and schizophrenia—a systematic literature review and meta-analysis. *Journal of Affective Disorders* 2016; 191:8–14.

Santelmann H, Franklin J, Bußhoff J, Baethge C. Test–retest reliability of schizoaffective disorder compared with schizophrenia, bipolar disorder, and unipolar depression—a systematic review and meta-analysis. *Bipolar Disorders* 2015; 17:753–768.

Chapter 20 (Tyler)

Hopkinson K, Cox A, Rutter M. Psychiatric interviewing techniques. III. Naturalistic study: Eliciting feelings. *British Journal of Psychiatry* 1981; 138:406–415.

Krebs G, Heyman I. Obsessive–compulsive disorder in children and adolescents. *Archives of Disease in Childhood* 2015; 100:495–499. [Free]

McKinley MB. The psychology of collecting. *National Psychologist* 2007 January 1. [Free at *http://nationalpsychologist.com/2007/01/the-psychology-of-collecting/10904.html*]

Rapp AM, Bergman RL, Piacentini J, McGuire JF. Evidence-based assessment of obsessive–compulsive disorder. *Journal of Central Nervous System Disease* 2016; 8:13–29. [Free]

Chapter 21 (Uma)

Biskin RS. The lifetime course of borderline personality disorder. *Canadian Journal of Psychiatry* 2015; 60:303–308. [Free]

Brüne M. Borderline personality disorder: Why 'fast and furious'? *Evolution, Medicine, and Public Health* 2016; 2016(1):52–66. [Free]

Hasler G, Hopwood CJ, Jacob GA, Brändle LS, Schulte-Vels T. Patient-reported outcomes in borderline personality disorder. *Dialogues in Clinical Neuroscience* 2014; 16:255–266. [Free]

Murray LK, Nguyen A, Cohen JA. Child sexual abuse. *Child and Adolescent Psychiatric Clinics of North America* 2014; 23:321–337. [Free]

Singh MM, Parsekar SS, Nair SN. An epidemiological overview of child sexual abuse. *Journal of Family Medicine and Primary Care* 2014; 3:430–435. [Free]

Timoshin N. Creativity and mental illness: Richard Kogan on Rachmaninoff. *Psychiatric Times* 2016 September 14. [Free at *www.psychiatrictimes.com/cultural-psychiatry/creativity-and-mental-illness-richard-kogan-rachmaninoff/page/0/1?GUID=0B63612F-423B-49DF-A7C8-D107BD91AB92&rememberme=1&ts=15092016*]

Chapter 22 (Vincent)

Rasmussen SA, Mazurek MF, Rosebush PI. Catatonia: Our current understanding of its diagnosis, treatment and pathophysiology. *World Journal of Psychiatry* 2016; 6:391–398. [Free]

Wilcox JA, Duffy PR. The syndrome of catatonia. *Behavioral Sciences (Basel)* 2015; 5:576–588. [Free]

Worku B, Fekadu A. Symptom profile and short term outcome of catatonia: An exploratory clinical study. *BMC Psychiatry* 2015; 15:164. [Free]

Chapter 23 (Whitney)

Cleckley H, Cleckley ES. *The mask of sanity.* 5th edition. [Free download at *https://cassiopaea.org/cass/sanity_1.pdf*

Cox A, Holbrook D, Rutter M. Psychiatric interviewing techniques. VI. Experimental study: Eliciting feelings. *British Journal of Psychiatry* 1981; 139:144–152.

Kessler RC, Chiu WT, Demier O, Walters EE. Prevalence, severity, and comorbidity of twelve-month DSM-IV disorders in the National Comorbidity Survey Replication (NCSR). *Archives of General Psychiatry* 2005; 62:617–627.

Rosengren, J. Losing it all. *The Atlantic* 2016 December; 66–78. [Free at *www.theatlantic.com/magazine/archive/2016/12/losing-it-all/505814*]

Chapter 24 (X)

Sharma P, Guirguis M, Nelson J, McMahon T. A case of dissociative amnesia with dissociative fugue and treatment with psychotherapy. *Primary Care Companion for CNS Disorders* 2015; 17(3):10.4088/PCC.14l01763. [Free]

Staniloiu A, Markowitsch HJ. The remains of the day in dissociative amnesia. *Brain Sciences* 2012; 2:101–129. [Free]

Chapter 25 (Yasmin)

Crews F. *Freud: The making of an illusion.* New York, Henry Holt, 2017.

Dollfus S, Lyne J. Negative symptoms: History of the concept and their position in diagnosis of schizophrenia. *Schizophrenia Research* 2017; 186:3–7.

Feighner JP, Robins E, Guze SB, Woodruff RA Jr, Winokur G, Muñoz R. Diagnostic criteria for use in psychiatric research. *Archives of General Psychiatry* 1972; 26:57–63.

Kosny A, MacEachen E, Lifshen M, Smith P. Another person in the room: Using interpreters during interviews with immigrant workers. *Qualitative Health Research* 2014; 24:837–845.

Velligan DI, Alphs LD. Negative symptoms in schizophrenia: An update on identification and treatment. *Psychiatric Times* 2014 November 24. [Free at *www.psychiatrictimes.com/schizophrenia/negative-symptoms-schizophrenia-update-identification-and-treatment*]

Chapter 26 (Zander)

Boylan M. The duty to rescue and the limits of confidentiality. *American Journal of Bioethics* 2006; 6:32–34.

Childress JF. A principle-based approach. In Kuhse H, Singer P, editors. *A companion to bioethics.* 2nd edition. Chichester, UK: Wiley-Blackwell, 2009.

Page K. The four principles: Can they be measured and do they predict ethical decision making? *BMC Medical Ethics* 2012; 13.10. [Free at *https://bmcmedethics.biomedcentral.com/articles/10.1186/1472-6939-13-10*]

Perez HR, Stoeckle JH. Stuttering: Clinical and research update. *Canadian Family Physician* 2016; 62:479–484. [Free]

Index

Note. Page numbers in italics indicate definitions, *t* following a page number indicates a table.

B

C

D

E

F

G

H

I

J

L

M

N

O

P

Q

R

S

T

U

V

W